Investigative Electrocardiography in Epidemiological Studies and Clinical Trials

Pentti Rautaharju and Farida Rautaharju

Investigative Electrocardiography in Epidemiological Studies and Clinical Trials

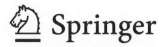

Pentti Rautaharju, MD, PhD
Wake Forest University School of Medicine
Winston-Salem, North Carolina
USA

Farida Rautaharju, PhD
Covance Cardiac Safety Services
Reno, Nevada
USA

British Library Cataloguing in Publication Data
Rautaharju, P. (Pentti)
  Investigative electrocardiography in epidemiological studies and clinical trials
  1. Electrocardiography   2. Heart – Diseases – Epidemiology   3. Clinical trials
  I. Title   II. Rautaharji, Farida
  616.1'207547
ISBN-13: 9781846284656
ISBN-10: 1846284651

Library of Congress Control Number: 2006926452

ISBN-10: 1-84628-465-1   eISBN 1-84628-481-3   Printed on acid-free paper
ISBN-13: 978-1-84628-465-6

9 8 7 6 5 4 3 2 1

Springer Science+Business Media
springer.com

TO:
Anu, Kristina, Mia
Satu
Sherene, Riza

Preface

This book on investigative electrocardiography is addressed to investigators who are using electrocardiology as a research tool in epidemiological or clinical research or in investigations on possible adverse responses of new pharmacological agents. The primary emphasis of the book is on prognostic implications of ECG abnormalities in the conditions covered, including the prevalence and incidence of ECG abnormalities in contrasting populations.

We excluded from our book cardiac disorders with a relatively low population prevalence that otherwise may be of great clinical interest. We also decided to exclude acute myocardial infarction because we had only limited resources available on this topic from our population studies and from those clinical trials in which we have personally participated in the classification of trial endpoints within the framework of an ECG research center.

Clinical trials are a relatively new area of electrocardiology. However, electrocardiography has become a most valuable research tool in clinical trials and in investigations on morbidity and mortality risk associated with various clinical and subclinical conditions. It has also become a crucial research tool in investigating adverse cardiac events associated with administration of new drugs. Evaluation of QT prolongation plays a central role in these investigations. As a possible marker of malignant arrhythmias, it is used by regulating agencies in their decision process for approval of new pharmacological agents.

Part 1 of this book begins with an account of ventricular excitation and repolarization (Chapter 1), followed by Chapter 2 composed to facilitate the understanding of ECG leads. Chapter 3 is a review of ionic channel functions in relation to ECG waveforms and their role in drug effects. Heart rate and heart rate variability evaluation is covered next (Chapter 4). Arrhythmic conditions selected include epidemiological aspects of atrial flutter and fibrillation and other atrial dysrhythmias (Chapter 5) and the role of ectopic ventricular complexes (Chapter 6). Chapter 7 provides insights and a critical evaluation of electrocardiographic left ventricular hypertrophy, and Chapter 8 covers ventricular conduction defects. The last three chapters cover epidemiological aspects of old myocardial infarction (Chapter 9), the importance of primary repolarization abnormalities (Chapter 10), and finally, a critical evaluation of QT prolongation and QT dispersion (Chapter 11). An important component in this last chapter is the establishment of appropriate adjustment functions for QT interval, to overcome critical problems associated with the traditional Bazett's formula and other power functions currently used for QT rate adjustment.

Each chapter starts with a synopsis summarizing the importance of the topic. The main text in each chapter covers the mechanism, classification problems, prevalence and incidence, and predictive value of the abnormality.

Part 2 of the book contains an extensive series of tables listing normal standards by gender, age (40–79 years), and ethnicity (Caucasian white and African–American), established from large groups of healthy North-American populations. No previous properly established normal standards are available for African–American men and women or for older white women, and only limited standards are available for vectorial parameters of ECG waves for any of these subgroups. These normal standards are presented as five sections: Section A, ECG intervals; Section B, ECG wave amplitudes; Section C, ECG vector components and spatial magnitudes at normalized time scale; Section D, ECG amplitudes at 10-ms intervals; and Section E, repolarization waveform vectors.

Many individuals have significantly contributed to the effort that was required for the completion of this book. The authors have closely collaborated for over a quarter of a century in operating a central ECG laboratory that has been in charge of computer analysis of major national health surveys conducted by the US National Center for Health Statistics and a series of large cardiovascular observational studies and clinical trials sponsored by the US National Heart, Lung, and Blood Institute. The authors wish to express their gratitude to the sponsors and participants of these studies, principal investigators, and their supporting staff. Our participation in several large clinical trials sponsored by the pharmaceutical industry has also been a valuable experience that has benefited the composition of this book.

The authors wish to acknowledge the collaborative efforts of the personnel of the central ECG laboratory that has operated in different locations under the name EPICARE. In particular, Dr. Ron Prineas, Dr. Zhu-Ming Zhang, and Charles Campbell, Wake Forest University, NC, and James Warren, Dalhousie University, have provided important support for this undertaking. The collaboration and friendship of Dr. Henry Blackburn since the earliest years of cardiovascular epidemiology has provided an important intellectual stimulus throughout these years.

Pentti Rautaharju and Farida Rautaharju

Contents

Part 1
Investigative Electrocardiography in Epidemiological Studies and Clinical Trials

1
Cardiac Excitation and Repolarization

Synopsis

P and QRS Waves

Atrial and ventricular action potential gradients at phase 0 upstroke initiate propagating wave fronts during cardiac excitation that generate sequentially the P and QRS waves of the electrocardiogram (ECG). Ventricular excitation follows atrial excitation after a delay in the atrioventricular (AV) node and conduction time through the His-Purkinje network. This delay permits completion of atrial contraction and ventricular filling before ventricular contraction.

ST Segment, T Wave and T Wave Polarity

Ventricular action potential gradients during phase 2 and phase 3 generate the ST segment and the T wave. Ventricular action potential duration (APD) shortens normally with excitation time (ET) more than the delay of the onset of excitation, at least in the lateral wall of the left ventricle where the sequence of repolarization is normally discordant, or reverse, with respect to the sequence of depolarization. After the initial phase, repolarization wave fronts propagate simultaneously in different segments of the ventricular walls and the septum, and as a consequence, the overall spatial repolarization sequence is semireverse rather than reverse. The spatial angle between the mean QRS and T vectors in normal adults is 76° in men and 62° in women, closer to 90° than to 0°.

The Role of M Cells

The M cells in intramural layers have been documented to have strongly rate-dependent APD that is longer than in the cells of subepicardial and subendocardial layers, particularly at slow stimulus rates. This suggests that the initial lateral transmural repolarization sequence should be from epicardial toward M cell layers at midwall and then from endocardial toward the M cell layers, and the T waves in lateral leads should be biphasic (positive/negative) rather than positive. The size of the M cell population may be too small and the effect of electrotonic interaction between repolarizing myocytes may potentially explain these observations. M cells may play a role in generation of the U wave, which overlaps the tail end of the T wave.

Abbreviations

APD – action potential duration
AV – atrioventricular
ECG – electrocardiogram
ET – excitation time
RT – repolarization time
SA – sino-atrial
Ta – atrial T wave
Tend – time point of the end of the T wave
Tp – time point of the peak of the T wave

1.1 Cardiac Excitation/ Repolarization Cycle

Cyclic transients of transmembrane potentials of the excitable myocardial cells generate the cardiac action potentials (Figure 1.1). Potential differences between already excited and still resting cells create potential gradients that generate the electrocardiogram (ECG) (Figure 1.2). Living cardiac myocytes maintain concentration gradients of certain ions (sodium, potassium, and calcium) across the muscle membranes when the ventricular myocytes are at rest during the diastolic period from the end of the T wave to the beginning of the next P wave, after having recovered from the previous cycle. There is no net ionic current flow across the membrane during the diastolic resting period (phase 4), and there is a steady resting potential of $-90\,\text{mV}$, the inside of the muscle cells being negative (i.e. at lower potential) with respect to the outside. Phase 4 corresponds to the TP segment of the ECG.

When the excitation cycle begins, cardiac cell membranes are rapidly depolarized (phase 0). In ventricular myocytes, the transmembrane poten-

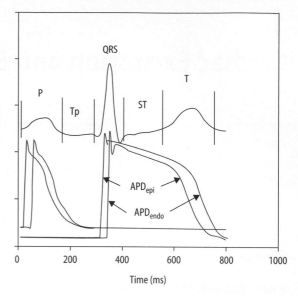

FIGURE 1.2 Schematic of ventricular action potential at the left lateral wall subendocardial and subepicardial myocyte zones. If epicardial excitation time is 30 ms longer than endocardial excitation time, then epicardial action potential duration (*APDepi*) has to be more than 30 ms shorter than endocardial action potential duration (*APDendo*) for a reverse transmural repolarization and positive T waves in left lateral leads to occur.

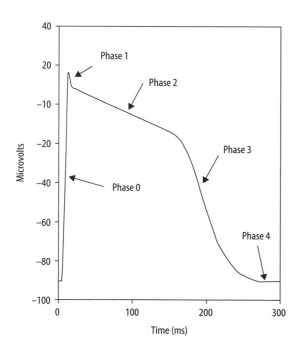

FIGURE 1.1 Schematic of the action potential of ventricular subendocardial myocytes.

tial difference reverses to a slightly positive value (phase 1 or the overshoot). Depolarization of atrial myocytes generates the P wave, and depolarization of ventricular myocytes the QRS complex of the ECG and the corresponding mechanical systolic state. After depolarization, the transmembrane potential difference settles to a relatively steady value during the systolic state, with a gradual decrease towards zero potential difference or slightly negative value during this slow phase of repolarization, phase 2 of the action potential. Phase 2 corresponds to the ST segment of the ECG. Phase 2 is followed by phase 3, the fast phase of repolarization that generates the T wave. This event signals the end of the systolic phase of the excitation/repolarization cycle, and the diastolic resting period begins.

Cardiac excitation is a propagated response. Once the myocytes are triggered into activity by firing of the terminal branches of the Purkinje network (described later) at the septal and endocardial surfaces of the ventricles, excitation spreads from cell to cell. Ventricular depolariza-

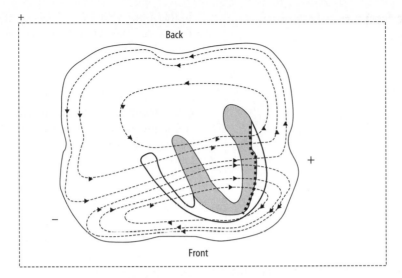

FIGURE 1.3 Schematic of the current lines (*light broken lines with arrows*) in a horizontal plane cross-section of the human thorax at the time point when the left ventricular excitation front has reached its maximum area at approximately 35 ms from the onset of ventricular excitation. Note how the current flow from the source is directed from the already excited part of the lateral ven-tricular wall to the still unexcited part, reaches the left lateral body surface, then bends and travels tangentially to the body boundary and returns to the source. Isopotential lines (not shown) are per-pendicular to the current lines and generate one potential maximum (+) and one minimum (−) on the body surface.

tion starts at the left side of the ventricular septum. The cardiac source generates electric currents flowing in the body, a three-dimensional volume conductor.

The schematic in Figure 1.3 shows the excita-tion current lines in a horizontal plane cross-section of the human thorax at the time point when the left excitation front has reached its maximum area at approximately 35 ms from the onset of ventricular excitation. The current "loops" in the schematic generate one potential maximum and one minimum on the body surface in locations indicated by + and − as isopotential lines in body surface maps would reveal. Body surface potentials with respect to a common refer-ence potential (like the central terminal described in the context of lead vectors) produce an ECG at every pick-up point, or node, at the body surface, such as the standard chest leads V1–V6.

Detailed examination of body surface maps has revealed multipolar distributions (i.e. more than one maximum and minimum) at some instances of the cardiac excitation/repolarization cycle, mainly at the end period of ventricular excitation when the early onset of slow ventricular repolar-ization overlaps with ventricular excitation.

1.2 Atrial Excitation

The P wave of the ECG is the manifestation of depolarization of the atria. Atrial repolarization generates an ECG wave that is the counterpart of the T wave of ventricular repolarization. It is called the atrial T wave (Ta). Ta is as a slow deflec-tion in the PR segment of the ECG with the polar-ity opposite to that of the P wave.

The sino-atrial (SA) node is the pacemaker of the heart that triggers the excitation/repolariza-tion cycle of the atrial cells and normally also the ventricular cells. The action potential of the SA node cells shown in Figure 1.4 has a rounded peak and no plateau, as in the action potential of the ventricular myocytes. The minimum resting potential is −60 mV. Phase 4 has a positive slope called pacemaker potential. Once the SA node pacemaker potential threshold level is reached, the pacemaker fires and starts the excitation/repo-larization cycle of cardiac cells.

The SA node is located in the wall of the right atrium at the junction of the superior vena cava and the right atrium. The node is about 2 cm long, with an extension of its tail section running down on the crista terminalis and from its head upwards

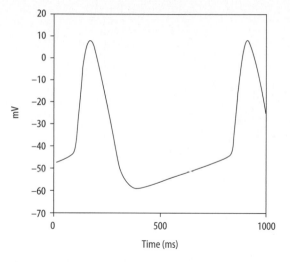

Time (ms)

FIGURE 1.4 Schematic of the SA node action potential. Note the broad rounded peak and the absence of the plateau. SA node cells start depolarizing again during phase 4 (pacemaker potential) and reach the firing threshold at −50 mV level.

along the lateral–dorsal aspects of the superior vena cava.

Atrial excitation isochrones in superior SA node rhythm in a superior view of the atria are shown in Figure 1.5, sketched from simulation data from an early computer model.[1] Excitation spreads faster along the fiber direction in thicker wall structures, around the holes in the walls, and around the membranous parts and foramen ovale

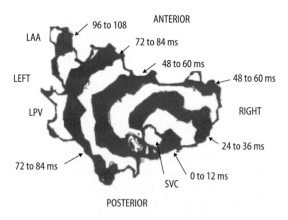

FIGURE 1.5 Schematic of excitation isochrones in normal sinus rhythm in a superior view of the atria sketched at 12-ms time intervals using data from an older computer simulation model. Every second excitation interval is shaded black. *LAA* left atrial appendix, *LPV* left pulmonary vein, *SVC* superior vena cava.

in the septal wall. Isochrones on the atrial surface reflect the existence of these preferential pathways. These reflect simultaneously propagating and often colliding wave fronts during the excitation of the atria. At the right atrial surface seen in a superior and a posterior view, excitation proceeds from the area surrounding the SA node to the right and downwards. Left atrial excitation propagates from the upper part of the atrium to the left and downwards, and after septal excitation, inferiorly to the left from the coronary sinus area. The last part of the atria that is excited is the left atrial appendix. There is temporal overlap between the right and the left atrial excitation. The main part of the right atrial excitation is finished at the time when the left atrial excitation fronts are still prominent.

The initial P vector at time point one-tenth of the P wave has an anterior component in 96% of normal male subjects. In two-thirds of the subjects, the direction is normally either right–anterior–up (41%) or right–anterior–down (25%). In the remaining third, the direction is left–anterior, either down or up.

The main ECG features during atrial excitation in SA node rhythm are seen in frontal and horizontal plane phase diagrams of the P wave vectors in Figure 1.6. The frontal plane view (on top) shows that the main direction of atrial excitation is downwards and to the left. The horizontal plane view (below) shows that the initial half of atrial excitation is directed anteriorly. The direction shifts to the left, and during the terminal half the direction is to the left and posteriorly. The biphasic P wave in lead V1 reflects this directional shift in the horizontal plane, as seen in Figure 1.6. Total excitation time (ET) of the adult human atria is approximately 90–100 ms.

Average excitation–conduction times shown in Figure 1.7 indicate the normal delays in various parts of the conduction system.[2] It takes, on average, 35 ms from the time the SA node cells reach the firing threshold to the start of the right atrial excitation and the first notable signs of the P wave in ECG. Then it takes, on average, 37 ms for excitation to reach the bottom part of the right atrium and the atrioventricular (AV) node. The delay in the AV node until excitation enters the bundle of His is on average 77 ms, and finally it takes approximately 40 ms for the conduction in the His bundle and the main bundle branches to reach the Purkinje network at the left and right sides of the ventricular septum. Thus, according to these average figures, the total interval from the start of SA node excitation to the start of ventricular excitation is 189 ms.

The mean PR interval from computer measurements in normal adults is 165 ms, with upper and lower 2% normal limits 122 and 228 ms. The wide normal range indicates the variability in the conduction times in various parts of the conduction system. The conduction time from the SA node to the AV node also varies widely, depending, in

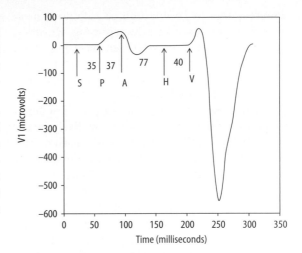

FIGURE 1.7 Excitation conduction from the SA node to the left septal branches of the Purkinje network in the ventricles. The arrows indicate the onset of excitation of the SA node (*S*), right atrium (*P*), AV node (*A*), His bundle (*H*), and the ventricles (*V*). Lead V1 shows a biphasic P wave arising from sequential excitation of the right and left ventricles.

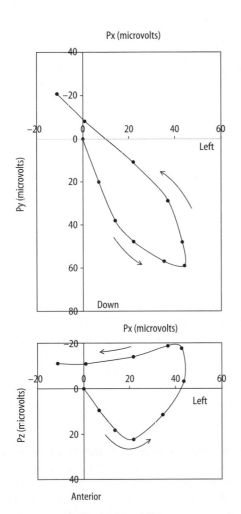

FIGURE 1.6 Projections of the spatial P wave vectors of normal adult men in frontal plane (*top*) and horizontal plane (*below*) projections at ten equally spaced time instants of time-normalized P wave duration.

part, on the originating impulse in various parts of the SA node and the conduction velocity in atrial fibers. In clinical practice, a PR interval 220 ms or longer is considered to indicate an abnormal AV conduction delay, or first-degree AV block.

1.3 Atrial Repolarization and the Baseline for Electrocardiographic Measurements

Atrial action potentials are relatively uniform in duration throughout atrial structures. As a consequence, atrial cells that depolarize earliest repolarize earliest, and the atrial repolarization process follows the same time course and direction as atrial depolarization, i.e. repolarization is concordant with depolarization so that the polarity of the Ta wave is opposite to that of the P wave.

In comparison with the other ECG waves, the Ta wave has received little attention in electrocardiography. The end of the P wave and the onset of the Ta wave overlap. As a consequence, it is difficult to determine the true end of the P wave and the onset of the Ta wave. The Ta wave is usually ignored, and no Ta duration or amplitude measurements are used in ECG reporting. However, the presence of a Ta wave can have important consequences for ECG amplitude measurements (Figure 1.8). The question about the selection of an appropriate baseline arises.

During the period when the low frequency response of ECG amplifiers was relatively inadequate because of filtering to avoid baseline drift, three different baselines by taking the baseline closest to the wave were used for ECG wave amplitude measurements: (1) the TP baseline for P wave amplitudes; (2) the PR baseline for QRS and ST measurements; and (3) the TP segment for T wave measurements. Presently, the PR segment preceding QRS onset is most commonly used as the baseline for all ECG wave amplitude measurements. The PR baseline is often depressed in the leads with a prominent P wave and a negative Ta wave, as shown in Figure 1.8. When the PR segment is taken as a common baseline, P wave amplitudes appear larger than the true P amplitudes, the difference being equal to the difference between TP and PR baselines. The ST segment may appear elevated, and the measured ST depression is reduced by the amount of the difference between

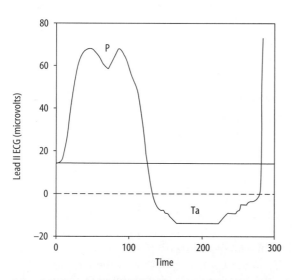

FIGURE 1.8 The effect of baseline selection on P wave and other ECG amplitudes as seen in lead II ECG of a subject with a first-degree AV block. Atrial T wave (*Ta*) amplitude is substantially larger when measured from the TP baseline (*heavy line*) than from the PR baseline (*broken line*). Note that the Ta wave polarity is opposite to that of the P wave.

the TP and PR baseline. T wave amplitudes may be larger, and the end of the T wave often does not return to the PR baseline. This may cause QT interval measurement problems, depending on the type of algorithm used.

1.4 Ventricular Excitation

The specialized ventricular conduction system is a continuous structure that provides a relatively fast pathway for cardiac excitation to propagate from the lower part of the right atrium to the ventricular myocardium at the left and right endocardial zones of the interventricular septum. The specialized ventricular conduction system consists of the following components: (a) the AV node,[3] which provides the connection between the right atrium and the ventricles; (b) the bundle of His;[4] and (c) the right and the left main bundles, which branch and end up as a network of thinner fibers known as the Purkinje network, described as early as 1845.[5a]

1.4.1 Ventricular Conduction System

Ventricular specialized conduction system components are the AV node, the bundle of His, the left and right bundle branch, and the Purkinje network.

1.4.1.1 The Atrioventricular Node

Fibrous connective tissue in septum between the atria and the ventricles prevents excitation spread from the atria to the ventricles except through the AV node and the bundle of His. The AV node is located in the atrial septum near the tricuspid valve. The functional importance of the AV node is to produce a delay so that atrial contraction is finished and the ventricles are fully filled before ventricular systole starts. The AV node structure is shaped like a funnel. Atrial excitation fronts arrive at the AV node via the crista terminalis and atrial septum at the wide base of the funnel in the AV node transitional cells. The conduction

---

[a] Check scientist Jan Evangelista Purkyné. Purkinje is the German version of his name.

velocity in the central part of the node is slow until excitation reaches the His bundle fibers at the narrow end part of the funnel-like structure.

1.4.1.2 The His–Purkinje Conduction System

The short common AV bundle divides into two branches. The left main bundle penetrates the upper part of the interventricular septum to the left endocardial side at the septal surface. The right branch terminates as the Purkinje network at the lower part of the right side of the ventricular septum and the apex of the right ventricle. Both main branches divide and terminate at the endocardial surface as the Purkinje network.

Conduction through the His–Purkinje system provides a second level of delay in the synchronization process of atrial and ventricular excitation and pumping action. It takes approximately 50 ms for excitation to propagate in the left main bundle branch from the bifurcation to the Purkinje fibers. The Purkinje network also synchronizes the initiation of ventricular excitation at ventricular endocardial zones including the papillary muscles, so that these structures contract first to protect the AV valves from prolapsing into the atria. On the left side, the Purkinje fibers are topographically located in the lower and middle two-thirds of the ventricular septum as a mesh of subendocardial fiber strands. From these strands ventricular activation spreads as a propagated response to the rest of the ventricles.

There have been a variety of differing descriptions of the topography of the fascicles and the branching tree of the Purkinje system ever since the early description by Tawara. A simplified concept of the patterns was introduced by Rosenbaum in the 1970s. He promoted the concept of the "hemiblocks" that he attributed to conduction defects in the left anterior or posterior fascicles.[6]

Extensive histological studies by Demoulin and Kulbertus have shown a great deal of variation in the topology of the specialized conduction system arising from the left main bundle in human hearts.[7] These investigators made a strong case for the existence of a midseptal fascicle in their initial report on 20 human hearts. Their later observations on 49 normal human hearts[8] were summarized as follows: in addition to a thin anterior

fascicle and a wider posterior fascicle, there was an easily identifiable sub-branch of midseptal fibers in 65% of the hearts. The midseptal branching arose in 10% of the hearts from the posterior fascicle and in the remaining 25% of the hearts consisted of a complicated anastomosing network, presumably originating from both main fascicles. These observations support the existence of a principally trifascicular arrangement of branching of the left main bundle in a substantial fraction of hearts. Demoulin and Kulbertus also suggested the possibility of a midfascicular block in addition to the left anterior and posterior fascicular blocks.

1.4.2 Initial Ventricular Septal Excitation

Detailed observations on initial ventricular excitation were reported by Durrer et al.[9] during the late 1960s. These investigators used transmural mapping of the left ventricular excitation in the Langendorf preparation of isolated human hearts removed in cardiac transplantation. They demonstrated that normal ventricular excitation starts practically simultaneously at three areas on the septal surface of the left ventricle: (a) superior anterior paraseptal region; (b) posterior lower paraseptal area approximately one-third the distance from the apex to the base; and (c) the central area of the left septal surface.

When assessing the spatial direction of the initial left ventricular septal excitation, it is important to note that the septum in a horizontal cross-section is not in the frontal plane. It is oriented obliquely, as shown in Figure 1.9. The long axis of the left ventricular cavity is oriented from the mitral ring at the base to the apex in a superior–right–posterior to inferior–left–anterior direction.

A schematic of the ventricular conduction system on the left side of the septum in Figure 1.10 shows the left bundle branch branching into three fascicles, which each branch into the Purkinje network. The heavier lines in the schematic indicate the three main areas of the Purkinje fiber branching where the septal excitation starts earliest. The central area of initial excitation comes from the midseptal fascicle, from the branching of the posterior fascicle, or from a more complex network arrangement depending on the topography of the branching.

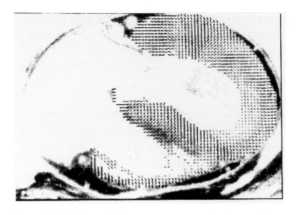

FIGURE 1.9 Horizontal plane cross-section of a human heart viewed from above. Note that the ventricular septum is oriented obliquely at a nearly 45° angle. The apex is also shifted so that the long axis of the left ventricular cavity from the mitral ring to the apex is oriented from a superior–right–posterior to an inferior–left–anterior direction. (Source: The National Library of Medicine, National Institutes of Health. www.nlm.nih.gov/research/visible/vhpconf2000/AUTHORS/SACHSE/TEXTINDX.HTM, 2005.)

The right bundle branches into the Purkinje network in the subendocardial right ventricle at the lower right anterior septal surface and the entire free right ventricular wall. The earliest right ventricular excitation occurs near the base of the anterior papillary muscle and the surrounding free wall. About a third of the lower anterior right interventricular septum is excited from the right side of the septum. During early periods of septal excitation, the wider septal excitation front left to right perpendicular to the left septal endocardial surface produces the dominant component of the net cardiac dipole. The two excitation fronts propagating in opposite directions in the septum gradually weaken the net septal dipole. The right ventricular anterior paraseptal epicardial breakthrough occurs at 25 ms from the onset of ventricular excitation, approximately 10 ms before the left ventricular anterior and posterior epicardial breakthroughs.

1.4.3 Ventricular Excitation Isochrones

Figure 1.11 shows the excitation isochrones at 10-ms intervals in an isolated human heart reproduced from the report of Durrer et al.[9] Essential

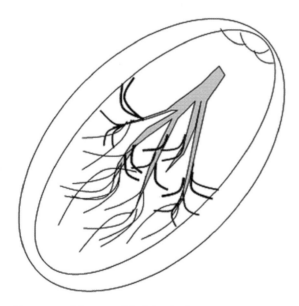

FIGURE 1.10 Schematic of the left side of the ventricular septum in an oblique view in right–anterior direction. The sketch shows the left main branch penetrating to the left side of the septum below the aortic valves and branching into the left anterior, the left posterior, and the midseptal fascicles, which each branch into the Purkinje network. The branches with thicker lines indicate the fibers in the three left septal areas excited earliest.

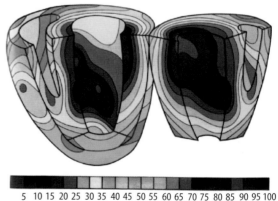

5 10 15 20 25 30 35 40 45 50 55 60 65 70 75 80 85 90 95 100

FIGURE 1.11 Excitation isochrones at 10-ms intervals in an isolated human heart viewed in oblique cross-sections along the right and left ventricular cavities after cutting and hinging a slice of the ventricles and turning it open to the left side. See text for details. (Source: Durrer et al.[9] Circulation 1970;41:899–912. © 1970 American Heart Association, Inc. Reproduced with permission from Lippincott, Williams & Wilkins.)

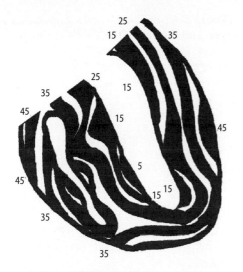

FIGURE 1.12 Summary schematic of the approximate sequential timing of excitation in a longitudinal oblique cross-section of the septum and the left ventricle.

the midwall and epicardium. At 20–25 ms excitation fronts circle the midwall of the left ventricle. Excitation reaches the epicardial surface of the left ventricular free wall in various hearts approximately 45 ms after the onset of septal excitation.

A summary schematic of the sequential timing of excitation in a longitudinal oblique cross-section of the septum and the left ventricle is shown in Figure 1.12.

1.4.4 Terminal Ventricular Excitation

The location of the latest ventricular region excited varies, being the top zones of the interventricular septum, crista supraventricularis, or the outflow tract of the right ventricle at the pulmonary cone. The timing of the latest ventricular excitation also varies, in parallel with the QRS duration.

information from this figure can be extracted by viewing the left side of the figure, which shows an oblique cross-section along the right and the left ventricular cavities. The isochrones in a cross-section of the septum show excitation proceeding from left to right and after some delay from right to left. The figure shows that in the left lateral wall, excitation spreads concentrically from endocardium to epicardium and, in this heart, diagonally slightly downwards from an area near the base (mitral ring area) towards

1.4.5 Ventricular Excitation and Body Surface Potential Distribution

Isopotential lines calculated from recorded body surface potential maps were demonstrated as early as 1963 by Taccardi in his classic report.[10] The figure reproduced here shows the isopotential lines at the time point of maximum ventricular excitation wave front in the left ventricle (Figure 1.13).

FIGURE 1.13 Isopotential lines on body surface at time point of maximum ventricular excitation wave front. (Source: Taccardi B.[10] Circ Res 1963;12:341–52. © 1963 American Heart Association, Inc. Reproduced with permission from Lippincott, Williams & Wilkins.)

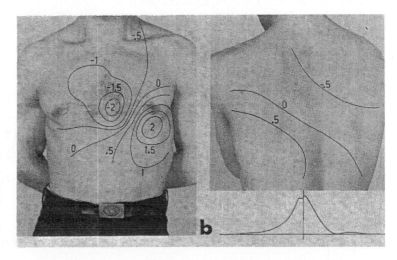

It is relatively easy to comprehend ECG manifestations of the early septal excitation in terms of the isochrones of excitation spread and a single net cardiac dipole. Deduction of the ECG manifestations from the isochrones of ventricular excitation at later time points is more complex. The source is best characterized as a set of distributed dipoles, which add up to one net dipole. Distance from the source dipoles to body surface recording locations and other factors influencing lead vectors dominate the net result. Refined computer models of the excitation and repolarization of the human heart in an inhomogeneous torso have made it possible to simulate realistic body surface potential distributions by solving the so-called forward problem.[11]

The approach introduced by van Oosterom[12,13] determines body surface potential distribution as matrix multiplication **AS**, where matrix **S** represents the source dipoles at sequential steps of excitation and repolarization, and matrix **A** contains the coefficients for calculating the surface potential at each node on the body surface ($n = 64$) for 257 epicardial source node locations. For a single dipole source, the three elements of the row vector **A** are equivalent to the lead vector for the node for a specific dipole location. At each excitation step at each source node, the dipole strength is uniformly taken equal to the change in transmembrane potential (100 mV). The beauty of the model is that the resulting equivalent source matrix **S** is determined solely by timing of local excitation and repolarization, i.e. the time point of the onset of excitation and action potential duration. If epicardial potential distribution is determined first, body surface potential at each body surface node can be visualized by the solid angle subtended by the excitation front at any time instant.

1.4.6 Orientation of the QRS Vectors in Normal Subjects

The overall patterns of the frontal and horizontal QRS vector loops shown in Figure 1.14 were derived from combined normal male and female subjects to demonstrate the relationships between QRS vectors. The QRS vector directions in the frontal plane (on top) are fairly uniform, oriented

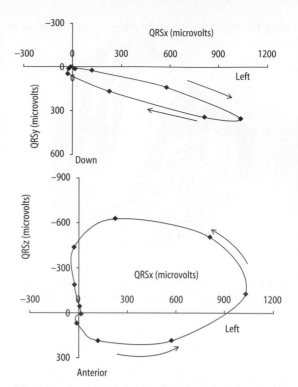

FIGURE 1.14 Mean QRS vectors of combined normal male and female subjects at ten equally spaced time points in frontal plane (*top*) and horizontal plane (*below*) projections. The direction of rotation of QRS vectors in time is indicated by the two curved arrows.

to the left and inferiorly. The horizontal plane projections (below) of the QRS vectors show anterior and left rotation until the point when the QRS amplitudes reach the maximum at four-tenths of QRS, corresponding approximately to the left free wall epicardial breakthrough. After this time point, QRS vectors rotate gradually more posteriorly during the second half of ventricular excitation. Terminal vectors after the 70-ms time point are directed posteriorly and to the right, corresponding to the late excitation.

1.4.7 Normal Variations in the Direction of the Initial Ventricular Excitation

Directional distributions of the QRS vectors shown in Table 1.1 identify spatial variations of ventricular excitation at various time points. This information was derived from Table C4 in Section C of Part 2 of this book. The directional distribu-

TABLE 1.1 Directional distributions (%) of the QRS vectors at ten equally spaced time points of QRS of 11,707 normal men and women.

	Time point as a fraction of QRS interval									
Direction	1/10	2/10	3/10	4/10	5/10	6/10	7/10	8/10	9/10	10/10
AR	**45**	**19**	0	0	0	0	0	0	1	9
AL	**20**	**56**	**31**	4	0	0	0	0	2	**16**
L	2	12	**54**	**72**	**62**	12	2	2	6	9
ILA	7	9	11	8	**19**	1	0	1	6	**23**
PL	0	1	3	**13**	4	**42**	30	23	17	5
PR	0	0	0	0	1	**27**	**47**	**44**	**21**	6
IP	1	1	1	3	9	14	14	18	**26**	14
SLP	0	0	0	0	3	2	2	2	5	3
SRP	1	0	0	0	1	1	4	9	10	4
R	4	1	0	0	1	0	1	1	3	5
IRA	8	0	0	0	0	0	0	0	0	0
SA	13	2	0	0	0	0	0	1	3	8

AR anterior–right, *AL* anterior–left, *L* left, *ILA* inferior–left–anterior, *PL* posterior–left, *PR* posterior–right, *IP* inferior–posterior, *SLP* superior–left–posterior, *SRP* superior–right–posterior, *R* right, *IRA* inferior–right–anterior, *SA* superior–anterior. The spatial directions corresponding to the acronyms are shown in Figure 1.15. Bold-faced numbers indicate the two most prominent directions for each time point.

tions are described using 12 symmetrical spatial reference directions of equal area as shown in Figure 1.15.[14] Normal directional variations of QRS at the initial one-tenth time point of QRS in Table 1.1 indicate the directional distribution of the initial ventricular septal excitation. There are two dominant directions in normal subjects: anterior right in 45% and anterior left in 20%. In addition, the direction is superior–anterior in 13%, inferior–right–anterior in 8% and inferior–left–anterior in 7%. These five directions, all with an anterior component, occupy 92% of the 12 spatial directions.

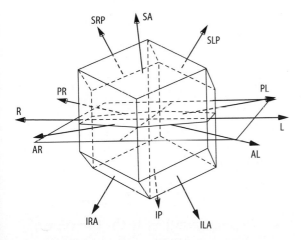

FIGURE 1.15 Twelve symmetrical spatial reference directions for summarizing directional distributions of ECG vectors. The letters in the acronyms denote the directions in order of the closeness to left (*L*), right (*R*), inferior (*I*), superior (*S*), anterior (*A*) and posterior (*P*) directions of the *x*, *y* and *z* axis. (Source: Rautaharju et al.[14] Circulation 1973;48:541–8. © 1973 American Heart Association, Inc. Reproduced with permission from Lipincott, Williams & Wilkins.)

1.4.8 Shifting Dominant Directions during the Time Course of Ventricular Excitation

As seen in Table 1.1, the dominant direction shifts from anterior–right to anterior–left and then to the left during the initial three-tenths of QRS. Then the orientation stays in the left direction for four-tenths of QRS and the midpoint of ventricular excitation, five-tenths of QRS. During the second half of excitation, the dominant direction shifts to posterior–left at six-tenths of QRS and to posterior–right at seven-tenths of QRS.

1.4.9 Dominant Directions During Terminal Ventricular Excitation

At the time point of nine-tenths of QRS, the dominant direction is inferior–posterior or posterior–right in 47% of normal subjects, and the rest of the directions are mainly to posterior–left or superior–right–posterior. The dominant directions during the last one-tenth of QRS (the J-point) are inferior–left–anterior, anterior–left and inferior–posterior. This directional distribution of the J-point vectors is in an apparent conflict with visual J-point measurement data that show the highest J amplitudes in V1 and V2. The reason is that the computer algorithm defines the end of QRS using amplitude thresholds for the composite spatial magnitude curve rather than separate thresholds for each ECG lead. The apparent J-point elevation in V1–V2 is generally due to enhanced early slow ventricular repolarization overlapping with late ventricular excitation.

1.5 Ventricular Repolarization

Ventricular repolarization often begins before ventricular excitation is completed. The first part of ventricular repolarization corresponds to phase 2 of ventricular action potential and the ST segment of the ECG, and is properly called the slow phase of ventricular repolarization. The fast phase of ventricular repolarization generates the T wave and corresponds to phase 3 of the ventricular action potential. The transition from the slow to the fast phase of ventricular repolarization is gradual, and the beginning of the T wave is often difficult to discern from the ECG.

1.5.1 Slow Phase of Ventricular Repolarization and the ST Segment

The action potential phase 2 plateau is not exactly horizontal. It slopes slightly down towards zero or slightly more negative values. The downslope of the subepicardial myocytes is slightly steeper than that of the subendocardial myocytes. This generates a potential gradient with a gradually increasing magnitude during phase 2 in the direction from endocardium to epicardium. Considering the potential gradient in the lateral wall of the left ventricle, the ST segment in lateral leads will be upsloping. The normal dominant directions of the mean ST vector are inferior–left–anterior, left, or posterior–left.

1.5.2 Fast Phase of Ventricular Repolarization and the T wave

The spatial directions of repolarization vectors are shown in Figure 1.16 in frontal (top) and horizontal plane (below) projections. The T wave vector directions are remarkably uniform compared with the wide variation of the QRS vectors, particularly in horizontal plane projections as shown in Figure 1.14. A summary of the spatial relationships between normal mean QRS and T vectors in Table 1.2 shows that the dominant directions of the mean QRS vector are left, posterior–left, inferior–posterior and inferior–left–anterior. The four directions occupy 97% of the distribution. Three dominant mean T vector directions occupy 96% of the distribution: anterior–left, inferior–left–anterior and left.

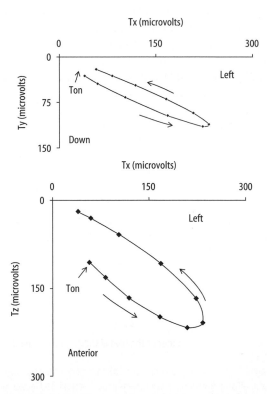

FIGURE 1.16 Mean T vectors of normal adult men and women at successive 10-ms time points in frontal plane (*top*) and horizontal plane (*below*) projections. Note that the T onset amplitude (*arrow*) as well as the T end amplitude deviate from zero when QRS onset is used as the baseline level.

TABLE 1.2 Joint distribution of the directions of the mean QRS and T vectors by the four dominant direction categories of each vector.

		Mean T vector direction				
		AL (52%)	ILA (8%)	L (11%)	Other (29%)	Percent
Mean	L (43%)	52.7	32.5	10.6	4.2	100
QRS	PL (37%)	50.5	33.0	12.3	4.2	100
Vector	IP (9%)	52.6	32.0	11.8	3.6	100
Direction	ILA (8%)	53.8	32.9	9.9	3.5	100

Percentages in brackets indicate dominant directions of the QRS and T vectors, other percentages joint distributions of the two vectors. The acronyms are defined in Table 1.1 and the spatial directions corresponding to the acronyms are shown in Figure 1.15.

1.5.3 The Degree of Discordance of Ventricular Repolarization

The direction of repolarization is in general reverse with respect to the direction of depolarization, an observation that has intrigued electrocardiographers for a century. The present generation of electrocardiographers tend to think that repolarization is uniformly reverse to excitation, a concept that holds for the left lateral free wall of the left ventricle but not so when the other regions of the ventricles repolarize.

The spatial angle between the mean QRS and mean T vectors is 62° in normal women and 76° in men, closer to 90° than to 0°, and repolarization and depolarization processes, on the average, are nearly perpendicular to each other (Table 1.3). The isochrone lines in the free left ventricular wall in the human heart in Figure 1.12 showed that the ET difference across the wall is approximately 30 ms. This means that the action potential duration (APD) at the epicardial layers should be over 30 ms shorter than that at the endocardial surface for a reverse repolarization sequence to occur and a positive T wave in the left lateral leads, as was

noted at the beginning of this chapter (Figure 1.2). There is actually a scarcity of documented information that such large APD differences between subepicardial and subendocardial cells exist. Taking spatial aspects of ECG manifestations of the depolarization and repolarization process into consideration, repolarization is neither concordant nor fully reverse. It is semidiscordant or semireverse, and the degree of discordance varies with repolarization time (RT). In the horizontal plane projection, the initial half of repolarization appears to be largely reverse and the latter half largely concordant, as can be deduced by inspecting Figures 1.14 and 1.16.

A further complication in the concept of the reverse repolarization sequence is that a certain proportion of M cells with long APD have been reported to be present in the hearts of several species.[15–17] The distribution of M cells in canine hearts varies in various myocardial segments. In the lateral wall, M cells are predominantly located in the layers between the subepicardium to midmyocardium and in the anterior wall predominantly between the subendocardium and midmyocardium.[16]

TABLE 1.3 Mean, standard deviation and the upper and lower second and fifth percentile ranges of the spatial QRS/T angle (°) in normal men and women.

	Men ($n = 4,726$)	Women ($n = 6,981$)	Gender groups combined ($n = 11,707$)
Mean	76	62	68
Standard deviation	29.7	27.8	29.5
Second to 98th percentile range	31 $\rightarrow$ 130	21 $\rightarrow$ 113	17 $\rightarrow$ 139
Fifth to 95th percentile range	39 $\rightarrow$ 116	29 $\rightarrow$ 98	22 $\rightarrow$ 126

The M cell layers potentially play an important role in determining the direction of transmural repolarization. As will be discussed in Chapter 10 on QT interval (shown in Figure 10.2), in canine ventricular myocardium RT in subepicardial layers increases initially slowly from epicardium to deeper subepicardial layers, then suddenly starts increasing faster, apparently at the M cell transitional zone. After this jump, subepicardial RT is approximately equal to the RT in the subendocardial layers. The RT increases progressively in subepicardial as well as in subendocardial layers towards the M cell layers, which have the longest APD and RT.

Antzelovitch points out that the existence of myocardial cells with M cell type characteristics have not been verified in vivo in several studies, suggesting methodological differences such as the use of anesthetics that preferentially block late sodium current in M cells.[17]

The overall effect of the M cells will depend on two factors: (a) the size of the M cell population; and (b) the potential effect of electrotonic interaction between repolarizing myocytes. Taggart et al. evaluated activation recovery intervals from the electrograms in 21 patients during routine coronary artery surgery in five transmural locations in the left ventricular wall.[18] RT gradients were uniform across the wall, and no maximum RT was present in the midsection.

There used to be a longstanding debate whether repolarization is a propagated response. Simultaneous repolarization wave fronts can coexist in different myocardial regions as determined by the RT distribution in the whole ventricular myocardium. The current understanding is that repolarization is not a propagated response although it appears as if it were because of the rather regular repolarization sequence.

1.6 The U Wave

Numerous hypotheses have arisen over time to explain the generation of the U wave. The discovery of the M cells appears to offer a plausible mechanism.[19] The M cell APD is strongly rate-dependent. The M cell APD prolongation with decreasing stimulus rate is substantially more pronounced than that in epicardial or endocardial cells.

Recently, RitZsema van Eck et al. emphasized that the effect of varying distance of various transmural layers on an ECG lead's sensitivity (lead vector strength) has to be considered.[20] U waves overlapping the tale end of the T wave became apparent when incorporating the distance effect from various transmural layers on lead sensitivity and varying distance from the epicardium to the potential pick-up point in their infinite homogeneous volume conductor model.

References

1. Eifler WJ, Macchi E, Ritsema van Eck HJ et al. Mechanism of generation of body surface electrocardiographic P-waves in normal, middle, and lower sinus rhythms. Circ Res 1981;48:168–82.
2. Marriott HJL, Boudreau MH. Advanced Concepts in Arrhythmias. St. Louis, Toronto, London: C.V. Mosby Company, 1983.
3. Tawara S. Das Reizleitungssystem des Saugetierherzens. Eine anatomisch-histologische Studie über das Atrioventrikularbündel und die Purkinjeschen Fäden. Jena: Gustav Fischer Ferlag, 1906.
4. His W Jr. Die Tätigkeit des embryonalen Herzens und deren Bedeutung für die Lehre von den Bewegungen beim Erwachenen. Arkiv medizinishe Klinik Leipzig 1893;20:14–50.
5. Purkinje JE. Mikroskopisch neurologische Beobachtungen. Archiv für Anatomie, Physiologie und wischenshaftliche Medicin 1845;12:281.
6. Rosenbaum MB. The hemiblocks: diagnostic criteria and clinical significance. Mod Concepts Cardiovasc Dis 1970;39:141–6.
7. Demoulin JC, Kulbertus HE. Histopathological examination of concept of left hemiblock. Br Heart J 1972;34:807–14.
8. Demoulin JC, Kulbertus HE. Pathological findings in patients with left anterior hemiblock. In: Hoffman I (ed). Vectorcardiography 3. Amsterdam, Oxford: North Holland Publishing Company, 1976, pp 123–7.
9. Durrer D, van Dam R Th, Freud GE et al. Total excitation of the isolated human heart. Circulation 1970;41:899–912.
10. Taccardi B. Distribution of heart potentials on the thoracic surface of normal human subjects. Circ Res 1963;12:341–52.
11. Horáček BM, Warren JW, Feild DQ et al. Statistical and deterministic approaches to designing transformations of electrocardiographic leads. J Electrocardiol 2002;35(Suppl):41–52.

12. van Oosterom A, Oostendorp TF. ECGSIM: an interactive tool for studying the genesis of QRST waveforms. Heart 2004;90(2):165–8.
13. Huiskamp GJM, van Oosterom A. The depolarization sequence of the human heart surface potentials computed from measured body surface potentials. IEEE Trans Biomed Eng 1988;35:1047–58.
14. Rautaharju PM, Blackburn H, Warren J, Menotti A. Waveform patterns in the Frank-lead rest and exercise electrocardiograms of healthy elderly men. Circulation 1973;48:541–8.
15. Sicouri S, Antzelovitch C. A subpopulation of cells with unique electrophysiological properties in the deep subepicardium of the canine ventricle: the M cell. Circ Res 1991;68:1729–41.
16. Yan GX, Shimizu W, Antzelocitch C. Characteristics and distribution of M cells in artificially-perfused canine left ventricular preparations. Circulation 1998;98:1921–7.
17. Antzelovitch C, Zygmunt AC, Dumaine R. Electrophysiology and pharmacology of ventricular repolarization. In: Gussak I, Antzelovich C (eds). Cardiac Repolarization. Bridging Basic and Clinical Science. Totowa, New Jersey: Humana Press, 2002, pp 63–89.
18. Taggart P, Sutton PMI, Opthol T et al. Transmural repolarization in the left ventricle in humans during normoxia and ischemia. Cardiovasc Res 2001;50:454–62.
19. Antzelevitch C, Sicouri S. Clinical relevance of cardiac arrhythmias generated by afterdepolarizations. Role of M cells in the generation of U waves, triggered activity and torsades de pointes. J Am Coll Cardiol 1994;23:259–77.
20. RitZsema van Eck HJ, Kors JA, van Herpen G. The U wave in the ECG: a new view on its genesis. Int J Bioelectromagnetism 2003;5:309–11.

2
Electrocardiographic Lead Systems

Synopsis

Electrocardiogram Leads and Lead Vectors

An electrocardiogram (ECG) lead is defined by the electrode locations on the body surface and the specifications of the node network used for the lead. Body surface ECGs in standard 12-lead locations are, as a first approximation, adequately represented by their model-based lead vectors and a single fixed-location cardiac source dipole, varying in orientation and magnitude in the course of the cardiac excitation/repolarization cycle.

Electrocardiogram Lead Triangles

Algebraic relationships between all six limb leads can be deduced from a triangle formed by the lead vectors of leads I, II and III. The shape of this scalene lead vector triangle deviates considerably from that of Einthoven's equilateral lead vector triangle with the cardiac dipole in the center of his homogeneous, symmetric, spherical volume conductor model.

Lead Vectors and Source Dipoles

The lead vectors of leads I, II and III and other so-called "bipolar" leads are represented in the image surface counterpart of the human torso surface obtained by mapping lead vectors for a defined source dipole location. Lead vectors for leads involving an ECG node network, such as the augmented aV leads and chest leads V1–V6, are characterized by lead vectors between a node inside the image surface of the torso in image space and the pick-up electrode locations on the image surface. The lead vector describes how the ECG in that lead is related to the cardiac source dipole of unit magnitude excited in X, Y and Z directions in a selected fixed location in the cardiac area within the volume conductor representing the human torso. The lead vector strength of various ECG leads varies with torso geometric factors and inhomogeneities (fiber orientation, distance from the source, torso resistivity).

Electrocardiogram Models

The X, Y and Z components of the heart vector (E) at any time instant and the lead vector of a lead can be used to represent the ECG in that lead as the scalar product $L \bullet E$ between the lead vector (L) and the heart vector E. $L \bullet E$ is the product of the absolute magnitudes of vectors L and E multiplied by the cosine of the spatial angle between them. More sophisticated ECG models make use of distributed cardiac dipole sources in various cardiac locations, each with its own set of lead vectors.

Abbreviations and Symbols

aVR – Goldberger's augmented lead from reference node GR to right arm
EASI – Dower's quasiorthogonal ES, AS and AI leads
ECG – electrocardiogram
E – heart vector (the net cardiac source dipole)

18

F – left leg (electrode location)
L – lead vector
LA – left arm (electrode location)
P – current dipole moment
RA – right arm (electrode location)
WCT – Wilson's central terminal
Z – transfer impedance vector

2.1 Introduction

An electrocardiogram (ECG) is a recording of the potential difference between two ECG electrodes, between an electrode and a network node, or between two network nodes. An ECG lead is defined by the location of the ECG electrodes on the body surface and the electrical network of the node or nodes used for recording of that lead. The lead-off electrode is connected to the positive terminal and the node to the negative terminal of the electrocardiograph. (Because even a single lead-off point is connected through the input network of an ECG amplifier, even a single electrode lead-off point can in fact be considered as a node.)

A familiar node is the Wilson's central terminal (WCT). This node is formed by connecting the right arm (RA), left arm (LA) and the left leg (F) electrodes to a network node with equal resistors and equal weighting of the potentials, so that the potential of the node is equal to the average of the potentials at RA, LA and F. Another familiar set of nodes are the Goldberger's reference terminals. These consist of three pairs of electrodes (LA and F, RA and F, RA and LA), each connected to their node with equal weighting for recording Goldberger's leads aVR, aVL and aVF.

Twelve ECG leads are generally recorded in clinical electrocardiography. In research applications, as many as 200 or more body surface ECGs are sampled simultaneously. Research on body surface potential maps has revealed that body surface potential distributions are mainly dipolar, with a single maximum and a single minimum present at each instant of cardiac activity. At some instances of cardiac excitation, potential distributions show two maxima (or one with a saddle point).

Principal component analysis (singular value decomposition) of the standard 12-lead ECG indicates that, in normal subjects, nearly all of the QRS energy (amplitude variance) and practically all of the T wave amplitude variance can be attributed to a single dipolar source. The average magnitude of nondipolar voltage within the QRS complex of the 12-lead ECG of normal subjects is $48\,\mu V$, accounting for 0.14% of the QRS amplitude variance. In T waves, the magnitude of the average nondipolar voltage in normal adult subjects is $11\,\mu V$, accounting for just 0.25% of the T wave amplitude variance.[1] Consequently, the manifestations of cardiac activity in standard ECG leads can be represented by their lead vectors in image surface and the cardiac source dipole, first introduced by Burger and van Milan.[2-4] The concept was operationally formulated in terms of a current dipole and transfer impedance by Schmitt.[5] The lead vector concept was extensively explored by Frank[6,7] and several other investigators, and more recently quantified with extensive documentation by Horáček et al.[8,9]

2.2 ECG Lead Vectors

Lead vector properties of body surface ECG leads are of interest to noninvasive electrocardiography. Electrocardiographic investigators in the period after the Second World War used homogeneous torso tank models. A calibrated voltage dipole was activated in the heart region sequentially in three perpendicular (X, Y and Z) directions, and then the X, Y and Z components of the lead vectors of various ECG leads were measured.

The most important practical result from these empirical torso tank experiments was the development of the so-called orthogonal lead systems. One of these orthogonal lead systems has survived until today, namely the lead system developed by Frank.[7] The design objective of these orthogonal lead systems was to represent the activity of the cardiac source occurring in the X, Y, and Z directions with equal sensitivity in the X, Y and Z leads so that for instance lead X would respond to cardiac source dipole excited only in the X direction.

Detailed computer models of the human heart and torso with inhomogeneities (lungs, intracavitary cardiac blood masses) have greatly facilitated examination of the properties of various ECG leads. The strength and direction of lead vectors depend strongly on the location of the source dipole, and both are modified by the inhomogeneities of the torso.[8,9] Points connecting the lead vectors representing various body surface points form the so-called image surface. It should be noted that an image surface is valid for a specific representative source dipole location. If this location is changed, a new image surface needs to be determined. A lead field for a dipole located near the centroid of the heart is commonly used to express general properties of different ECG leads in terms of the direction and magnitude of the lead vectors.

A cardiac electric source dipole in an electrolytic tank is characterized by the current dipole moment P, a vector with magnitude P and units of ampere-meters (amp.m). The potential difference V generated in an ECG lead is a scalar quantity. The magnitude of V is determined by P and another vector Z that Schmitt called transfer impedance.[5] The units of Z are ohms/meter (ohm.m^{-1}). The potential difference V (volts) is then the scalar product between P and Z:

$$V = P \bullet Z = P^*Z^*\cos\theta = Px^*Zx + Py^*Zy + Pz + Zz$$

where P and Z refer to the absolute magnitudes of P and Z, and υ is the spatial angle between P and Z. Px, Zx, Py, Zy, and Pz, Zz are the X, Y, and Z coefficients of P and Z.

The following brief notes summarize key properties of the image surface and image space, perhaps helping to interpret questions often asked by electrocardiographers, such as where is WCT located. The understanding of these notes is facilitated by viewing Figure 2.1, a simplified sketch of the image space cross-section in the frontal (X,Y) plane.[10]

• In image space, the intersection of the spatial XYZ coordinate system is the reference point for evaluating ECG lead properties. Surface S' (heavy line) in Figure 2.1 is the counterpart of body surface S in torso topography. Points RA', LA' and F' on the image surface represent anatomical points RA, LA, and F. On the image surface, the corners RA', LA' and F' determine the form of the scalene lead vector triangle of the frontal plane leads. (In image space, the triangle is not exactly in the frontal plane because

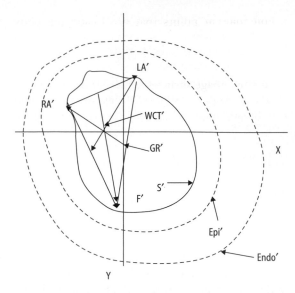

FIGURE 2.1 Schematic of the frontal plane counterpart of the human torso in convoluted image space. The limb lead recording points on body surface (S), R, L and F are located on the image surface counterpart of the body surface (S') in locations R', L' and F', and network nodes external to the body surface, such as Wilson's central terminal (WCT) and the negative pole of Goldberger's aVR lead (GR) are inside S', labeled as WCT' and GR'. Because the sensitivity of the ECG leads increases profoundly with shorter distance from the cardiac source, the image surface of the epicardium (Epi') is outside S', and the endocardial image surface (Endo') is even further out. (Source: Rautaharju PM.[10] J Electrocardiol 2005;38:128–9. Copyright © 2005. Reproduced with permission from Elsevier.)

of the image surface convolution with respect to the anatomic torso surface.)
• The length of each lead vector, for instance of lead I (from RA' to LA') corresponds to the sensitivity of the lead and its direction indicates the direction for which the lead is most sensitive for recording cardiac electrical activity.
• Lead vector properties in image space have been determined for a specified fixed location of the cardiac dipole in the cardiac region. This point, the center of the dipole location Q, is at point Q' at the intersection point of the spatial XYZ reference frame in image space, taken as zero reference potential.
• The location of the node of a network external to the body surface such as WCT is at location WCT' inside the image surface. A vector from Q' to WCT' indicates the potential of WCT with respect to the zero reference potential.

- Potentials at points that are inside the body surface increase in magnitude the closer they are to the dipole activated at point Q (inverse square of the distance relationship). Consequently, image surfaces corresponding to endocardial and epicardial surfaces are convoluted in image space so that they are both outside the image surface of the body surface, and the image surface of the endocardium is further out than that of the epicardium, as depicted in Figure 2.1.

The importance of lead vectors for the understanding of the relationships between ECG leads and the relationships between cardiac source events and the recorded body surface potentials cannot be adequately emphasized. The characteristics of commonly used ECG leads will be discussed next.

2.2.1 Einthoven's Limb Leads I, II and III

These are the leads that Einthoven used in the early 1900s for recording ECGs with his famous invention, the string galvanometer electrocardiograph.[11] Einthoven illustrated the relationship between his leads using as a reasonable approximation, an equilateral triangle in an unbounded infinite homogeneous volume conductor.

The lead vector directions and magnitude of the limb leads of the so-called Burger's triangle in image surface differ considerably from those of Einthoven's equilateral triangle (Figure 2.2). The deviations occur because the cardiac source is asymmetric within the human torso, and the human torso is an inhomogeneous volume conductor bound by the body surface. Inhomogeneities in tissue resistivity (blood, lungs) influence the direction of current flow and the direction of lead vectors, as does the asymmetry of the location of the heart within the thorax and the distance from the source to the lead-off points on the body surface.

2.2.2 Wilson's "Unipolar" and Goldberger's Augmented Limb Leads

In 1934, Wilson et al. introduced his central terminal and the "unipolar" leads. Wilson reasoned

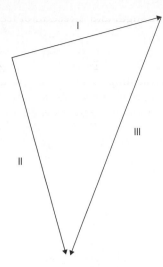

FIGURE 2.2 Lead vectors of standard limb leads I, II, and III. Note that the shape of this scalenic triangle differs substantially from that of Einthoven's equilateral triangle. However, vector addition rules are valid for any shape of the vector triangle. The resultant vector by adding lead vectors of leads I and III is: **I + III = II**. This implies that the ECG in lead II is the sum of leads I and III at any instant of the cardiac excitation/repolarization cycle.

that these leads recorded potential variations just under a single, "active" or "exploring" electrode,[12] while the potential in his central terminal was 0. WCT was obtained by connecting RA, LA, and LL electrodes through a network of equal resistors to the reference (negative) input terminal that recorded the average potential of RA, LA and LL. Each of the limb electrodes was then connected sequentially (in a single-channel galvanometer electrocardiograph) to the positive input to record leads VR, VL and VF, and also the chest leads V1–V6.

The problem with Wilson's limb leads was that their amplitudes were small. Eight years later, Goldberger introduced a method of augmenting Wilson's limb leads.[13] He achieved the augmentation by connecting sequentially each pair of limb electrodes, for instance LA and LL, through a network of equal resistors to the reference electrode that thus recorded the average potential of LA and LL at Goldberger's reference node for the augmented VR lead (aVR). The remaining limb RA was then connected to the positive terminal. Like Wilson, Goldberger also considered his reference electrode connection to represent zero

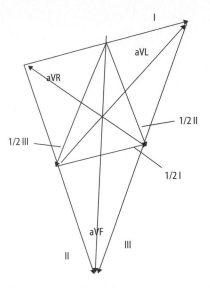

FIGURE 2.3 An ancillary vector triangle drawn by connecting midpoints of lead vectors **I**, **II** and **III**, with sides equal to 1/2**I**, 1/2**II** and 1/2**III**. A variety of equivalent expressions for the relationships between the limb lead ECGs summarized in Table 1.1 can be deduced from the diagram without resorting to trigonometric calculations just by following vector addition rules. A vector with negative sign is used when traversing in a direction opposite to the direction of the lead vector. As an example, **aVL** = 1/2**I** − 1/2**III**, or 1/2**II** − **III**, or −1/2**III** + 1/2**I**.

potential and the leads as augmented unipolar leads.

The lead vectors of Wilson's and Goldberger's limb leads show that the augmentation achieved by Goldberger with respect to Wilson's VR leads is 50%, for instance the lead vector **aVL** = 3/2 **VL** (Figure 2.3). As mentioned above, WCT records the average potential of RA, LA, and LL. WCT is located at the intersection of the lead vectors aVR, aVL, and aVF at the centroid of the lead vector triangle of leads I, II and III in the frontal plane of the image surface.

2.3 Common Misconceptions about ECG Leads

These misconceptions are numerous, and the most common are considered next:

1. Since there are two poles in each ECG lead, an ECG represents two potentials or "views" of cardiac electrical activity. However, an ECG is not a potential; it is a potential difference, and the difference of two "views" is one view and one view only.

2. An active or exploring electrode like V1 represents the potential "under" the exploring electrode. This is a misconception popularized by Wilson. Each electrode reflects at any time point the contribution to the potential of the excitable cells from all regions of the heart that are electrically active at each time point. The contribution is weighted by the distance and other factors influencing current flow and potential distribution within the torso.

3. Contributions to the potential difference from various parts of the heart are proportional to their projection on the axis of the lead. This is partly correct, but the projections in question are only on the portion of the lead axis between the two nodes in question. For instance, the projection on the axis of lead V1 is on the portion of the V1 axis between the WCT and V1 location, and not on the portion between the WCT and the point on the back opposite to V1. This portion of the posterior wall activity is not obtained merely by inverting the V1 lead. It could be recorded in a lead from WCT to the point on the back of the chest.

4. The potential at Wilson's central terminal is zero and thus it is an "indifferent electrode". This is the concept promoted by Wilson. Kirchhoff's laws do not make any claims that the potential in a node like WCT is zero. Although relatively low, it is not zero, and its potential does not remain constant throughout the cardiac electrical activity cycle.

5. There is also a great deal of confusion prevailing about the location of nodes such as WCT, with claims that it is located within the anatomic cardiac source. This question needs consideration of the location of the central terminal node in relation to the origin of the XYZ reference point in image space counterpart of the anatomical torso. Network node locations that are physically outside the body surface are inside the image surface of the torso in image space, and they exist in image space only, with their location defined in relation to the origin of the reference coordinate system.

2.3.1 The Importance of Lead Vector Relationships

The set of 12 standard ECG leads has only eight independent components. If any two of the six limb leads are recorded simultaneously, the remaining four can be calculated from the pair using trigonometric relationships between the lead vectors. This is because there are only two independent components in the six limb leads. ECG acquisition systems generally sample only two of the six limb leads, in pairs such as I and II, or I and aVF (Table 2.1).

A simple schematic is helpful for understanding the relationships of all limb leads without the need to resort to trigonometric calculations (Figure 2.4). The schematic has an ancillary vector diagram obtained by connecting the midpoints of lead vectors I, II and III, with sides equal to 1/2 I, 1/2 II and 1/2 III. Note that the midpoints of this new vector diagram again divide the above half-

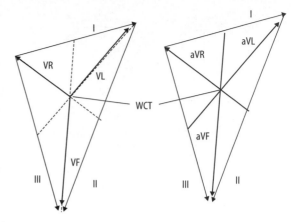

FIGURE 2.4 Wilson's central terminal (*WCT*), lead vectors of Wilson's "unipolar" leads VR, VL, VF (*left*), and Goldberger's augmented limb leads aVR, aVL and aVF (*right*) shown together with lead vectors for Einthoven's leads I, II and III. WCT is at the intersection of the lines connecting the half points of lead vectors **I**, **II** and **III** to the corners of the lead vector triangle. WCT is also the point of intersection of lead vectors aVR, aVL and aVF. Note that the lead vectors of Wilson's limb leads are 2/3 of the length of Goldberger's aV leads, i.e. the augmentation factor for aV leads is 3/2 compared to Wilson's limb leads.

TABLE 2.1 Primary equivalent expressions of limb lead relationships. The table includes expressions sufficient for calculating the remaining four leads when only leads I and II, or only leads I and aVF are recorded.

Lead	Reference connection	Positive connection	Primary equivalent expressions
I	RA	LA	$I = II - III$ $= -2/3\,aVR + 2/3\,aVL$
II	RA	LL	$II = I + III$ $= -2/3\,aVR + 2/3\,aVF$ $= 1/2\,I + aVF$
III	LA	LL	$III = -I + II$ $= -2/3\,aVL + 2/3\,aVF$ $= -1/2\,I + aVF$
aVR	1/2 (LA + LL)	RA	$aVR = 1/2\,III - II$ $= -1/2\,III - I$ $= -1/2\,I - 1/2\,II$
aVL	1/2 (RA + LL)	LA	$aVL = -1/2\,II + I$ $= 1/2\,II - III$ $= -1/2\,III + 1/2\,I$ $= 3/4\,I - 1/2\,aVF*$
aVF	1/2 (RA + LA)	LL	$aVF = 1/2\,I + III$ $= -1/2\,I + II$ $= 1/2\,II + 1/2\,III$

* This and other less obvious lead vector relationships can be deduced from the lead vectors in Figure 2.3. For aVL, traveling from the aVL lead vector starting point following the vector path 1/4 I, −1/2 aVF, 1/2 I we get aVL = 3/4 I − 1/2 aVF.

vectors into halves, with length equal to 1/4 of lead vectors **I**, **II** and **III**. The midpoints of the new vector triangle also divide the lead vectors of the aV leads into halves, and the halves within the new vector triangle are again divided at the point of the central terminal in proportion 2/3 and 1/3.

The lead vector of each limb lead can be expressed in several ways by traveling various vectorial paths of vector triangles. (The minus sign must be included whenever a vector component is added by traveling in the direction opposite the direction of the lead vector.) Thus, as an example, $aVL = -\frac{1}{2}II + I$, or $aVL = \frac{1}{2}II - III$.

2.3.2 Standard 12-Lead Electrocardiograms

Standardized locations of the lead-off points of the chest leads can be referenced to the thoracic landmarks of the human torso (Figure 2.5). V1 and V2 are located at the right and left sternal border at the fourth intercostal space. V4 is at the intersection of the fifth intercostal space and a meridian drawn from the midclavicular bend, and V6 is at the left midaxillary line at the horizontal

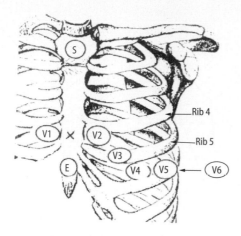

FIGURE 2.5 Locations of Wilson's chest leads V1–V6 in the reference frame of the left side of the bony thorax, specified in detail in the text. The figure also indicates the locations S and E of the EASI lead system.

level of V4. V5 is half-way between V4 and V6, and V3 is half-way between V2 and V4. S and E indicate the locations of two of the four electrodes in the EASI lead system of Dower. The location of electrode A is in the left midaxillary line at the location of V6 and electrode I is at the symmetric location in the right midaxillary line (not shown).

The lead vectors of the chest leads V1–V6 are mainly in the horizontal (XZ) plane of the image space. When viewed in the horizontal plane projection shown in Figure 2.6, V1 points mainly to anterior–right, V2 anterior, V3 anterior–left, V4 left–anterior, V5 is to the left, and V6 to the left and slightly posterior. In terms of their lead strength or sensitivity, V1 and particularly V2, V3 and V4 are strong, and they can be expected to produce large ECG amplitudes, provided that excitation or repolarization cardiac dipoles have adequately strong components in their directions and not perpendicular to them.

Electrocardiographers have used model-based and statistical procedures for determination of transformation coefficients for predicting standard 12-lead ECG from various orthogonal and semi-orthogonal ECG leads ever since Burger introduced his image surface concept. Dower used image surface data of Frank to determine transformation coefficients used in an analog resistor network to "synthesize" standard 12-leads from the XYZ leads.[14] Wolf et al. evaluated the

accuracy of the standard leads derived using Dower's coefficients in comparison with statistically derived coefficients from the Frank leads using 14 simultaneously recorded bipolar leads in a group of 113 subjects.[15] The authors concluded that there are considerable differences between ECG amplitudes, waveforms, and diagnostic classification obtained by the two sets of lead transformations. As expected, individual transformations produced a better fit than that with global (average) coefficients.

Transformations from six independent bipolar components of the lead-off points of the Frank leads produced a more satisfactory fit. Derivation of the Frank leads from the standard 12 leads produced a better fit than the reverse transformation, as can be expected from a transformation using a larger number of independent variables. Some earlier investigators have reported a good agreement between clinically significant features of the original and derived leads.[16,17] More recent investigations in larger sets of data from body surface maps have produced more accurate predictions of the standard leads from the Frank leads.[9]

When body surface maps are available, any set of orthogonal leads or subsets of the leads of interest can be calculated. Considering unit vectors **x**, **y** and **z** as basis vectors in X, Y and Z

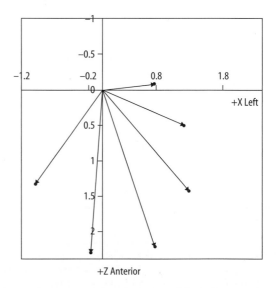

FIGURE 2.6 Horizontal plane projections of the lead vectors of the standard leads V1–V6.

TABLE 2.2 Transformation coefficients for the standard 12-lead ECG derived as the mean lead field of 1,239 cardiac source locations in a torso model with lungs and cardiac blood masses.

	Cx	Cy	Cz
I	0.80	−0.12	0.00
II	0.66	1.30	0.04
III	−0.14	1.42	0.04
aVR	−0.73	−0.59	−0.02
aVL	0.47	−0.77	−0.02
aVF	0.26	1.36	0.04
V1	−0.98	−1.44	−1.33
V2	−0.17	−0.76	−2.30
V3	0.77	−0.35	−2.22
V4	1.29	0.12	−1.43
V5	1.21	0.20	−0.50
V6	0.77	0.16	0.08
WCT	0.07	0.00	0.21

Source: Horáček et al.[9] J Electrocardiol 2002;35:41–52. © 2002. Reproduced with permission from Elsevier.

directions, the amplitudes of X, Y and Z leads can be taken to represent the components of the net cardiac dipole at successive instants of time. These can then be used to calculate the least-squares estimate of the x, y and z coefficients of the lead vectors of any ECG lead, including the standard 12 leads. Then, lead $V = Cx^*x + Cy^*y + Cz^*z$ (Table 2.2).

It should be noted that the original orthogonal lead systems were designed for a homogeneous human torso. Inhomogeneities influence lead vector properties in such a way that for instance the X, Y and Z components of the Frank leads are not exactly equal in their sensitivity and they also deviate to some extent from orthogonality.

2.3.3 Standard 12-lead ECG Derived from the EASI Leads

Standard 12-lead ECGs derived from quasi-orthogonal EASI leads have recently received considerable attention because of the practicality of obtaining these leads in emergency monitoring applications. The application of the EASI leads is based on the original patented invention of Dower.[18] The EASI leads consist of three bipolar leads: ES, AS and AI. The locations of the S and E electrodes are shown in Figure 2.5. The location of the A electrode is the same as that of V6, and electrode I is in a symmetrical location in the right

midclavicular line. Three quasi-orthogonal lead components are obtained from these bipolar leads, and global lead transformation coefficients are then used to derive the approximated standard 12-lead ECG.

Recent investigations in larger sets of data from body surface maps have produced reasonably satisfactory accuracy for monitoring purposes for standard leads derived using various sets of improved EASI lead coefficients.[9,19–24] For some of the improved lead sets, the average correlation coefficients for instance for the chest leads ranged from 0.91 to 0.94.[19] In spite of these high correlations, the differences in waveform patterns can occasionally be profound, for instance in some patients with myocardial infarctions. It should be noted that the EASI leads have been approved for monitoring purposes only and not as a substitute for the standard ECGs because of these occasional large differences in ECG waveforms.

The standard 12-lead ECG and the XYZ leads can be derived from the EASI leads. The coefficients for transformation of the standard 12 leads from the EASI leads shown in Table 2.3 were derived by Horáček et al.[9]

A different strategy for improving information yield from special ECG leads is to derive so-called regional aimed ECG leads.[25] These, in principle,

TABLE 2.3 Transformation coefficients for derivation of the standard 12-lead ECG and X, Y and Z leads from the EASI leads ES, AS and AI.

Lead	ES	AS	AI
I	0.026	−0.174	0.701
II	−0.002	1.098	−0.763
III	−0.028	1.272	−1.464
aVR	−0.012	−0.462	0.031
aVL	0.027	−0.723	1.082
aVF	−0.015	1.185	−1.114
V1	0.641	−0.391	0.080
V2	1.229	−1.050	1.021
V3	0.947	−0.539	0.987
V4	0.525	0.004	0.841
V5	0.179	0.278	0.630
V6	−0.043	0.431	0.213
X	0.068	−0.022	0.794
Y	0.004	1.056	−0.900
Z	−0.650	0.418	−0.421

Source: Feild et al.[19] J Electrocardiol 2000;35(Suppl):23–33. © 2002. Reproduced with permission from Elsevier.

should enhance the sensitivity of detecting ischemic injury in specific myocardial regions.

2.3.4 ECG Leads for Exercise Stress Testing

Standard lead ECGs during stress testing suffered from excessive muscle noise if the limb electrodes were kept in their standard positions. In 1966, Mason and Likar introduced a modification in the limb lead positions in order to alleviate the noise problem during exercise.[26] RA and LA electrodes were placed in the right and left infraclavicular fossae 2 cm below the lower border of the clavicle and medial to the border of the deltoid muscle. The LL electrode was placed initially in the left anterior axillary line midway between the rib margin and the iliac spine. This modification of the limb electrode positions was commonly used for exercise stress testing, although the LL electrode was usually placed on the left iliac crest. Modified arm electrode positions have been commonly used in intensive care applications.

It was later shown that the Mason–Likar modification induced substantial differences in the limb lead amplitudes and waveforms.[27,28] Limb lead waveform changes show an average of 16° shift of the mean QRS axis to a more vertical position. The changes in the frontal lead QRS amplitudes and waveforms are mainly due to directional changes in the lead vectors of leads II and III, resulting in increased R wave amplitudes in these leads. The lead vector of lead I is also considerably shortened so that the R amplitude in lead I is reduced.

The interindividual changes in the limb lead waveforms differed substantially depending on the mean QRS axis, and no universal group transform could be derived to correct or reconstruct limb lead ECGs for the changes. The modification of the position of the LA electrode has a more pronounced influence on the changed waveforms than that of the RA, due to the closer proximity of the LA electrode to the cardiac source. The critical exercise leads V5–V6 were not notably influenced.

Because the V5 lead appeared to be the standard chest lead with most pronounced ST depression during exercise, special sets of exercise ECG leads were sought that would resemble V5. This was particularly important at the time when recording capacity was limited to three simultaneous ECG leads. These leads, called bipolar exercise leads, used the V5 electrode connected to the positive terminal of the amplifier. The commonly used exercise leads had their negative terminal connections at the right shoulder (lead RV5), right subclavicular space (CV5), or the manubrium (MV5). (Confusingly, these leads were labeled as CR5, CC5 and CM5, respectively.)

An examination of Figure 2.7 reveals that the lead vector RV5 is equal to V5 + 2/3 aVR, so that RV55 = V5 + 2/3 × inverted aVR. This figure shows that all of these bipolar exercise leads are more sensitive than chest lead V5. The directions of RV5 and V5 nearly coincide in image space (both directly to the left, nearly horizontal) so that their waveforms are closely similar. Lead CV5 is slightly more vertical in comparison with V5, and lead MV5 is approximately 30° more vertical than V5, so that their waveforms can be expected to deviate to a certain degree from that of V5. Overall, the placement variations of the negative electrode of the bipolar exercise leads have a fairly predictable effect on the ECG strength and waveform. As noted before, the placement of the LA electrode

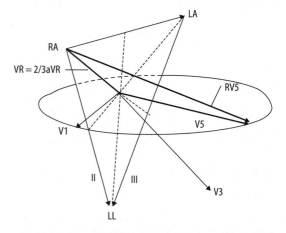

FIGURE 2.7 Lead vector RV5 for an exercise test lead RV5 from the RA to V5 location. $RV5 = 2/3 \times (-aVR) + V5$, indicating the amplitude of RV5 = V5 + (2/3 × inverted aVR). Note that VR is the lead vector for Wilson's lead VR, from the central terminal to RA. If the RA electrode is placed on the right subclavicular space (exercise lead CV5), the lead vector CV5 differs slightly from RV5 because of the small potential difference between RA and the subclavicular (C) locations. The lead vector differences for all limb leads are more pronounced if all limb lead connections are in modified electrode positions such as with Nehb's leads.

into the subclavicular location causes more pronounced and unpredictable changes (interindividual variations) in the limb lead waveforms.

While the use of the proximal placement of the limb electrodes alleviates noise problems, the recording of all six chest leads during exercise also causes technical problems due to noise and artifacts and problems with lead placement, particularly in women. Recording of the limb leads in modified Mason–Likar positions with a reduced subset of chest leads such as V1 and V5 and deriving the missing leads from the rest has been proposed.[29] The rationale for this choice is that the V2 location is the preferred echocardiogram transducer location, and V3–V4 the preferred location for a defibrillator pad. V1 is retained for its content of valuable arrhythmic information.

Newlan et al. evaluated the feasibility of reconstruction of the 12-lead ECG from a variety of combinations of the subsets of the eight independent components of the 12-lead ECG.[30] The authors concluded that global coefficients allow reconstruction of one or two precordial leads reasonably well and subject-specific coefficients allow reconstruction of up to four leads. It remains to be seen how well the standard leads derived from the EASI leads will perform in exercise testing in comparison with the original leads.[29]

References

1. Rautaharju PM. Why did QT dispersion die? Cardiovasc Electrophysiol Rev 2002;6:295–301.
2. Burger HC, van Milan JB. Heart vector and leads, I. Br Heart J 1946;8:157–61.
3. Burger HC, van Milan, JB. Heart vector and leads, II. Br Heart J 1947;9:154–60.
4. Burger HC, van Milan JB. Heart vector and leads, III. Br Heart J 1948;10:229–33.
5. Schmitt OH. Lead vectors and transfer impedance. Ann NY Acad Sci 1957;65:1092–109.
6. Frank E. The image surface of a homogeneous human torso. Am Heart J 1954;47:757–68.
7. Frank E. An accurate, clinically practical system for spatial electrocardiography. Circulation 1956;13:737–49.
8. Horáček MB. Lead theory. In: MacFarlane PW, Lawrie TDV (eds). Comprehensive Electrocardiology. New York: Pergamon Books, Ltd, 1988, pp 291–314.
9. Horáček BM, Warren JW, Feild DQ, Feldman CL. Statistical and deterministic approaches to designing transformations of electrocardiographic leads. J Electrocardiol 2002;35(Suppl):41–52.
10. Rautaharju PM. Elusive understanding of electrocardiographic lead networks. J Electrocardiol 2005;38:128–9.
11. Einthoven W, Fahr G, De Waart A. Über die Richtung und manifeste Grösse der Potentialschwankungen im menschlichen Herzen und Über den Einfluss der Herzlage auf die Form des Elektrokardiograms. Pflügers Arch 1913;150:275–315.
12. Wilson FN, Johnston FD, MacLeod AG, Barker PS. Electrocardiograms that represent the potential variations of a single electrode. Am Heart J 1934;9:447–58.
13. Goldberger E. A simple, indifferent, electrocardiographic electrode of zero potential and a technique of obtaining augmented, unipolar, extremity leads. Am Heart J 1942;23:483–92.
14. Dower GE. A lead synthesizer for the Frank system to simulate standard 12-lead electrocardiogram. J Electrocardiol 1968;1:101–16.
15. Wolf HK, Rautaharju PM, Unite VC et al. Evaluation of synthesized standard 12 leads and Frank vector leads. In: Abel H (ed). Electrocardiology, Advances in Cardiology. Basel: S. Karger Publishing Co, 1976, pp 87–97.
16. Pipberger HV, Bialek SM, Perkoff JK, Schnaper HW. Correlation of clinical information in the standard 12-lead and in corrected orthogonal 3-lead ECG. Am Heart J 1961:61:34–43.
17. Dower GE, inventor. Method and apparatus for sensing and analyzing electrical activity of the human heart. US Patent No 4, 850, 370;7/1989.
18. Dower GE. EASI 12-Lead Electrocardiography. Point Roberts, WA: Totemite Publishers, 1996.
19. Feild DQ, Feldman CL, Horáček BM. Improved EASI coefficients: their derivation, values, and performance. J Electrocardiol 2002;35(Suppl):23–33.
20. Drew BJ, Adams MG, Pelter MM et al. Comparison of standard and derived 12-lead electrocardiograms for diagnosis of coronary angioplasty-induced myocardial ischemia. Am J Cardiol 1997;79:639–44.
21. Drew BJ, Loops RR, Adams MG, Dower GE. Derived 12-lead ECG. Comparison with the standard ECG during myocardial ischemia and its potential application for continuous ST-segment monitoring. J Electrocardiol 1994;27(Suppl):249–55.
22. Drew BJ, Schneinman MM, Evans GT Jr. Comparison of a vectorcardiographically derived 12-lead electrocardiogram with the conventional electrocardiogram during wide QRS complex tachycardia,

and its potential application for continuous bedside monitoring. Am J Cardiol 1992;69:612–18.

23. Rautaharju PM, Zhou SH, Hancock EW et al. Comparability of 12-lead ECGs derived from EASI leads with standard 12-lead ECGs in the classification of acute myocardial ischemia and old myocardial infarction. J Electrocardiol 2002;35(Suppl): 35–9.

24. Feldman CL, MacCallum G, Feold QD, Hartley LH. Comparison of direct and vectorcardiographically derived (EASI) electrocardiograms recorded during exercise. In: Liebman J (ed). Electrocardiography '96. From the Cell to the Body Surface. Singapore: World Scientific Publishing, 1996, pp 577–80.

25. Hyttinen J. Development of regional aimed ECG leads especially for myocardial ischemia diagnosis. Doctor of Technology thesis, Tampere University of Technology Publications #138, 1994.

26. Mason RE, Likar I. A new system of multiple-lead exercise electrocardiography. Am Heart J 1966;71: 196–205.

27. Rautaharju PM, Prineas RJ, Crow RS, Furberg C. The effect of modified limb electrode positions on electrocardiographic wave amplitudes. J Electrocardiol 1980;13:109–14.

28. Pahlm O, Haisty WK Jr, Edenbrandt L et al. Evaluation of changes in standard electrocardiographic QRS waveforms recorded from activity-compatible proximal limb lead positions. Am J Cardiol 1992;69: 253–57.

29. Drew BJ, Pelter MM, Brodnick DE et al. Comparison of a new reduced leads set ECG with the standard ECG for diagnosing cardiac arrhythmias and myocardial ischemia. J Electrocardiol 2002; 35(Suppl):13–21.

30. Newlan SP, Kors JA, Meij SH et al. Reconstruction of the 12-lead ECG using reduced sets for patient monitoring. In: Schlij MJ, Janse MJ, van Oosterom A, Wellens HJJ, van der Wall EE (eds). Einthoven 2002. 100 Years of Electrocardiography. Leiden, The Netherlands: The Einthoven Foundation, 2002, pp 545–51.

3
Normal and Arrhythmogenic Ionic Channel Mechanism

Synopsis

Generation of Action Potential

Steady-state transmembrane ionic gradients in living cardiac muscle cells at rest generate a potential difference or voltage across the membrane called resting potential.

Resting Potential

The resting potential in ventricular muscle cells is −90 mV, inside negative with respect to outside, and is dependent on membrane permeability and ion concentrations (activities) in the cytoplasm inside and in the extracellular fluid outside. Active transport (ionic pumps) and countertransport systems (ion exchangers) contribute to the maintenance of the resting potential.

Transient Ionic Currents

The action potential of excitable cardiac cells is generated by a transient flow of ionic currents through ion-specific channels that contain molecular structures called gates. Ionic current flow in some channels is easier inward or outward (rectifier channels). The magnitude of the transient flow of each ion is dependent on the potential and concentration gradients and the conductance of the channel. Voltage-gated ionic channels are activated and inactivated in a characteristic time course along the excitation/repolarization cycle, with the gates opening and closing at specific voltage thresholds.

Phase 0 and Phase 1

Normal ventricular excitation starts at the terminal branches of the Purkinje fibers as a propagated response in the electrically coupled syncytium when depolarized by electrotonic interaction to the threshold of the I_{Na}-channel activation potential of approximately −55 mV. This inward excitatory current is largely responsible for ventricular depolarization (phase 0). It is followed by an overshoot to a positive polarization of 20 mV or more (phase 1) where subepicardial and intramural M cells have a notch. Phase 1 notch is generated by the early transient outward current I_{to}. From its two components, I_{to1} is carried through a voltage-gated potassium channel, and I_{to2} is considered to be a calcium-activated chloride current. I_{to} currents activate fast during early depolarization and then inactivate.

Phase 2 and Phase 3

Phase 1 is a transition point to a quasi-stationary state (phase 2), commonly called plateau although more appropriately denoted as the slow phase of ventricular repolarization. In human ventricular cells, the voltage-gated Ca^{2+} current I_{Ca-L} is activated during phase 0 at threshold $\approx$ −20 mV. I_{Ca-L} is a long-lasting current that is important for membrane voltage balance during phase 2, for release of calcium from the intracellular stores and excitation–contraction coupling, and at the end of phase 2, for initiation of the fast phase of repolarization (phase 3) by the Ca^{2+}-dependent inactivation and spontaneous closure of this

29

channel. A number of other ionic channels play an important role in ventricular repolarization by regulating potassium flux, including delayed rectifier I_K currents I_{Kr} and I_{Ks}.

Temporal Sequence of Repolarization

The temporal sequence of the normal ventricular repolarization is spatially remarkably uniform. This suggests that intrinsically longer action potential durations of the intramural M-type cells are largely moderated by electrotonic coupling to the surrounding myocardial syncytium or that potential gradients generated by diffuse clusters of M cells are largely cancelled spatially. Physiological, pathophysiological and pharmacological agents that prolong QT interval with only minor changes in T waveform act primarily by producing a homogeneous uniform delay of the onset combined with an unaltered slope of phase 3 and unaltered normal spatial/temporal dispersion of action potential duration. Delayed onset of phase 3 occurs with I_{Na}-blocking agents that reduce the slope of phase 0, with I_{to} agonists that broaden the notch, and with all agents that cause prolongation of phase 2. Altered T waveform, T amplitude increase or decrease, biphasic T or changed T wave polarity indicate increased or decreased dispersion of the onset or the end of phase 3 (or both) or altered phase 3 slope.

Cardioactive Agents and Ionic Channels

A variety of ionic channel mechanisms are involved in antiarrhythmic and other effects of cardioactive pharmacological agents. The main differences in drug actions are in their agonistic or antagonistic effect on different receptors, pumps and ionic channels, the affinity and strength of their action, as well as their rate- and voltage-dependence and the kinetics in relation to onset and release of the channel block at various phases of the action potential.

Abbreviations and Acronyms

APD – action potential duration
ATP – adenosine triphosphate
AV – atrioventricular
DAD – delayed afterdepolarizations
DRT – dispersion of repolarization time
EAD – early afterdepolarizations
EMIAT – European Myocardial Infarct Amiodarone Trial
FDA – Food and Drug Administration
HVA – high-voltage activated
LQTS – long QT syndrome
LVA – low-voltage activated
PKA – phosphate kinase
SA – sino-atrial

3.1 Cardiac Action Potential

3.1.1 Resting Membrane Potential in Cardiac Cells

Cardiac muscle cells, like other living cells, have a potential gradient across the cell membrane. In excitable cardiac muscle cells at the resting phase, the transmembrane voltage, commonly called the resting potential, is dependent on the permeabilities of ionic channels to the flow of each ion and ion concentrations (activities) in the cytoplasm inside and outside in the extracellular fluid. Active transport (ionic pumps) and countertransport systems (ion exchangers) contribute to the maintenance of the resting potential. In ventricular muscle cells, the resting potential is −90 mV, inside negative with respect to the outside. Among the ATP-dependent ionic pumps in the sarcolemma are the Na/K pump and the calcium pump. The Na/K pump generates a small steady outward current throughout the excitation/repolarization cycle (three Na^+ out , two K^+ in). This ionic pump is blocked by digitalis. $I_{Na/Ca}$ current is generated by the Na/Ca countertransport system. The Na/Ca exchanger is the main mechanism for Ca^{2+} efflux through the sarcolemma, inwards or outwards depending on the membrane potential and gradients of Na^+ and Ca^{2+}.

Intracellular and extracellular ion concentration differences (Table 3.1) produce large concentration gradients. Sodium is kept outside by the Na^+ pump. Potassium permeability and influx is high and practically all potassium is intracellular. Extracellular potassium with a concentration of 4 mM makes up only 2% of total body potassium.

TABLE 3.1 Normal intracellular and extracellular ion concentrations (mmol/l) in resting ventricular muscle cells. Potassium permeability is high and its chemical potential gradient is equal and opposite to the transmembrane potential gradient.

	Intracellular	Extracellular
Potassium	140	3.5–5
Calcium	0.0001	2
Sodium	10	140
Chloride	30	140

Potassium maintains electroneutrality so that the transmembrane potassium K^+ chemical concentration gradient potential (inside positive) is equal and opposite to the transmembrane potential gradient (inside negative). Thus, the transmembrane resting potential gradient (denoted as resting potential) is normally equal to the K^+ equilibrium potential. The intracellular calcium concentration is only 0.0001 mM. In spite of this, very minor variations in the availability of free intracellular calcium from intracellular stores have a major modifying effect on ionic currents.

3.1.2 Action Potential Transients

Transient ionic currents through ionic channels in the membrane generate the action potentials of cardiac ventricular and atrial myocytes, of cardiac pacemaker cells, and of the specialized His–Purkinje conduction system of the ventricles. The ion-specific channels contain molecular structures called gates. The opening and closing of the gates is regulated by the transmembrane voltage in the voltage-gated channels. When the gates are open, specific ions flow in these channels so that the concentration gradients across the membranes change. In addition to the voltage-gated channels, there are so-called rectifying channels that conduct channel current to a variable degree easier inwardly or outwardly across the membrane. The activity of the numerous ionic channels is carefully orchestrated in normal physiological conditions. Each channel is activated and inactivated, opening and closing at different times, changing concentration gradients and charge separation across the membrane, and thus generating the normal action potential.

Electrophysiological investigations including the long QT syndrome (LQTS) have advanced our understanding of the physiological and pathophysiological mechanisms involved in normal and derailed ionic channel functions, including the mechanism of action of cardioactive drugs.[1] A 1991 treatise of the Task Force of the Working Group on Arrhythmias of the European Society of Cardiology contains a review of the ionic channel mechanisms in relation to drug actions on arrhythmogenic mechanisms.[2] A recent monograph on cardiac repolarization contains notes on the molecular biology of ionic channels and on the electrophysiology and pharmacology of ventricular repolarization, with an extensive list of references in various chapters.[3]

The following notes pertain primarily to ionic channel mechanisms of the ventricular fibers. The characteristics of the action potentials of the sinoatrial (SA) node pacemaker cells, the atrioventricular (AV) node, the specialized ventricular conduction system and the Purkinje fibers are different, and some of their specific features will be pointed out separately.

Functional characteristics of the ionic channels change in the course of growth and maturation. There are species differences in the distribution and characteristics of the ionic channels. This brief description will be largely limited to major ionic channels found in mammalian hearts. The list of references is very short, and the reader is advised to consult extensive sources in electrophysiological literature, including references 1–3 cited above.

3.2 Ionic Channel Mechanisms that Regulate Action Potentials

The time course of activation and inactivation of ionic currents associated mainly with the generation of normal ventricular and atrial action potentials is illustrated in Figure 3.1.

3.2.1 Ionic Channel Currents and Ventricular Action Potential

3.2.1.1 Inward Excitatory Sodium Current

Inward current flow through voltage-gated sodium channels generates phase 0 of the ventricular

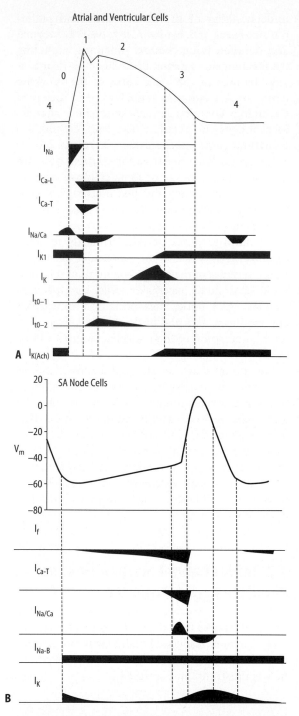

FIGURE 3.1 Main normal ionic currents involved in generation of normal ventricular and atrial action potentials (*top*) and the SA node action potential transients (*below*). (Source: Task Force of the Working Group on Arrhythmias of the European Society of Cardiology.[2] Circulation 1991;84:1831–51. Copyright © 1991 American Heart Association. Reproduced with permission from Lippincott, Williams & Wilkins.)

action potential. Normal ventricular excitation starts at the terminal branches of the Purkinje fibers as a propagated response in the electrically coupled syncytium when depolarized by electrotonic interaction to the threshold of the I_{Na}-channel activation potential of approximately $-55\,mV$. Once activated, the current through the sodium channels is intense. I_{Na} channels have a fast time course of activation and inactivation. In spite of their early closure, some of the sodium channels remain potentially available during a time window for a transition back to the open state. Such a reversible inactivation at a certain level of membrane potential may generate a so-called window current and become one of the determinants of action potential duration (APD) by contributing to the maintenance of relatively steady-state equilibrium during phase 2.

3.2.1.2 Early Outward I_{to} Currents

Following the action potential overshoot to a positive polarization of $+20\,mV$ or more (phase 1), there is a quasi-stationary state (phase 2) commonly called plateau, although more appropriately denoted as the slow phase of ventricular repolarization. Subepicardial and intramural M cells have a notch at the transition point from phase 1 to phase 2. The notch is generated by the early transient outward current I_{to}. From its two components, I_{to1} is an outward current that is under modulating influence of neurotransmitters. It is carried through a voltage-gated potassium channel. I_{to2} is considered to be a calcium-activated chloride current. I_{to1} channels have a fast time course of activation and inactivation during early depolarization, and they are also called $I_{to,f}$, with subscript "f" denoting fast. I_{to1} channels recover fast from their inactivated state, meaning that they can be activated again after a short pause. I_{to2} channels also activate and inactivate fast, although slower than I_{to1} channels, and the time course of the recovery from the inactivated state is slower. These channels are also called $I_{to,s}$, with subscript "s" denoting slow.

3.2.1.3 Inward Calcium Current

Electrophysiological terminology used to describe voltage-gated channels, the calcium channel in particular, is often confusing. At times, the terminology is based on physiological–pharmacological time-dependent properties (subscript T referring to transient, short-duration and L to longer lasting), and at times, the terminology is based on activation voltage thresholds (with LVA referring to low-voltage activated, meaning that activation threshold voltage is high negative, and HVA referring to high-voltage activated, meaning that activation occurs at lower, less negative voltage). Calcium channels other than I_{Ca-L} and I_{Ca-T} are variously denoted by subscripts N (neither type L nor type T), P (Purkinje), or R (remaining types).

I_{Ca-T} channels are apparently not present or are scarce in mammalian ventricular myocytes. The transient T-type calcium current is carried through a different voltage-gated channel. It may be associated with abnormal automaticity in atria. The I_{Ca-L} current influx increases from the onset of phase 1 and reaches its peak at the time of the notch of phase 1, then declines slowly during phase 2.

I_{Ca} channels are activated when depolarization has reached a higher level and the activation is delayed with respect to the depolarizing I_{Na} current. Thus, I_{Ca} current does not make a notable contribution to phase 0. The activated phase is long lasting. I_{Ca} triggers intracellular Ca^{2+} release, important for excitation contraction coupling. The quasi-stationary equilibrium during phase 2 plateau is dependent to an important extent on the balance of Ca^{2+} influx and K^+ efflux. With fast inactivation of I_{Ca-L} channels, the outward K^+ current dominates the transmembrane ionic balance because of the high driving force for the efflux of K^+, and the fast phase of repolarization begins. Thus, I_{Ca-L} plays an important role in the generation of phase 3 and as a determinant of APD. I_{Ca-L} is strongly influenced by neurotransmitters and calcium channel blocker action. In AV and SA node cells, it produces depolarization.

3.2.1.4 Outward Voltage-gated Potassium Currents

There are a number of voltage-gated outward currents carried by diverse I_K channels. I_{K1}, called "inward rectifier", is carried through channels that have a high conductance when the membrane is polarized to a high negative value during phase 4. It plays an important role in establishing the resting potential of cardiac myocytes. The high conductance is sharply reduced at the onset of depolarization when the transmembrane potential increases above $-40\,mV$. In spite of low conductance, during the plateau it maintains the membrane potential in atrial and ventricular cells and also in AV nodal and His–Purkinje cells. The mechanism of this I_{K1} action is its contribution to outward K^+ current because the driving force for K^+ ions is markedly increased when the membranes are depolarized. I_{K1} channels are absent in the SA node, thus permitting pacemaker rate modulation by small pacemaker currents during phase 4.

I_{Ks} is a slowly activating delayed rectifier current that is mainly responsible for the fast phase of repolarization when the inward calcium channels are inactivated. I_{Ks} channels, some of them modulated by neurotransmitters, are turned off slowly after repolarization. These channels contribute to phase 4 depolarization in SA node cells.

I_{Kr} is a rapidly activating delayed potassium current. I_{Kr} block increases the dispersion of repolarization, at least in part by preferential prolongation of APD of the M cells. Kr block prolongs QT interval and produces a tall, broad-based T wave with or without a notch in the descending limb when the extracellular potassium ($[K^+]o$) is normal.[4]

$I_{K(ATP)}$ is a metabolically regulated potassium channel blocked by ATP and activated by ischemia, possibly producing APD shortening in myocardial ischemia. While most channel-active agents act by blocking ionic currents, the agents activating $I_{K(ATP)}$ increase outward potassium current. Experimentally administered antiarrhythmic drugs act either by increasing or decreasing $I_{K(ATP)}$ and thus either shorten or prolong repolarization.

Among other ionic channel currents are I_{Cl} and I_{NS}. The Cl^- current flow is usually small but is increased by adrenergic receptor activation, thus potentially contributing to repolarization if the $[Cl^-]_i$ concentration deviates from its normal equilibrium value.

I_{NS} is a current through a non-selective channel, and it is gated by Ca^{2+} and carried by Na^+. It may be activated in some abnormal conditions during the early phase of depolarization and also by Ca^{2+} release from the sarcoplasmic reticulum in Ca^{2+} overload. In these conditions, it may contribute to generation of delayed afterdepolarizations (DAD).

3.3 Ionic Currents that Regulate the Sino-Atrial Node

The ionic currents that regulate the SA node are functionally different from those regulating other cardiac structures, as shown in Table 3.2.

- The I_{Na} channel does not exist or its density is sparse in the SA node (like in the AV node), and it has no role in pacemaker action.
- I_{Na-B} is an inward sodium current carried through a voltage-independent channel in SA node cells. It generates phase 4 of the action potential in pacemaker cells (together with I_f).
- I_{Ca-L} current (with I_{Ca-T}) generates the upstroke of the action potential in the SA node (and the AV node) cells. The upstroke is slower than that generated by I_{Na} channels in phase 0 in ventricular cells.
- I_{Ca-T} is activated already at the end period of phase 4. It may participate in generating abnormal atrial automaticity.
- I_K produces SA node repolarization. It also produces a current that opposes inward sodium current at the early part of phase 4. After I_K

decay, I_{Na-B} generates phase 4 pacemaker potential of the SA node cells.
- I_{K-ACh} can produce hyperpolarization in SA (and AV) node cells.
- I_f is an inward Na^+ current through a channel that is activated at high polarized state (also present in AV node and His–Purkinje cells). It produces with I_{Na-B} phase 4 of the pacemaker potential. This channel is under a strong modulating influence of neurotransmitters.

Among other ionic channel currents in the SA node are the I_{pump} (Na/K pump and the calcium pump) current and $I_{Na/Ca}$, current generated by the Na/Ca countertransport system.

3.4 Electrolytes and Action Potentials

The effect of some electrolyte concentrations deviating from their normal values can cause notable changes in action potential waveforms, as shown in Table 3.3 and also in body surface ECGs, summarized in Table 3.4. At body surface ECG level, manifestations of changes in potassium concentrations are most readily visible, whereas calcium level variations are apparent in more severe cases only. Sodium or magnesium concentration effects on ECG are not notable in practical clinical electrocardiography. Only potassium effects summarized in Table 3.4 will be discussed here because they are most often associated with visible ECG manifestations.

3.4.1 Hyperkalemia

Hyperkalemia may occur clinically with the use of potassium sparing diuretics or ACE inhibitors, in kidney failure, acidosis and hyperkalemia with excessive administration of potassium supplements. With an increase in extracellular potassium, the resting potential becomes less negative and the action potential amplitude decreases. $(dV/dt)_{max}$ decrease in phase 0 decreases the conduction velocity in atrial and ventricular muscle cells. P wave and QRS broaden. Atrial cells are particularly sensitive. P wave amplitude decreases and at higher concentrations atrial cells become unexcitable. However, the SA node is little influenced, and AV conduction may modestly increase

TABLE 3.2 Major differences in the functional roles of the ionic channels in SA nodal and ventricular muscle cells.

	SA node cells	Ventricular cells
I_{Ca-L}	Generates with I_{Ca-T} phase 0	Minor role only in generating phase 0
I_{Ca-T}	Activated at end of phase 4. May induce abnormal atrial automaticity	Absent or density low in human ventricular cells
I_{Na}	Does not exist, or density sparse	Main channel generating phase 0 upstroke
I_{Na-B}	Inward sodium channel. Generates with I_f pacemaker potential	Not present
I_f	Activated at high depolarized state. Under strong influence of neurohormones. Regulates firing rate of the SA node	Not present

TABLE 3.3 Action potential waveform changes with serum potassium and calcium concentration.

	Hyperkalemia	Hypokalemia	Hypercalsemia	Hypocalsemia
Phase 0 $(dV/dt)_{max}$	Decreases	Decreases	Decreases	Increases
Phase 2	Shortens	Prolongs	Shortens	Prolongs
Phase 3	Shortens	Prolongs	Shortens	Prolongs
Phase 4 membrane potential	Decreases (becomes less negative)	Increases	No change	No change

(mild hyperkalemia) or decrease (moderate hyperkalemia). With shortening of phase 2 and phase 3, the QT interval shortens. Peaked, high amplitude T wave is the most sensitive ECG indicator of mild hyperkalemia. However, this ECG amplitude change in moderate hyperkalemia is relatively modest, approximately 20%.

A mild hyperkalemia may suppress ectopic latent focal pacemaker activity and it has a transient antiarrhythmic effect. Potassium chloride infusion has extremely potent electrophysiological effects. Slow infusion of potassium produces sinus bradycardia, ending up with sinus arrest, impaired AV conduction, idioventricular rhythm and asystole. Rapid infusion of potassium induces ectopic ventricular rhythms associated with depressed conduction and ends up with fatal ventricular fibrillation.

3.4.2 Hypokalemia

Like in hyperkalemia, $(dV/dt)_{max}$ and conduction velocity decrease in hypokalemia in atrial and

TABLE 3.4 Changes in ECG waveforms observed in elevated or decreased serum concentration of potassium.

	Hyperkalemia	Hypokalemia
P wave	Low amplitude, broad; vanishes at higher concentrations	Amplitude usually, increases wave broadens; may resemble P pulmonale
QRS	Broadens; at higher concentration QRS-T complex resembles a sine wave	Amplitude increases, wave broadens in severe hypokalemia
ST	Shortened with QRS prolongation, elevated or depressed; vanishes at higher concentrations	Depressed
T	Peaked, high T first ECG sign (although sensitivity low)	Decreased amplitude
U wave	Diminished	Prominent

ventricular muscle cells. P wave and QRS broaden with decreased conduction. The mechanism of P amplitude increase is not entirely clear. QT prolongs with prolongation of phase 2 and phase 3. The emergence of the prominent U wave, T-U fusion and decreasing T wave amplitude (at least the first half) suggests a profound increase of dispersion of ventricular repolarization by a differential effect on endocardial, epicardial, and M cell populations. Compared to the relatively low prevalence of typical ECG changes in hyperkalemia, the prevalence of ECG changes in moderate hypokalemia is high, 78% according to Surawicz et al.[5]

3.5 Neurohormones and other Receptor Stimulating Agents

The heart responds to demands for increased cardiac output during stress by increasing the heart rate and contractility. This occurs as a response to adrenergic neurohormones released at postsynaptic nerve terminals. A complex of proteins within the cardiac sarcolemmal membrane, including adrenergic receptors and an effector enzyme, adenylyl cyclase, initiate a series of biochemical processes. Among these processes as the end result of positive inotropic and chronotropic response is the synthesis of an intracellular second messenger cAMP and phosphorylation of protein kinase (PKA).

The receptors, categorized as α- and β-adrenergic, muscarinic, and purinergic types, modify the functions of various ionic channels and pumps through receptor–effector coupling systems. Activation of one type of receptor can also influence other receptor types. For instance, beta 1-adrenoreceptors and M2 muscarinic receptors have antagonistic features in their actions.

The autonomic nervous system, acting on the receptors, modulates cardiac rhythm and may contribute to the effects of antiarrhythmic or proarrhythmic agents. Modified receptor functions can influence impulse formation and initiation and propagation of action potentials.

3.5.1 Beta-adrenergic Receptor Stimulation

Beta-adrenergic receptor stimulation acts on various potassium channels (only I_{K1} is apparently not affected), on I_{Ca-L}, I_{Cl}, I_f (also sodium channels under some conditions), and it can enhance Na/K pump activity. Beta-adrenergic stimulation or agonist action can thus be expected to have a variety of manifestations under different conditions. Shift of the I_f activation curve towards a more positive potential produces a chronotropic effect in the SA node and enhances latent pacemaker activity at ectopic atrial and ventricular sites. Increased L-type Ca^{2+} current enhances contractility (increased intracellular Ca^{2+}) and it could also induce triggered activity due to early as well as late afterdepolarizations.

The effect of β-adrenergic receptor stimulation on potassium channels can be expected to shorten the refractory period. Spatial heterogeneity in the distribution of I_{to} channels (present in subepicardial and M cell regions only) could conceivably induce increased dispersion of the end of the refractory period. In the AV node, combined Ca^{2+} and K^+ effect may shorten AV node refractoriness and speed up AV conduction. In a healthy heart the conglomerate of the above actions will produce shortening of the QT interval, sinus- and at times ectopic supraventricular tachycardias.

Of the several subtypes of α-adrenergic receptor–effector coupling systems, subtypes of α_1-receptor are linked to effector systems that modulate impulse initiation and APD. Their stimulation effect on the Na/K pump may suppress the tendency to ectopic pacemaker-type activity in the atria. The potential role of β-adrenergic receptors in arrhythmogenic mechanisms in humans is unclear.

3.5.2 Muscarinic Cholinergic Receptor Stimulation

The M_2 muscarinic receptor is the main cardiac muscarinic receptor. It is particularly important in the atria where its density is five times higher than in the ventricles. Whereas the ventricles are dominantly under β-adrenergic control, the atria are strongly under vagal control. Vagal stimulation, muscarinic activation, and muscarinic agonist action (digoxin) have antagonistic adrenergic effects. Muscarinic effect is blocked by atropine. In the atria, muscarinic activation effects include a decrease in I_f and suppression of the SA node through increased conductance of the muscarinic K^+ channel, thus slowing down the heart rate. An increase in $I_{K(ACh)}$ hyperpolarizes atrial myocytes and shortens atrial APD. A decrease of the SA node impulse rate increases atrial APD in linear proportion, and the direct vagal effect has a simultaneous opposite effect by shortening atrial APD.

At the level of the AV node, the antiadrenergic effect of muscarinic activation on Ca^{2+} and K^+ currents contributes to decreased conduction. Muscarinic activation can be expected to be effective in supraventricular arrhythmias and arrhythmias involving the AV node. In humans, an antiarrhythmic effect at the ventricular level has not been documented.

3.5.3 A₁-purinergic Receptor Stimulation

The cardiac purinergic (adenosine) receptor–effector coupling system is called A_1. It apparently has the same effector coupling pathway as the muscarinic receptor. Adenosine is effective in terminating tachycardias where the AV node is in the re-entrant pathway. Adenosine A_1-receptor agonists increase the resilience of ventricular myocardium to ischemic injury even several hours after experimental coronary occlusion and reperfusion.

3.6 Antiarrhythmic Drugs

The major classes of antiarrhythmic agents are categorized within the framework of the most commonly used classification system described by Vaugham Williams, summarized in Table 3.5.[6] The system does not necessarily identify the critical "vulnerable parameter" like the so-called Sicilian Gambit classification.[2] The vulnerable parameter is associated with the mode of arrhythmic suppression action of the agents. The

TABLE 3.5 Major classes of antiarrhythmic drugs according to the scheme of Vaugham Williams. The categories are largely defined on the basis of QT-prolonging effect.

Class	Mechanism of action	Examples
I. Na^+ channel blockers		
IA	Widening of the notch, APD prolongation in epicardial cells; prolonged APD due to	Procainamide
Prolong QT	combined action with associated K^+ channel block	Disopyramide
	Quinidine	
IB	A selective blocker; at higher concentrations shortens epicardial APD due to	Lidocaine
Shorten QT	abolishment of the dome, with only a slight shortening of endocardial APD. No K^+	Mexiletine
	channel block	Tocainide
		Phenytoin
IC Little or no effect on QT	Decreased $(dV/dt)_{max}$, conduction velocity in atrial and ventricular muscle cells	Encainide
		Flecainide
		Propafenone
II. Beta-adrenergic blockers	Block catecholamine effects on Ca^{2+} and K^+ channels; prolong APD and slow AV node conduction.	Propranolol
		Esmolol
		Timolol
III. K^+ channel blockers	ADP prolongation, particularly in M cells; effect decreasing progressively with increased rate (reverse use dependence). APD prolongation is less notable in endocardial and epicardial cells. This difference is pronounced for I_{Kr} blockers. I_{Ks} blockers increase APD on all three types of ventricular cells	Ibulitide
		Bretylium
		Sotalol
IV. Calcium^{2+} channel blockers	Suppression of SA node and AV conduction (except nifedipine). Some bind to L-type channels (suppression of contractility), except mibefradil (T-type binding)	Verapamil
		Diltiazem
		Nifedipine

classification scheme of Vaugham Williams is largely based on the QT-prolonging effect of the drug. The major problem here is that QT prolongation does not necessarily indicate increased dispersion of repolarization and QT shortening does not necessarily indicate decreased dispersion of repolarization. An additional complication with any simple drug classification scheme is that commonly used antiarrhythmic drugs act on multiple ionic channels.

It is important to understand that dispersion of repolarization at cardiac level is a different entity from QT dispersion measured from the QT interval differences in different from body surface ECG leads. Dispersion of repolarization at cardiac level is an important physiological and pathophysiological phenomenon. QT dispersion is based on an unsubstantiated and unproven hypothesis, as will be discussed at the end of Chapter 11.

The following is a brief summary of conceptually reasonably rational expressions of the relationships between the quantities in question. Abnormal dispersion (increased or decreased) of ventricular repolarization can be local (for instance between Purkinje fibers and subendocardial cells or between M cells and subendocardial or subepicardial cells), regional (transmural in a wall section), or global (between myocardial regions).

Normal repolarization, both its onset and end, is always dispersed regionally and globally, otherwise there will be no T wave. Most critical abnormal dispersions are likely to be local or regional.

- Denoting the local or regional end of repolarization by RT (repolarization time, measured for instance from the onset of excitation), dispersion of repolarization can be expressed as dispersion of repolarization time (DRT).
- Change in APD decreases DRT in a given region only if the temporal gradient of APD decreases. This occurs, for instance, if the agent decreases APD of the cells that repolarize later more than that of the cells that repolarize earlier, or if the agent increases APD of the cells that repolarize earlier more than that of the cells that repolarize later in that region. In the latter condition, DRT may initially decrease and then increase again (as shown in Figure 11.2 in Chapter 11).
- Changes in the regional repolarization time or DRT will influence QT measurements in body surface ECG only under special circumstances. In most instances, DRT change will have no notable effect on QT, although it can always be expected to influence ST-T waveform to variable degrees.

- Prolonged repolarization as a response to the action of an agent can be detected from QT measurement in body surface ECG only if APD prolongation involves the cells in the region that repolarized last before the action of the agent, or if APD prolongation in some other region is pronounced enough so that this region now repolarizes last.
- Shortened repolarization can be detected from QT measurement only if APD shortening involves the region that repolarized last before the action of the agent.
- A uniform spatial global increase or decrease of APD increases and decreases QT without a change in DRT.
- There are two alternative conditions that are necessary for detection of local prolonged or shortened DRT from body surface ECG: (1), the presence of nondipolar components in T wave originating from the region that is repolarizing last that are above the threshold of Tend detection criteria; or (2), the presence of nondipolar components in T wave originating from some other local region that are sufficiently strong to modify the effect of the stronger dipolar components and thus to influence the end of T wave detection. The presence of nondipolar components of sufficient magnitude in the T wave for detection of the changes in local or regional DRT has not been demonstrated.
- Thus, detection of increased or decreased DRT is possible only in exceptional circumstances, and the establishment of the association between DRT and various subintervals of QT in time domain is problematic.
- T wave waveform in amplitude domain and its spatial characteristics can be expected to change whenever DRT increases or decreases. These T waveform changes also occur whenever action potential phase 3 slope changes differentially in various myocardial regions.

The relationships of the cardiac source events above are reiterated in Chapter 11.

3.6.1 Differences in Regional Response Characteristics of Ventricular Cells

Sodium channel blockers such as tetrodoxin, propranolol and flecainide, slow down ventricular conduction. They have a differential effect on subendocardial and subepicardial action potentials in canine ventricular myocardium.[7] In concentrations that reduce $(dV/dt)_{max}$ by approximately 40%, epicardial and M cell APD is prolonged, mainly because of the widening of the notch and the consequent delay of the onset of repolarization. In contrast, endocardial APD may even shorten. With a more pronounced sodium channel blocker action, phase 2 onset will shift to a lower, more negative potential. As a result, I_{Ca} is diminished and the outward ion currents may dominate, resulting in a pronounced decrease of epicardial APD and possibly an all-or-none repolarization at the end of phase 1. Endocardial APD may shorten only slightly. This may enhance the heterogeneity of ventricular repolarization.

Epicardial and endocardial action potentials differ in their response to parasympathetic and sympathetic agonists. Although vagal stimulation and acetylcholine are known to prolong the ventricular effective refractory period, acetylcholine has no notable effect on endocardial APD. In vivo acetylcholine effect has been thought to be strictly through antagonism of β-adrenergic tone. However, acetylcholine has a direct effect on subepicardial action potentials.[8] At low concentrations acetylcholine accentuates the notch of phase 1 and delays the peak of the dome, prolonging APD. At higher concentrations there is a marked abbreviation of the action potential. The direct acetylcholine effect is thought to be associated with the inhibition of I_{Ca} and/or activation of I_{K-ACh} (since acetylcholine does not influence I_{to}).

The APD of subepicardial cells shortens more with catecholamine than that of endocardial cells. Catecholamines enhance I_{Ca} and reduce the notch at the onset of the plateau. All major currents contributing to phase 1 and phase 3 (I_{to}, I_{Ca}, I_K, Ca- and cAMP-activated I_{Cl}) are influenced by β-adrenergic agonists.

The M cell action potentials differ in many aspects from both the endocardial and epicardial cells. The APD rate sensitivity of the M cells is higher than that of the endocardial and epicardial cells, and APD prolongation in response to class III agents is pronounced whereas there is a less notable response in endocardial and epicardial cells.[9] This difference is pronounced for I_{Kr} blockers. M cells may induce early afterdepolarizations

(EAD) with class III-type agents and DAD as a response to digitalis, catecholamines, and high calcium ion concentrations. The APD of the M cells increases markedly in response to I_{Ks} blockers and I_{Kr} channel blockers.

There are significant species differences in the presence, density, distribution, and functional properties of ionic channels.[9,10] Various disease conditions may cause profound alterations in electrophysiological functional properties of cardiac cells.[11]

3.7 Multifaceted Drug Effects on Ionic Channels

The Food and Drug Administration's (FDA) focus has been heavily on QT-prolonging effect as a surrogate endpoint in evaluating possible toxic effects of drugs in phases 1 and 2 of drug trials. As noted earlier, detection of localized dispersion of myocardial repolarization is possible from QT measurements only in special circumstances. Myocardial dispersion may have little effect on measured QT. The antiarrhythmic effect of class III and class IA agents is assumed to be associated with AP and QT prolongation. Excessive QT prolongation may become proarrhythmic. Class 1C drugs block Na^+ channels and decrease $(dV/dt)_{max}$ with no or little QT-prolonging effect. The sodium channel affinity of most antiarrhythmic drugs is relatively low in the repolarized state of the excitation/repolarization cycle. The affinity of class I drugs increases during the activated state of the channel, i.e. the block is phasic or use-dependent. The "use" occurs mainly when the channel is activated to the open state and increases with stimulus rate (heart rate). Some voltage dependence of sodium channel blocking drugs may be important, especially in the ischemic myocardium, where drugs such as lidocaine have a more pronounced effect on conduction in depolarized or partially depolarized cells.

Selective I_{to}-blocking agents (4-aminopyridine (4-AP) at low concentrations) abolish arrhythmic effects of ischemia and drugs and neurohormones (sodium channel blockers and acetylcholine) that increase dispersion of repolarization. Also quinidine inhibits I_{to}. Because of the early short-

duration nature of I_{to} currents, there seems to be some controversy on its influence on APD, for instance about the reported APD prolongation with downregulation of I_{to} channel density in heart failure.[11] I_{to} broadens the notch and decreases phase 2 plateau level and influences all active currents later in phase 2. Therefore, I_{to} inhibition or reduction of the current can be expected, at least in physiological conditions with normal intracellular ion levels. This will reduce APD in subepicardial and M cells, thus reducing the dispersion of the end of ventricular repolarization.

Chromandol 293B, one of the most specific I_{Ks} blockers, has an APD-prolonging action similar in all three types of ventricular cells. QT can be expected to prolong without a notable increase in DRT.

Most channel blockers have properties of several drug categories, and prediction of their effect on DRT is complicated. For instance, quinidine (class 1A) and amiodarone (class III) have functional properties of all four drug classes, and they also have additional actions. Quinidine, at lower doses, induces M cell APD prolongation with I_{Kr} block; at higher dose and a I_{Ks} block in addition to I_{Kr} block, M cell APD shortens while endocardial and epicardial APD prolongs. Thus, at lower doses of the drug, DRT can be expected to increase, and a decrease can be expected at higher concentrations, even at toxic doses.

The chronic amiodarone administration effect, although strongest on the K^+ channel,[2] is also multifaceted: β-blocking and blocking of sodium, potassium, and calcium channels. The combined action results in prolonged repolarization without notable increase in DRT. Amiodarone and quinidine, like some other commonly used drugs that have multiple modes of action (procainamide, disopyramide, sotalol), are effective in therapy of a broad range of arrhythmias. Amiodarone in oral form is used to convert atrial fibrillation and flutter into sinus rhythm and to suppress recurrence after conversion. Successful conversion has been achieved in approximately 50–80%.

With class III drugs, prolongation of repolarization is most pronounced at low stimulus (heart) rates, decreasing progressively with increased stimulation rate (reverse use dependence, the effect opposite to that of class 1A drugs). This has raised concern about the loss of efficacy of class

III antiarrhythmic drugs with increased heart rate.

Increased Na/K pump activity may hyperpolarize ventricular cell membranes especially if they are partially depolarized in ischemic states. This may influence the antiarrhythmic effect of drugs.

3.8 Antiarrhythmic Drug Classification

The so-called "Sicilian Gambit" antiarrhythmic drug classification scheme proposed by the European Society of Cardiology Task Force[2] specified the most likely "vulnerable parameter" for characterization of various mechanisms of drug action. The vulnerable parameter was defined as a property the alteration of which will be sufficient to terminate the arrhythmia or to prevent its initiation. Usually alteration of one such vulnerable parameter is most susceptible to a desired change with a minimum of undesirable cardiac effects.

The actual drug classification scheme of the European Task Force is reproduced in Table 3.6 with some modifications. Selected summary comments of various arrhythmogenic mechanisms and the terminology used by electrophysiologists are necessary to facilitate appreciation of the logic of this classification scheme.

3.8.1 Enhanced Normal Automaticity

This category includes the so-called inappropriate sinus tachycardia, atrial tachycardias, and some idioventricular rhythms. Inappropriate sinus tachycardia is a tachycardia of sinus origin persisting both during physical exercise and at rest. Enhanced normal automaticity is generally harmless and only rarely, if severe, may require therapeutic action. The antiarrhythmic effect on the vulnerable parameter is singly or combined a decreased phase 4 depolarization rate, increased maximum resting potential, hyperpolarization level, or the level of the firing threshold. The desirable therapeutic effect can be achieved by

TABLE 3.6 Categorization of arrhythmogenic mechanisms, desired antiarrhythmic effect on the most likely vulnerable parameter and ionic currents most likely to achieve the desired antiarrhythmic effect.

Mechanism of arrhythmia	Antiarrhythmic effect on vulnerable parameter	Ionic currents most likely to achieve desired effect
Enhanced normal automaticity	Decrease rate of phase 4 depolarization	Block I_f, I_{Ca-T} Activate $I_{K(ACh)}$
Abnormal automaticity	Increase (hyperpolarize) max diastolic potential or decrease rate of phase 4 depolarization in latent focus	Activate I_K; $I_{K(ACh)}$ Block I_{Ca-L}; I_{Na}
Triggered activity induced by EAD	Shorten APD	Activate I_K Block I_{Ca-L}; I_{Na}
Triggered activity induced by DAD	Reduce calcium overload or suppress DAD	Block I_{Ca-L} Block I_{Ca-L}; I_{Na}
Na channel-dependent re-entry with primary impaired conduction (long excitatory gap)	Decrease excitability and conduction	Block I_{Na}
Na channel-dependent re-entry with conduction encroaching on refractoriness (short excitatory gap)	Prolong effective refractory period	Block I_K
Ca channel-dependent re-entry	Decrease excitability and conduction	Block I_{Ca-L}
Reflection	Decrease excitability	Block I_{Ca-L}; I_{Na}
Parasystole	Decrease rate of phase 4 depolarization in automatic (Purkinje) focus	Block I_f (if max neg diastolic potential hyperpolarized)

EAD early afterdepolarizations, *DAD* delayed afterdepolarizations, *APD* action potential duration.
Source: Task Force of the Working Group on Arrhythmias of the European Society of Cardiology.[2] Circulation 1991;84:1831–51. Copyright © 1991 American Heart Association. Reproduced with permission from Lippincott, Williams & Wilkins.

β-adrenergic blocking agents or sodium channel blockers.

3.8.2 Abnormal Automaticity

Abnormal automaticity may arise in damaged, partially depolarized atrial, Purkinje, or other ventricular fibers that start exhibiting enhanced latent pacemaking activity. In damaged Purkinje fibers, phase 4 slope is determined by I_f, except when maximum diastolic potential is reduced to below $-55\,mV$ and the decay of K^+ currents determines the slope of phase 4. Muscarinic receptor M2 agonists, activation of I_K or I_{K-ACh} may have a remedial effect on the vulnerable parameter in this situation, and I_{Ca-L} or I_{Na} block on phase 4 repolarization.

3.8.3 Triggered Activity

Triggered activity refers to depolarization events associated with afterdepolarizations. They are oscillatory variations in membrane potential that occur when preceding repolarization is not completed, called early afterdepolarizations (EAD), or that occur later on during phase 4, called delayed afterdepolarizations (DAD).

3.8.3.1 Early Afterdepolarizations

The schematic in Figure 3.2 illustrates some possible patterns of EAD and DAD. Several ionic mechanisms may be associated with the mechanism of EAD. It is thought that EAD may be the triggering mechanism in Torsades de Pointes. Facilitating factors for EAD (likely vulnerable parameters) include slow heart (stimulus) rate or a pause, decreased extracellular K^+ concentration, and the actions of drugs that prolong APD (I_K, I_{K1} block). Consequently, the desirable therapeutic approach is to consider withdrawal of drugs that prolong APD and/or the use of β-agonists or vagolytic agents to increase heart rate. Triggering inward currents may be suppressed by calcium or sodium channel blocking agents, β- or α-adrenergic receptor blocking drugs.

3.8.3.2 Delayed Afterdepolarizations

Delayed afterdepolarizations are associated with intracellular calcium overload. Inward, depolar-

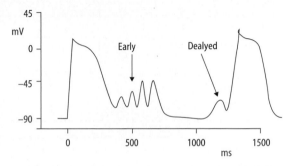

FIGURE 3.2 Schematic of afterdepolarizations. Early afterdepolarizations occur primarily at slow heart rates and prolonged action potential duration, and may result in repetitive oscillations and under certain circumstances in abnormal automaticity-like activity or possibly Torsades de Pointes. Delayed afterdepolarizations may arise from oscillatory repetitive release of calcium from sarcoplasmic reticulum in calcium overload and they may trigger ventricular ectopic complexes and tachycardias.

izing currents are caused by repetitive release of calcium from intracellular stores. Arrhythmic events most likely to be initiated by DAD are ectopic ventricular complexes (not necessarily premature), tachycardias associated with digitalis overdose, and some tachycardias related to catecholamine effect. Reduction of calcium overload (the vulnerable parameter), for instance by calcium channel blocking agents, may abolish clinically significant tachycardias in this category. Delayed afterdepolarizations may also be suppressed by agents that block the nonselective inward sodium channel current (I_{Ns}).

3.8.4 Re-entry

A model of re-entry was originally introduced by Schmitt and Erlanger, who as early as 1928 produced experimental evidence for the condition (Figure 3.3).[12]

Two models of re-entry are described in Figure 3.4. The model on the left was proposed by Schmitt and Erlanger to explain the mechanism of ventricular ectopic complexes with fixed coupling. In the model, the normal excitation arrives from the AV node in D and enters two branches of the Purkinje fibers, which connect to the ventricular muscle fibers below. One branch conducts normally but the other branch has a unidirectional block between A and B. By the time ventricular excitation arrives at B, the fiber has regained its

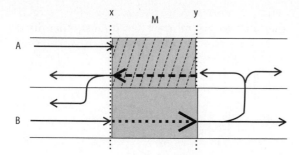

FIGURE 3.3 Schematic of re-entry from a 1928 model by Schmitt and Erlanger. A segment between x and y subjected to KCl poisoning and pressure injury produced a unidirectional block in fiber A and strongly slowed conduction through fiber B. Excitation exits fiber B after a delay, excites fiber A in both directions and re-enters back to fibers A and B.

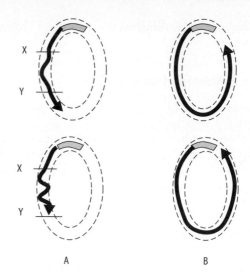

FIGURE 3.5 Schematic of the re-entry and circus movement. Black arrows indicate the portion of the circuit that is absolutely refractory, and the gray area at its tail is in the relative refractory phase. The region inside the smaller dotted ellipse is a nonconducting anatomical or functional barrier that prevents short circuiting of the propagating wavefront in the loop. At *top left* in **A**, there is a long excitatory gap between the head of the circulating wavefront and its tail, and there is an impaired conduction in the segment between lines X and Y. Further depression of conduction by drug action (*bottom left* in **A**) may block the circulating wavefront. At *top right* in **B**, the excitatory gap is short. Prolongation of the refractory period of the circulating wavefront may block re-entry at the heavy line in **B** (*bottom right*).

excitability and excitation propagates retroactively from B to A and then from the bifurcation to C, eliciting the ectopic complex.

The model on the right in Figure 3.5 illustrates the mechanism of an accessory pathway eliciting reciprocating tachycardia by re-entry involving the AV node.

3.8.5 Circus Movement and Excitable Gap

A circus movement with re-entry can occur in a circuit of cardiac tissue. In re-entrant arrhythmias, the path of circus movement has to be longer than the wavelength of the excitatory wave in the circuit that is determined by the effective refractory period and conduction velocity. The circuit path can also have a nonconducting boundary,

anatomical or functional, on both sides because otherwise there will be a short circuit. An excitatory gap is considered to be present in the circuit if an external stimulus can enter the circuit and elicit an excitatory response. A premature stimulus or overdrive pacing (at a rate higher than the intrinsic arrhythmic rate) may terminate a re-entrant arrhythmia.

If the excitatory gap is long like that shown on the left in Figure 3.5, drugs that depress conduction further in the segment of the circuit susceptible to a block may induce a block and terminate the circuit movement. If the excitatory gap is short like that shown on the right in Figure 3.5, prolonging the refractory period of the traveling wavefront in the circuit may terminate re-entry when the head approaches the tail of the circuit. Prolongation of the refractory period can be achieved by reducing the excitatory current.

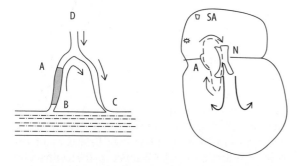

FIGURE 3.4 Schematic of a model for the mechanism of ventricular ectopic complexes with fixed coupling (*left*) and the mechanism of an accessory pathway eliciting reciprocating tachycardia by re-entry involving the AV node (*right*).

3.8.6 Atrial Fibrillation

In atrial fibrillation, multiple excitatory wavefronts are present simultaneously. Their pathways are frequently blocked or altered by fibers that are in absolute or relative refractory phase. Drugs that prolong the effective refractory period may reduce the number of wavefronts below a critical point and they may achieve the desired therapeutic effect. Defibrillation shock may terminate fibrillation, at least temporarily. Atrial fibrillation and flutter will be discussed in Chapter 5.

3.8.7 Parasystole

Ventricular or atrial parasystole is an ectopic complex arising from a focus where entrance block prevents its excitation from normal regularly timed wavefront until escape complexes occur. Their occurrence is at constant time intervals (or at multiples of the shortest interval). The coupling interval from the regular complexes is variable. The condition is rare and harmless except possibly in ischemic myocardium. Desirable therapeutic action may be achieved, if considered necessary, by a decrease in the rate of phase 4 depolarization by I_f block if maximum membrane negative diastolic repolarization level is high.

3.9 Antiarrhythmic Therapy with Channel Blockers

The medical community became acutely aware of the possibility of unexpected detrimental effects of cardioactive drugs when the results of the Cardiac Arrhythmia Suppression Trial (CAST) were published in 1989.[13] The class 1C ventricular ectopic suppressing drugs flecainide and encainide were associated with a substantial excess (2.5-fold) mortality. Roden, in 1994, classified encainide and flecainide as agents that increase mortality and moricide associated with a short-term increased mortality and possibly with long-term mortality.[14] Other drugs identified as possibly associated with increased mortality were disopyramide and mexiletine. Only β-adrenergic blockers were identified to be associated with

reduced mortality, amioradone in the category that may reduce mortality, and most other drugs as having inadequate data to conclude a significant mortality-reducing effect.

A large number of new drugs have been introduced since 1994, including the class 3 drug amiodarone. More recent developments include class 3 drugs that prolong QT by selectively blocking the delayed rectifier K^+ channel or its fast component I_{Kr} (dofelitide). They may also have reverse rate dependence, possibly through increased I_{Ks} at rapid rates. Some other newer drugs (ibulitide) are effective in reverting atrial fibrillation into sinus rhythm by prolonging APD through activation of the slow inward Na^+ current. There are inadequate data available from controlled clinical trials to demonstrate the safety of these newer drugs. In principle, class 3 drugs with enhanced effectiveness at high rates should be effective in preventing arrhythmias and reducing mortality.

The European Myocardial Infarct Amiodarone Trial (EMIAT) reported a 35% reduction ($p = 0.05$) of the risk of arrhythmic deaths in the amiodarone group compared to the placebo group, although there was no significant difference in all-cause and cardiac mortality, the primary endpoints of the trial.[15] The trial enrolled 1,486 myocardial infarction patients with left ventricular ejection fraction <40%. The authors concluded that although amiodarone is not indicated for systematic use in post-myocardial infarction patients with impaired left ventricular function, it reduces arrhythmic deaths with no proarrhythmic effect and has only a few minor side effects.

The Amiodarone Trials Meta-Analysis investigators evaluated the effect of prophylactic administration of amiodarone on mortality in patients with acute myocardial infarction or congestive heart failure or both.[16] The total number of patients included from 13 eligible studies was 6,500. To reduce bias in the analysis, the investigators used data from individual patients from each study rather than pooled summary statistics. Of the two statistical models used, the random effects model had an odds ratio 0.85 (0.71–1.02) and the fixed effects model an odds ratio 0.87 (0.78–0.99). The random effects model assumes that each study may have a different outcome, and the fixed effects model that all studies have the same basic effect of the drug on the outcome. The fixed effects model demonstrated no effect on noncardiac deaths but a substantial, 29%, decrease in arrhythmic/sudden death (odds ratio 0.71 (0.59–0.85)). Adverse noncardiac effects were more common with amiodarone, including pulmonary toxicity, thyroid and liver dysfunction, and peripheral neuropathy.

Beta-adrenergic blocking agents block catecholamine effects on Ca^{2+} and K^+ channels, prolong the refractory period, and slow the conduction of action potentials in the AV node cells. These agents will have an antiarrhythmic effect mainly on those arrhythmias where the AV node is involved and that are influenced by the functional state of the AV node. (In atrial fibrillation, β-adrenergic blocking agents slow ventricular response. In Wolf-Parkinson-White tachycardia, they slow the AV node pathway.)

References

1. Roden DM, Lazzara R, Rosen M et al. Multiple mechanisms in the long-QT syndrome. Current knowledge, gaps, and future directions. Circulation 1996;94:1996–2012.
2. Task Force of the Working Group on Arrhythmias of the European Society of Cardiology. The Sicilian Gambit. A new approach to the classification of antiarrhythmic drugs based on their actions on arrhythmogenic mechanisms. Circulation 1991;84: 1831–51.
3. Gussak I, Antzelovitch C (eds). Cardiac Repolarization. Bridging Basic and Clinical Science. Totowa, New Jersey: Humana Press, 2003.
4. Yan GX, Antzelovitch C. Cellular basis for the normal T wave and the electrocardiographic manifestations of the long-QT syndrome. Circulation 1998;98:1928–36.
5. Surawicz B, Braun HA, Crum WB et al. Quantitative analysis of electrocardiographic patterns in hypopotassemia. Circulation 1957;16:750–63.
6. Vaugham Williams EM. Classification of antiarrhythmic drugs. In: Sandoe E, Flensted-Jensen E, Olesen K (eds). Cardiac Arrhythmias. Sõdertälje, Sweden: Astra, 1981, pp 449–72.
7. Krishnan SC, Antzelovitch C. Sodium channel blockade produces opposite electrophysiologic effects in canine ventricular epicardium and endocardium. Circ Res 1991;69:277–91.
8. Litovsky SH, Antzelovitch C. Differences in the electrophysiological response of canine ventricular subendocardium and subepicardium to acetylcholine and isoproterenol. A direct effect of acetylcholine in ventricular myocardium. Circ Res 1990;67: 615–27.
9. Antzelovitch C, Zygmunt AC, Dumaine R. Electrophysiology and pharmacology of ventricular repolarization. In: Gussak I, Antzelovitch C (eds). Cardiac Repolarization. Bridging Basic and Clinical Science. Totowa, New Jersey: Humana Press, 2003, pp 63–89.
10. Nerbonne JM, Kass RS. Physiology and molecular biology of ion channels contributing to ventricular repolarization. In: Gussak I, Antzelovitch C (eds). Cardiac Repolarization. Bridging Basic and Clinical Science. Totowa, New Jersey: Humana Press, 2003, pp 25–62.
11. Armoundas AA, Tomaselli GF. Electrical and structural remodeling of the ventricular myocardium in disease. In: Gussak I, Antzelovitch C (eds). Cardiac Repolarization. Bridging Basic and Clinical Science. Totowa, New Jersey: Humana Press, 2003, pp 127–52.
12. Schmitt FO, Erlanger J. Directional differences in the conduction of the impulse through heart muscle and their possible relation to extrasystolic and fibrillatory contractions. Am J Physiol 1928;87: 326–47.
13. The Cardiac Arrhythmia Suppression Trial investigators. Preliminary report: effect of encainide and flecainide on mortality in a randomized trial of arrhythmia suppression after myocardial infarction. N Engl J Med 1989;32:406–12.
14. Roden DM. Risks and benefits of antiarrhythmic therapy. N Engl J Med 1994;331:785–91.
15. Julian DG, Camm AJ, Frangin G et al. Randomized trial of effect of amiodarone on mortality in patients with left ventricular dysfunction after recent myocardial infarction: EMIAT. European Myocardial Infarct Amiodarone Trial investigators. Lancet 1997;349:667–74.
16. The Amiodarone Trials Meta-Analysis investigators. Effect of prophylactic amiodarone on mortality after acute myocardial infarction and in congestive heart failure: meta-analysis of individual data from 6500 patients in randomized trials. Lancet 1997;350:1417–24.

4A
Heart Rate and Heart Rate Variability

Synopsis

Significance

High resting heart rate (HR) is in generally considered as a nonspecific indicator of poor health. Reduced HR variability (HRV) has been associated in numerous studies with mortality risk.

Mechanism

Faster components of normal HRV with cycle length <2.5s are associated with periodic variations in the tonic reciprocal vagal and sympathetic activity. It coincides with the periodicity of respiration that normally has a cycle length 2.5s or longer. Lower frequency HRV with cycle lengths between 2.5s and 25s are assumed to be oscillations associated with sympathetic modulation or with the combined influence of both sympathetic and parasympathetic activity. Reduced HRV reflects impaired neural control and impaired sympathovagal balance. HRV is reduced after acute myocardial infarction (MI), followed by a partial recovery of normal sympathovagal balance (reduction of low frequency [LF] and increase of high frequency [HF] power) 1–6 months after acute phase.

Classification Problems

Numerous measures of HRV have been introduced, many of them of limited value or inadequately validated. From time-domain variables, standard deviation of the RR intervals of normally conducted sinal QRS complexes (SDNN), and from frequency-domain variables, HF and LF power are most often used. Lower limits for normal HRV are strongly dependent on age, gender and heart rate. All components of HRV decrease with age, and their magnitude is significantly lower in younger women than in younger men. The age difference disappears in older age groups.

Confounding Factors

Age, HR, and common cardiovascular disease (CVD) risk factors are confounding factors. LF, HF power and SDNN decrease exponentially with increasing HR, and HR may be a significant confounder in models evaluating the prognostic value of HRV.

Mortality Risk

High HR is associated with in-hospital and peri-hospital (6-month) mortality in patients hospitalized for acute MI. Reduced HRV is associated with a significant increase in mortality risk in general populations, in diabetics, and in survivors of acute MI. The power-law regression slope is an important independent marker of excess mortality risk. SDNN has been identified as one of the primary time-domain mortality predictors. Improved sympathovagal balance induced by β-blockade in survivors of acute MI may mediate the beneficial effect of the β-blockers in post-MI patients. Comparative assessment of various risk reports is often difficult because the prevalence of various abnormal HRV strata associated with excess risk is not indicated.

Acronyms and Abbreviations

$\alpha 1$ – short-term scaling exponent

APD – action potential duration

ApEn – approximate entropy

ARIC – Atherosclerosis Risk in Communities Study

β – power-law regression slope

BHAT – Beta-Blocker Heart Attack Trial

CAD – coronary artery disease

CAPS – Cardiac Arrhythmia Pilot Study

CHD – coronary heart disease

CVD – cardiovascular disease

GISSI – Gruppo Italiano per lo Studio della Streptochinasinellâ Infarto miocardico

GUSTO – Global Utilization of Streptokinase and Tissue Plasminogen Activator to Treat Occluded Arteries

HF – high frequency

HR – heart rate, complexes or cycles per minute (cpm)

HRV – heart rate variability

LF – low frequency

MI – myocardial infarction

MPIP – Multicenter Post-Infarction Program

NHANES – National Health and Nutrition Examination Survey

pNN50 – proportion of successive NN interval differences >50 ms

RMSSD – square root of mean squared forward differences of successive NN intervals

SD – standard deviation

SDANN – standard deviation of the averaged NN intervals in all 5-min segments

SDNN – standard deviation of normally conducted RR intervals

TINN – width of triangular approximation to NN interval frequency distribution

ULF – ultra low frequency

VLF – very low frequency

4A.1 Heart Rate

In medical terminology, heart rate (HR) refers to the average number of ventricular complexes over some time interval, ranging from as few as two or three RR intervals to all complexes in a typically 10-s ECG record. The units of HR commonly used are beats per min (bpm) because non-ECG procedures evaluate pulse rate as a mechanical event. In electrocardiography, an appropriate term for HR units is cycles per min (cpm). The average number of complexes in a given interval is obtained as an inverse function of the average interval between the QRS complexes included in the estimate HR = 60/RR, where RR is the average RR interval in seconds.

The variability of the HR estimate is large if only a short evaluation interval is used. This has implications for instance to errors in QT rate adjustment. It is generally desirable to obtain the HR estimate from the whole 10-s period usually available for standard ECG analysis.

In clinical electrocardiography, commonly used lower and upper limits for normal HR are 60–100 cpm, respectively. As shown in Table 4A.1, these limits are arbitrary and inappropriate in adult men and women.[1,2] With 60 cpm as the lower normal limit for HR, one out of five to one out of three normal adult men and one out of ten to one out of five normal adult women in various age groups will be classified as having sinus bradycardia.[1] Similarly, 100 cpm is clearly too high for all age groups of adult men and women. For older men (over 40 years of age) and older women (over 50 years of age), 50 cpm is recommended for sinus bradycardia, and 90 cpm as a limit for sinus tachycardia.

The normal firing rate of the SA node is controlled by regulatory feedback mechanisms that are closely related to blood pressure control systems. Under ordinary conditions in normal sinus rhythm, HR is regulated by the sympathetic and parasympathetic divisions of the autonomic nervous system acting ordinarily in a reciprocal, coordinated fashion. If both divisions are blocked, the sinus rate in young adults is approximately

TABLE 4A.1 Practical heart rate limits for sinus bradycardia and tachycardia in adults based on lower and upper second percentile distribution of heart rate in normal men and women.

Condition	Gender	Age (years)	Heart rate (cpm)
Sinus bradycardia	Males and females	Adults	≤ 50
Sinus tachycardia	Males	24–40	≥ 95
		≥ 40	≥ 90
	Females	24–50	95
		≥ 50	≥ 50

105 cpm (the intrinsic HR). Vagal control by acetylcholine release acts fast, with a short delay after stimulation. Its action also dissipates fast. Vagal control dominates at resting conditions. Sympathetic adrenergic control acts and dissipates more slowly than the fast vagal HR control.

4A.1.1 Impact of Heart Rate on Electrical Activity of the Heart

Changes in the rate and irregularities of the rate and rhythm have a significant impact on both the electrical functions and the contractile process of the heart.[3] Key aspects of the dependence of action potential duration (APD) on the basic firing rate were discussed in Chapter 3, in connection with the ionic channel mechanisms. Action potential duration and refractory period shortening with increasing firing rate differ in different myocardial regions and in different types of myocardial cells. After a long rest or at long stimulus intervals, endocardial and epicardial APDs are similar, and at higher firing rates endocardial APD shortens less than epicardial APD. Subendocardial APD may even initially prolong when stimulated after a resting period, as demonstrated by Cohen et al. in 1976 in sheep ventricular muscle preparations.[4] Myocytes from M cell regions have the longest APD at all stimulus rates, and their rate response is more pronounced than that of the other types of cells.[5] Longer APD in subendocardial than in subepicardial regions may actually play some protective role against possible erratic activity (afterpotentials) arising at the Purkinje fibers, by blocking what Nobel et al. called "back conduction".[6]

Action potential shortening and the subsequent shortening of the mechanical systole at higher HR serves an important physiological role. This secures adequate diastolic filling time for the ventricles at higher activity levels when the metabolic demands are high.

4A.1.2 Heart Rate and Life Expectancy

In mammals, the total number of heart beats per life time is remarkably constant in all species, for a wide range of life expectancy and HR.[7]

Levin comments that because the energy consumption/body atom/heart beat is the same in all animals, HR is a universal marker of the metabolic rate.[8]

4A.2 Heart Rate and Mortality

4A.2.1 Population Studies

There have been several reports on the association between resting HR and coronary heart disease.[9-13] A significant association has been observed between HR and cardiovascular and non-cardiovascular mortality in middle-aged men. In univariate analyses, cardiovascular and non-cardiovascular disease mortality in general increases with increasing HR. Representative examples from various studies will be described next.

4A.2.1.1 NHANES1

Gillum et al. examined the association between HR and cardiovascular disease (CVD) incidence and death using the data from the first National Health and Nutrition Examination Survey (NHANES I) Epidemiologic Follow Up.[14] NHANES I was performed from 1971 to 1975. The sample persons were 25 to 74 years old. The follow-up period was 6–13 years. Risk of death from all causes and from CVD associated with HR was increased in white and African–American men and in white and African–American women, independent from other risk factors. The association between increased HR and CVD mortality adjusted for other risk factors was strongest in African–American women, with relative risk 3.3 (95% confidence limits) (1.46, 6.28).

4A.2.1.2 Finland's Health Survey

Finland's Social Insurance Institution's study in four regions of the country (5,598 men and 5,119 women aged 30–59 years at baseline) with an average of 23 years follow-up found a significant association between increased HR and mortality from all causes, from CVD, and from natural non-cardiovascular, nonmalignant causes of death.[15] The authors concluded that the strong association between HR and blood pressure explained the increase in CVD mortality with high HR and that the increased mortality risk associated with high blood pressure related mainly to noncardiovascular diseases.

4A.2.1.3 French Population Study

Benetos et al. examined the association between HR and mortality in a large French population sample of men and women.[16] Heart rate, stratified at four levels (HR1 <60 cpm; HR2, 60–80 cpm; HR3, 80–100 cpm; and HR4, >100 cpm), was a significant predictor of noncardiovascular mortality in both men and women. Relative risks for CVD in men after adjustment for age and other risk factors with HR1 as the reference group were 1.35 (1.01, 1.80), 1.44 (1.04, 2.00), and 2.18 (1.37, 3.47), respectively, in various HR strata. Heart rate was not significantly associated with CVD mortality in women.

4A.2.1.4 Chicago Area Studies

Epidemiological studies in three Chicago area populations examined associations between HR and coronary heart disease (CHD), CVD, and all-cause mortality in white middle-aged men with varying follow-up periods.[12] In multivariate Cox regression controlling for other risk factors (age, blood pressure, serum cholesterol, cigarette smoking, and relative weight), HR had a significant association with sudden CHD and non-CVD death in two of the three populations studied. The authors concluded that whereas HR may be an independent risk factor for sudden CHD death, the associations with other mortality endpoints appeared to be secondary to the associations between HR and other CVD risk factors.

In a more recent report from an over 22-year follow-up in one of the Chicago area populations (the Chicago Heart Association Detection Project in Industry), a 12-cpm increment (one standard deviation, SD) in HR was associated with a moderate increase in excess risk for CHD death in younger and middle-aged adult men and in middle-aged women.[17] A higher HR was associated with all-cause mortality in younger and middle-aged men and in middle-aged women. Heart rate was also associated with cancer mortality in middle-aged men and women.

4A.2.1.5 The Framingham Study

Heart rate and mortality risk was evaluated over a 30-year follow-up in the Framingham study cohort of 5,070 men and women free of CVD at entry.[13] Age-adjusted death rates (direct method) were compared by gender in age groups 35–64 years and 65–94 years. Multiple logistic regression analysis was performed to predict the risk over each biennial cycle among the survivors of the originally healthy cohort. Age and other cardiovascular risk factors at the beginning of each cycle were included as simultaneous covariates in the model. This study covered a wide range of age and HR because of the long study period.

As expected, HR distributions were skewed toward higher rates. There was a significant progressive increase in overall mortality with higher HR, with a steeper gradient in men than in women. The overall mortality retained a significant association with HR in men and in women in the multivariate regression models after adjusting for age and other coexisting cardiovascular risk factors evaluated. Independent association of HR with excess sudden coronary death was significant only in men and the association was strong particularly in men 35–64 years old. The fraction of deaths due to CVD did not increase with HR, and there was an excess of noncardiovascular deaths at higher HR. The authors concluded that the relationship between higher HR and mortality may not be specific to CVD (except regarding sudden death), and that several mechanisms may be involved in causing high HR as an index of general poor health.

4A.2.1.6 An Older European Population

Palatini et al. examined the association between HR and mortality in a cohort of older subjects with isolated hypertension using data from the Systolic Hypertension in Europe Trial.[18] The study population consisted of 4,695 subjects (1,557 men and 3,138 women) 60 years old and older. Systolic blood pressure in the study group ranged from 160 to 219 mmHg, and diastolic pressure was below 95 mmHg. Of the subjects, 41 % had ECG evidence of left ventricular hypertrophy. The study group was randomized to treatment (double-blinded) with active medication or to placebo (untreated) groups. The study group was recruited over 8 years, so that the report covered a follow-up period from 1 to 97 months. In multivariate analysis of the placebo group comparing subjects in the top quintile of the HR with those in the lower four quintiles, mortality risk for fatal endpoints was 1.89 (1.33, 2.68) with adjustment for sex, age, current smoking, drinking status, systolic blood pressure, previous cardiovascular complications, diabetes, and hemoglobin level. Heart rate was not predictive of any of the nonfatal endpoints. Heart rate from 24-hour ambulatory ECG did not have a stronger association with mortality than the clinic HR, and when both HR measurements were added simultaneously into risk prediction models, only the clinic HR retained a significant association with mortality.

4A.2.1.7 Japanese Men

Trends similar to those in the above study were found in an 18-year follow-up study of a Japanese general male population sample.[19] Elevated HR was the strongest predictor of age-adjusted all-cause mortality. The death rate was 2.68 times higher in men with HR ≥ 90 cpm in comparison with those in the HR stratum 60–69 cpm, and the increase in risk appeared graded.

4A.2.1.8 Italian Men

In another low risk population, a cohort of 2,533 Italian men aged 40–69 years, HR and other risk data were collected between 1984 and 1993 and vital status updated to the end of 1997.[20] Heart rate was associated with an independent risk of all mortality endpoints. Comparing the highest with the lowest quintile of HR, the risk increase was over twofold for all-cause mortality and CVD mortality.

The overall impression from the above studies is that increased HR is a nonspecific indicator of general poor health. It is not possible to draw any conclusions about a causative association between HR and mortality. It is difficult to separate HR effect from the effects of factors like impaired hormonal-neural balance, ionic channel functions, blood pressure, aging, and reduced level of fitness, arterial stiffness, metabolic abnormalities like glucose intolerance, respiratory problems, etc. Heart rate is increased in many diseases and in conditions with impaired health when HR

increase may reflect compensatory mechanisms attempting to maintain adequate oxygen delivery to vital organs.

4A.2.2 Heart Rate and Prognosis in Myocardial Infarction

4A.2.2.1 Acute Myocardial Infarction

The heart rate as a prognostic indicator in patients with acute myocardial infarction (MI) was assessed in Gruppo Italiano per lo Studio della Streptochinasinellà Infarto miocardico (GISSI-2).[21] Heart rate at hospital admission in a general hospital population with MI was evaluated in 1,815 patients treated with fibrinolysis for in-hospital mortality and HR at hospital discharge in 7,831 patients for 6-month mortality. Excluded were patients not in sinus rhythm and those having a second or third degree AV block. In-hospital and 6-month mortality increased progressively with increasing HR. In multivariate analysis, HR retained its independent association with mortality.

4A.2.2.2 Heart Rate and Progression of Coronary Atherosclerosis in Young Myocardial Infarction Patients

A study from Sweden in a small group of male patients ($n - 56$) who had had their first MI before the age of 45 years found that a high minimum 24-hour HR was correlated with angiographic scores of global severity of diffuse atherosclerosis and stenotic lesions.[22] High minimum 24-hour HR was also associated with the progression of coronary lesions quantified in two examinations 4–7 years apart. It was noted that in addition to a high minimum HR, the ratio of low and high density lipoproteins was an independent predictor of progression. Factors such as hypertension, smoking, and treatment with β-adrenergic blockade did not help in discriminating between patients with and without disease progression.

4A.2.3 Heart Rate Response to Exercise and Mortality Risk

Abnormal HR recovery after cessation of an exercise test is clinically defined as a HR decrease ≤ 18 cpm during the first minute after the end of the test if it involves a low level load during the post-exercise adaptation phase and $\leq 12\,cpm$ otherwise.[23] Impaired HR recovery after exercise has been shown to be predictive of mortality, including persons with and without CHD.[24,25] In a 6-year follow-up of 2,935 patients who had exercise stress tests and coronary arteriograms for suspected coronary artery disease (CAD), an abnormal HR recovery was associated with increased mortality risk (hazards ratio 2.5 [1.6, 2.6]).[26] This increased risk was additive to the risk associated with the severity level of CAD (no interaction). One quarter of the study population was women. An abnormal HR response was associated with excess mortality risk (adjusted hazard ratio 1.5 (1.2, 1.9), even after adjusting for age, CAD severity, functional capacity, ejection fraction, smoking, use of aspirin, and end-stage renal disease.

4A.3 Heart Rate Variability

The emphasis has generally shifted from HR to evaluation of the risk associated with heart rate variability (HRV). Heart rate is not constant even in normal sinus rhythm. There can be substantial variations in the basic level of the HR, relatively abrupt changes and nonstationary periods, more or less random variations, periodic variations

TABLE 4A.2 Some time-domain variables used for estimation of heart rate variability.

Variable (units)	Definition
SDNN (ms)	SD of all NN intervals* in the recording
SDAN	Mean of SDs of NN interval averages in 5-min periods of the recording
RMSSD (ms)	Square root of the mean of the squared forward differences of successive NN intervals
pNN50 (%)	Proportion of successive forward differences of NN intervals >50 ms
Triangular index	Height to width ratio of triangular approximation to the frequency distribution of NN intervals on a discretized interval scale (bins)
TINN (ms)	The width of the triangular approximation

* NN interval is the interval between normally conducted QRS complexes of sinus origin (preferably excluding intervals preceding and following ectopic complexes).

modulated by various physiological control systems, periodic diurnal variations with the sleep–awake cycle, and circadian variations with seasons and temperature.

4A.3.1 Statistical Estimates of Heart Rate Variability

Several statistical measures have been proposed for estimation of HRV in time domain as well as in frequency domain, listed in Tables 4A.2 and 4A.3. Some of the time-domain variables are

TABLE 4A.3 Some frequency-domain variables used for estimation of heart rate variability from RR interval sequences.

Variable (units)	Definition
Long recording period*	
Total power (TP) (ms^2)	Variance of NN intervals (highest frequency $\approx 0.4\,Hz$)
Ultra low frequency (ULF) power (ms^2)	Power in range ≤ 0.0033
Very low frequency (VLF) power (ms^2)	Power in range $0.0033–0.004\,Hz$
Low frequency (LF) power (ms^2)	Power in range $0.04–0.15\,Hz$
High frequency (HF) power (ms^2)	Power in range $0.15–0.4\,Hz$
Power-law slope $(\beta)^{\dagger}$	Slope from linear interpolation of the ln power density distribution vs ln frequency from 0.0004 to 0.02 Hz
Short recording period‡	
LF/HF power ratio	Calculated over a shorter period (e.g. 5 min) or as an average of several or all shorter periods
Normalized LF (LFn) (%)	100*(LF/TP–VLF)
Power-law regression slope (β)	Slope of the plot of ln (power spectral density) vs ln frequency over the low range of frequencies up to near 0.1 Hz
Scaling exponent (α)	Slope of ln of detrended interval variance over progressively increasing interval length plotted against ln interval length ("box size")
Approximate entropy (ApEn)	A measure of the irregularity or unpredictability of a sequence-ordered time series

* Entire 24-hour period or separately from day-time and night periods. The recommended duration of the recording is at least ten times the lowest frequency in the band of the spectral component investigated.

† Power-law regression slope is at times denoted by α. It is labeled here as β to avoid confusion with the scaling exponent $\alpha 1$.

‡ ULF components are not obtained from short-term recordings.

highly correlated (for instance, RMSSD and SDNN in Table 4A.2 are practically identical).

From the frequency-domain variables, the high frequency (HF) power reflects primarily vagal control of HR during the respiratory cycle. The low frequency (LF) power expresses collectively both the sympathetic and parasympathetic HR modulation. Parasympathetic modulation is thought to be the principal factor in very low frequency (VLF) power, which reflects composite activity of physiological control systems (peripheral vasomotor, thermoregulatory and renin-angiotensin systems). Ultra low frequency (ULF) power comprises the very slow components of HRV associated with circadian variation, variations in the activity of neuroendocrine systems, etc.

Some methodological considerations of HRV analysis are presented in Chapter 4B. These include descriptions of nonlinear measures of HRV, including the power-law slope and two newer nonlinear measures of HRV of interest to the assessment of the risk of adverse cardiac events, the approximate entropy and the short-term scaling component.

4A.3.2 Correlations Between Heart Rate Variability Measures

Bigger et al. demonstrated that the correlations between log-transformed short-term and 24-hour RR variability were relatively high.[27] For instance, for 15-min day-time segments, the correlations were 0.78, 0.88 and 0.85 for lnVLF, lnLF and lnHF, respectively, and even for 2-min segments, 0.80 and 0.79 for lnLF and lnHF, respectively. (VLF power cannot be determined from 2-min segments, and ULF power only from 24-hour records.) In another study using the same material, Bigger et al. evaluated correlations between time-domain and frequency-domain measures of RR variability, both determined from 24-hour ambulatory recordings.[28] Some of the time-domain measures had a very high correlation ($r \geq 0.90$) with frequency-domain variables in various frequency ranges: ULF power with SDNN and SDANN index, VLF and LF power with SDNN index, and HF power with RMSSD. In contrast, associations between time- and frequency-domain variables

and established clinical post-infarction risk factors were "remarkably weak". The authors concluded that selected pairs of the time-domain and frequency-domain variables were essentially equivalent. Like the frequency-domain variables, particularly those time-domain measures that are strongly related to ULF and LF power were strong, independent predictors of death after MI.

4A.3.3 Clinical Limits for Reduced Heart Rate Variability

Published cutpoints to define abnormally reduced HRV are <0.75% for pNN50, <15 ms for RMSSD, <20 or <30 ms for SDNN Index, <40 ms for SDANN, and <50 ms for SDNN.[29] The medians and lower 25th and 5th percentile limits were listed in the Framingham report for age groups 30, 50 and 70 years for HR 50, 70 and 90 cpm for eight HRV measures in the healthy subset of the study population.[30] The healthy subset was considered free of coronary and cerebrovascular disease, congestive heart failure, and diabetes mellitus. Those receiving cardioactive medication were excluded. The lower limits were determined from linear regression, adjusted for age and HR, with natural-logarithmic transformed data that were then transformed back to ordinary linear scales. The lower limits and the medians of all HRV variables retained their dependence on HR. Selected values reproduced in Table 4A.6 suggest clearly that normal limits should be determined from rate-adjusted HRV data.

4A.3.4 Dimensions of Heart Rate Variability – a Suggestion

In HRV analysis, power is a measure of variance. However, electrocardiographers are used to expressing the variability of ECG variables as standard deviation rather than as variance. It is true that in mathematics power denotes the square of any quantity. In physics, power denotes a quantity with an ability to perform work. Frequency-domain HRV variables expressed in units (ms) rather than ms^2 will make these measures more comprehensive in practical applications in electrocardiography. This can be appreciated by reviewing Table 4A.6 where the square-root transformed values of the frequency-domain "power" variables are listed in brackets.

4A.4 Determinants of Heart Rate Variability

A variety of factors are involved as determinants of heart rate variability.

4A.4.1 Heart Rate Variation with Respiration

Although HRV with respiration is normal, ECG interpretation reports call it "respiratory sinus arrhythmia". At least one full cycle of this variation is present even in a 10-s ECG recording, and it is usually easily recognized. Reduced HRV may be abnormal and it has been associated with increased risk of adverse cardiac events in a variety of abnormal clinical conditions.

Respiratory variation is the main HF component of the HRV spectrum. Its peak coincides with respiratory frequency, with a period normally 2.5s or longer. This relatively fast periodic variation is dominated by the discharge rate of vagal efferent fibers. Vagal activity is inhibited during inspiration and facilitated during expiration. When stimulated, vagal nerve terminals release acetylcholine acting on the receptors at the SA node cells and slowing down the SA node firing rate. The SA node has an abundance of cholinesterase, an enzyme that hydrolyzes acetylcholine very fast, as soon as vagal fibers stop firing. This is the reason why vagal components of HRV form the HF part of the HRV spectrum. Low frequency variations with cycle length between 2.5 and 25s are assumed to be oscillations associated with sympathetic modulation or induced both by sympathetic and parasympathetic activity.

4A.4.2 Gender Differences in Heart Rate Variability

There are significant gender differences in HRV.[29-33] Pikkujämsä, from Huikuri's research group, documented HRV measures of RR interval dynamics in healthy middle-aged men and women, reproduced in Table 4A.4.[31] These HRV measures were calculated from 15-min periods in controlled supine position. Sex differences were significant for all of these measures except for LF and HF power when calculated in absolute units (not shown). When LF and HF power was calculated in normalized units (as a proportion of total power in the corresponding band), the normalized LF power was significantly lower and the normalized HF power significantly higher in women than in men. The short-term scaling exponent ($\alpha1$) was significantly lower and the approximate entropy (ApEn) significantly higher in women than in men, although the total overall variance was decreased. The author concluded that HRV dynamics in healthy middle-aged women compared to men reflects more complex, fractile-like characteristics. The persistence of the sex differences after multivariable adjustment also suggests that hormonal and genetic factors may play an important role in the mechanism of the healthy state of cardiovascular control systems in women.

Earlier reports by Huikuri et al. evaluated the reproducibility and circadian rhythm of heart rate variability in healthy subjects. In addition, gender differences in baroreceptor sensitivity were evaluated using HRV calculated from 15-min supine and resting periods and with the Valsalva manoever.[34,35] The baroreceptor sensitivity was significantly lower in women than in men. Comparing sex differences in responses to upright posture,

TABLE 4A.4 Mean values (standard deviation) of various measures of RR interval dynamics in healthy middle-aged men and women.

Variable	Men ($n = 192$)	Women ($n = 202$)	p value
RR interval	864 (136)	866 (107)	ns
ApEn	1.10 (0.14)	1.15 (0.14)	<0.001
LF power (ms^2)	805 (714)	671 (532)	ns
LF power, normalized	68 (17)	64 (14)	<0.01
HF power (ms^2)	357 (541)	351 (344)	ns
HF power, normalized	25 (11)	31 (10)	<0.001
LF/HF power ratio	3.4 (2.0)	2.5 (1.5)	<0.001

ApEn approximate entropy, *HF* high frequency, *LF* low frequency.
Source: Pikkujämsä S.[31] Heart rate variability and baroreflex sensitivity in subjects without heart disease. Doctoral thesis. Acta Universitatis Ouluensis, Series D, Medica 520. Copyright © 1999 Oulu University Library, Oulu, Finland. Reproduced with permission.

women had a smaller decrease in HF power and an attenuated HR response. Gender differences remained significant after adjustment for differences in mean HR, blood pressure, and alcohol consumption. The overall results suggest that compared to men, the tonic vagal activity is augmented in women.

4A.4.3 Heart Rate and Age as Determinants of Heart Rate Variability

Umetani et al.[29] evaluated five time-domain measures of IIRV by age and gender in 260 healthy men and women over an age range of nine decades. All HRV measures decreased with age to a varying degree. The decline, 5.7 ms per decade, was linear for SDNN Index ($r = -0.63$). The correlation with age was lower than for SDNN Index for the other four measures of time-domain HRV. The decline had a linear and quadratic component in the regression. This indicates that the decrease was faster in younger age groups and tended to level off after middle-age. All HRV measures were significantly lower in younger women (<30 years of age) than in age-matched men. Gender differences decreased with varying rates for different HRV measures and disappeared for all after the age of 50 years.

Mean values of various 24-hour time-domain measures of HRV reported by Umetani et al. in Table 2 of the report are reproduced in Figure 4A.1, and the upper and lower 95% confidence limits from Table 3 of Umetani's report are reproduced in Figure 4A.2. These figures show that SDNN, SDANN, and SDNN Index were all strongly influenced by age.

The rate- and age-dependence of various time- and frequency-domain variables was evaluated in a comprehensive report by Tsuji et al.[30] The data shown in Table 4A.5 were derived from 2-hour ambulatory recordings of the entire Framingham Heart Study population between ages 28 and 62 years participating in the biennial examinations between 1983 and 1987. Nonsinus rhythm, frequent premature complexes (>10% of total complexes), and subjects receiving antiarrhythmic medications were excluded from the data.

Stepwise regression analysis performed to identify important determinants of SDNN, LF and HF

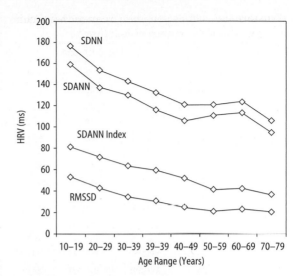

FIGURE 4A.1 Mean values of various HRV measures by decades of age. Note strong age-dependence of all measures of HRV. (Source: graphed from data in Table 2, Umetani et al.[29] J Am Coll Cardiol 1998;31:593–601. Copyright © 1998 The American College of Cardiology Foundation. Reproduced with permission.)

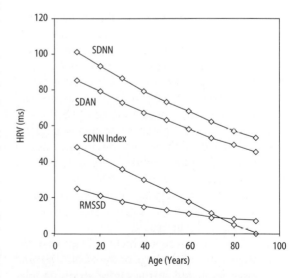

FIGURE 4A.2 Lower values of the 95% confidence limits for various HRV measures. Note the strong age-dependence of the lower limits. The effect of the equally strong HR dependence of the limits was not considered. (Source: graphed from data in Table 3, Umetani et al.[29] J Am Coll Cardiol 1998;31:593–601. Copyright © 1998 The American College of Cardiology Foundation. Reproduced with permission.)

TABLE 4A.5 Lower fifth percentile limits by age and heart rate in a healthy subset of the Framingham Heart Study.*

Variable	Age (years)	Heart rate (cpm)		
		50	70	90
RMSSD	30	40	24	15
	50	31	19	11
	70	24	14	9
2-Hour SDNN	30	113	80	56
	50	91	65	57
	70	74	53	46
VLF	30	4,248 (65)	1,848 (43)	804 (28)
	50	2,618 (53)	1,139 (34)	496 (22)
	70	1,614 (40)	702 (26)	305 (17)
LF	30	1,488 (39)	794 (28)	424 (21)
	50	718 (27)	383 (20)	204 (14)
	70	346 (19)	185 (14)	98 (10)
HF	30	373 (19)	181 (13)	88 (9)
	50	184 (14)	89 (9)	43 (7)
	70	91 (10)	44 (7)	21 (5)

HF high frequency, *LF* low frequency, *VHF* very low frequency, *RMSSD* root-mean-square successive differences, *SDNN* standard deviation of the normally conducted QRS complexes of sinus node origin. *The values in brackets for frequency-domain variables are those expressing variation in ms (square root of the corresponding power spectral density).
Source: Tsuji et al.[30] J Am Coll Cardiol 1996;28:1539–46. © 1996 The American College of Cardiology Foundation. Reproduced with permission.

revealed that HR and age were the primary determinants of all three HRV measures. There was a negative association with HR and age. Partial R-square values for age ranged from 0.218 for lnSDNN to 0.389 for lnLF and for HR between 0.125 for lnLF to 0.226 for lnSDNN. Thus, age and HR explained a substantial fraction of HRV variation. In addition, β-blocker use had a negative association with all three HRV variables, although the partial R-square values were substantially lower, ranging from 0.005 to 0.020. The data also suggested that if β-blocker use resulted in HR increase by more than 10 cpm, HRV variability measures actually increased.

The Framingham report included figures of the dependence on HR and age of the SDNN, HF and LF power predicted in the entire study population. The relationship of all HRV measures and HR is not linear but resembles closely an exponential function. This suggests that it should be possible to remove the HR dependence of SDNN by using lnSDNN instead of SDNN as a function of HR. This can be expected to produce lnSDNN

as a linear function of HR with closely identical slopes in each age group. Age differences can then be compared for instance by adjusting lnSDNN values to HR = 70. This was actually verified by digitizing the relevant graph in the Framingham report and converting SDNN to a log scale (not shown).

4A.4.4 Beta-blocker Medication and Heart Rate Variability

Beta-blockade has been shown generally to induce a significant increase in HRV in patients with CHD, although the Framingham study cited above[30] found a decreased HRV with subjects on blockers. In that study, the HRV reduction effect of β-blockers was similar to a 10 cpm increase in HR, and if β-blockers reduced HR by 10 cpm, HRV actually increased.

Niemelä et al. performed a randomized, placebo-controlled crossover study comparing two kinds of β-blockers (atenolol and metoprolol) in 18 patients with CHD.[36] Exclusion criteria included recent MI, congestive heart failure, and diabetes mellitus. The RMSSD of NN intervals increased by 70% after atenolol and by 62% after metoprolol, and 24-h HF variance increased by 64% and 62%, respectively; SDNN increased by 20% after atenolol and by 16% after metoprolol. Heart rate variability measures were not adjusted for HR. The mean RR interval increased with β-blockade by 30–33% during day-time hours and by 15–18% during night-time hours. The authors note that the enhancement of HRV with β-blockade occurs not only because of enhanced vagal activity but also because of reduced sympathetic β-receptor stimulation.

The study by Kamath and Fallen in MI patients during acute phase demonstrated that HF variance, otherwise reduced in MI, was significantly enhanced by β-blockade, especially between 7 a.m. and 3 p.m., and that the power spectral measures of HRV remained stable over 24 hours.[37]

Cook et al. evaluated the effect of the β-blocker atenolol and the calcium channel blocker diltiazem on HRV in 18 normal volunteers in a randomized, three-period, placebo-controlled crossover study.[38] The investigators found that the increase in pNN50, RMSSD and the HF component of HRV during atenolol treatment was significant for all, ranging from 61% to 84%. In addition to these HRV measures commonly considered to reflect tonic vagal activity, LF variance was also significantly increased (by 45%), suggesting that in addition to other factors, LF variance in healthy adults reflects tonic vagal activity during a 24-h period. It should be noted that the average NN interval increased by 23% during atenolol treatment in this study. In contrast to the β-blocker atenolol effect, the calcium channel blocker diltiazem had no effect on HR or any HRV measure.

A small subgroup of 184 patients (all men) of the study population from one of the study centers of the Beta-Blocker Heart Attack Trial (BHAT)[39] was evaluated with both frequency-domain and time-domain HRV measures. Holter recordings of adequate quality and recording length (>18 hours) at baseline and repeated 6 weeks later were used in the evaluation.[40] Two-way analysis of variance of repeated measures of the 6-week data was done to evaluate the effects of time and the interaction of time and β-blocker medication on HRV measurements. Log-transformed HRV parameters were used for statistical analyses. Ultra low frequency, VLF, and LF power all increased at 6 weeks from the start of the administration of β-blockers or placebo (8 weeks after acute phase onset) but the increase was not significantly affected by β-blockers. High frequency power increased in both groups but the increase was more pronounced in the β-blocker group ($p = 0.02$ for β-blocker effect above the effect time). The LF/HF ratio increased in the placebo group but decreased in the β-blocker group ($p < 0.01$). All time-domain HRV measures increased significantly over time during the 6-week period ($p < 0.01$). Like with HF power, there was a greater increase in faster time-domain measures pNN5 and RMSSD but not with SDNN concerning the propranolol effect above the effect of time.

4A.4.5 Diminished Heart Rate Variability in Survivors of Acute Myocardial Infarction

In a 1995 report, Bigger et al.[41] evaluated RR interval variability in 684 patients 2 weeks after an acute MI and in 274 healthy middle-aged persons 40–69 years old. The healthy group was used to establish normal limits to various HRV measures. The healthy group was also compared with measurements from 278 patients 1 year after the acute MI in order to determine the extent of recovery of HRV. Consistent with an earlier report,[42] HRV reduction was most pronounced in the subacute phase of MI compared with that 1 year after MI. The fractional distribution of total spectral power was similar in all three groups. Comparing probability distributions of log-transformed spectral power components in healthy subjects and the two CAD groups, the overlap with healthy subjects was smaller for the ULF component than that of any other component. From the MI group (2-week recordings), 60% were below the lower 2 SD point of the healthy subjects, but only 21% of the HF values. Similarly, 26% of the values of the CAD group without MI were below the lower normal limit, in comparison with only 12% of the HF values.

Reduction in HRV in acute MI recovers to a certain degree during the convalescent period, reaching a new plateau level within 6–8 weeks.[43,44]

4A.4.6 Prevalent Myocardial Infarction and Diminished Heart Rate Variability

The association of HRV with prevalent MI (by ECG or diagnosed by the person's physician) was evaluated in the ARIC study using 2-min ECG recordings of a stratified random sample of 2,243 men and women aged 45–64 years, 260 of them with a prevalent MI and the remaining 1,943 free of any manifestations of CHD.[45] The HF variance (in band 0.16–0.35 Hz) and the LF variance (band 0.025–0.15 Hz) were both significantly lower in the MI group than in the CHD-free group. Stratifying the variance into quintiles, the age-, race- and sex-adjusted odds ratios for the presence of lower levels of variance of HF and LF components comparing MI group with non-MI group were 1.52 (1.09, 2.10) and 1.54 (1.12, 2.10), respectively. When β-blocker use was included in the multivariate model, the odds ratios were no longer significant.

4A.4.7 Diminished Circadian Variation in Heart Rate Variability in Post-myocardial Infarction Patients

Kamath and Fallen showed that there are diurnal variations in HRV in patients during the acute phase of MI.[37] There was a significant increase in the LF component and a decrease in the LF/HF ratio from 3 p.m. to 11 p.m in patients not on β-blocker medication. The authors suggested that vagal tone may be more pronounced during late evening hours, with a shift to relative sympathetic dominance during early morning and mid-afternoon hours.

Other clinical studies have shown that the normal circadian variation in HRV patterns is lost or diminished in acute MI.[46-48] Vanoli et al. reported in 1995 that the differences in HF–LF relationships between MI patients and healthy subjects were particularly pronounced during nonrapid eye movement sleep.[49] In healthy subjects, the vagal dominance was pronounced and the contribution of the HF fraction to the total variance in the LF–HF band was relatively low. Relative sympathetic dominance in patients with a recent MI prevailed even in the nonrapid eye movement state and the HF fraction remained relatively low and the LF/HF ratio correspondingly high.

4A.4.8 Reduced Heart Rate Variability in Other Conditions

In 1996, the Task Force of the European Society of Cardiology and the North American Society of Pacing and Electrophysiology on HRV listed 21 studies (Table 4 of the report) selected to represent overt clinical disease with reduced HRV in conditions other than MI.[50] In general, the reduction observed has occurred because of diminished vagal tone and reduction in the HF component of HRV.

An enhanced LF component has been observed in hypertensive patients. Langewitz compared hypertensive ($n = 34$) and normotensive ($n = 41$) subjects and found reduced power in the HF (vagal) band as the most prominent difference in subjects with borderline hypertension and hypertensive subjects at rest and during various states of mental challenge.[51] Guzzetti et al. reported significant differences between hypertensive and normotensive subjects in circadian variation of frequency spectrum components.[52] The night-time resting LF power was greater in hypertensive than in normotensive subjects, and the difference between day-time and night-time LF power was progressively reduced with the severity of hypertensive state ($p < 0.05$).

Heart rate variability is reduced and there is an imbalance in autonomic tone in congestive heart failure.[53-57] With ACE inhibitor therapy, the HF component is enhanced following the initial reduced level. The clinically marked autonomic imbalance in congestive heart failure appears to be due to reduced vagal and dominating sympathetic tone, although alterations of HRV seem not so tightly linked to severity of congestive heart failure.

4A.5 Heart Rate Variability and Mortality Risk

4A.5.1 Reduced HRV and Mortality Risk in Community-based Populations

4A.5.1.1 Framingham, ARIC, and Rotterdam Studies

Representative reduced HRV measures and the risk of adverse events from three community-based population studies are compared in Table 4A.6. These studies used different ECG recording lengths for HRV analysis. The first report is from the Framingham Study, which used 2-hour Holter recordings from regular follow-up examination of the original Framingham cohort and the new Framingham Offspring study group.[58] The study population comprised 2,501 men and women free of apparent CHD and congestive heart failure at the time of the Holter recording. Five frequency-domain and two time-domain HRV measures from 2-hour recordings were evaluated for the risk of cardiac events (angina pectoris, unstable angina with transient ischemic changes in ECG, myocardial infarction, and coronary death – sudden or nonsudden) during the average 3.5-year follow-up. All HRV measures except LF/HF ratio and lnpNN50 had a significant association

TABLE 4A.6 The risk of adverse events for SDNN determined from ECGs with record lengths ranging from 10 seconds to 2 hours from three population studies.

	Framingham	ARIC	Rotterdam
Study group	Framingham original cohort + Offspring Study[59]	CHD-free men and women of ARIC[60]	Rotterdam Heart Study men and women[61]
Record length	2 h	2-min paper strip	10 s
Sample evaluated	2,501 (1,101 men, 1,400 women), free of CHD and CHF	2,252 CHD-free men and women and 137 incident CHD cases	Total study population of 5,272 (2,088 men, 3,184 women)
Follow-up	Mean 3.5 years	3 years	Mean 4 years
Endpoint evaluated	Incident CHD or CHF	Incident CHD	Cardiac mortality
Variable evaluated	lnSDNN decrement by 1 SD	Lowest quartile of HF (0.16–0.35 Hz) variance compared to 3 upper quartiles	SDNN
HR (95% CI or p)	1.47 (1.13, 1.85)	1.72 (1.17, 2.51)	Lowest vs 3rd quartile: 1.8 (1.0, 3.2) Highest vs 3rd quartile: 2.3 (1.3, 4.0)
Adjustment	Age, sex, laboratory and clinical factors including medication use, cigarette smoking, diabetes, systolic blood pressure	Age, race, gender, education level, diabetes mellitus, hypertension, and beta-blocker medication	Age, sex; additional adjustment for a variety of possible confounders did not notably change estimated risk
Comments	HR significant also for lnVLF, lnLF, lnHF with HR 1.38 for each ($p < 0.05$) but not when mean HR was included	HR not significant for LF, HF/LF power ratio or RMSSD	Study population not stratified by CHD status

CHD coronary heart disease, *CHF* congestive heart failure, *HF* high frequency, *HR* hazard ratio, *LF* low frequency, *SDNN* standard deviation of RR intervals of normally conducted QRS complexes.

with incident cardiac events after adjustment for all relevant clinical risk factors in a multivariate model. (It is not clear whether HRV measures were used in the multivariate model one-by-one or if all were entered together with clinical risk factors.)

One SD decrement in 2-hour SDNN was associated with a hazard ratio 1.47 (1.13, 1.85). Logarithmic measures lnVLF, lnVF and lnHF all had hazard ratio 1.38, with p values ranging from 0.0139 for lnVLF to 0.0341 for lnLF. An interesting finding was that when the HR was included in the multivariate model, 2-hour SDNN remained the only HRV measure with a significant association with the risk of cardiac events. This observation speaks strongly in favor of always including the HR as a covariate in HRV evaluation of the risk associated with HRV.

In an earlier report on a smaller sample of 736 subjects of the original Framingham cohort at the 18th biennial examination,[59] the association between five frequency-domain and three time-domain HRV measures and mortality risk was evaluated. Analysis of HRV was done from a

2-hour Holter recording, excluding records with nonsinus rhythms, frequent (>10%) ventricular ectopics, and records of patients on antiarrhythmic medication. The follow-up time was 4 years. Four frequency-domain measures (VLF power, LF power, HF power, and total power) and one time-domain measure (SDNN) were significant predictors of total mortality in univariate models adjusted for clinical factors. When all eight HRV measures were entered together into a multivariate stepwise regression model simultaneously with clinical risk factors, LF power was the only HRV variable with an independent risk of all-cause mortality ($p < 0.001$). One SD increment in ln-transformed LF power was associated with a hazard ratio 1.70 (1.37, 2.09) in a 2-min paper strip recording using a digitizing table to extract RR interval sequences.

The second report in Table 4A.6 comes from one of the ARIC HRV studies in a random sample of 2,252 participants free of CHD.[60] The study used a 2-min paper strip recording and a digitizing table to extract RR interval sequences. The risk analysis evaluated the association of SDNN and various frequency-domain HRV variables with a 3-year incidence of CHD (hospitalization for MI, CHD death, or cardiac revascularization procedure). Comparing the lowest quartile of HF variance with the higher three quartiles, the relative risk of incident CHD was 1.72 (1.17, 2.51). It was not significant for the other measures of HRV evaluated (LF variance, HF/LF variance ratio and RMSSD). The authors concluded that lower parasympathetic activity as manifested in lower variance of HF components in a 2-min ECG recording is associated with the risk of developing CHD.

The third report in Table 4A.6 is from the Rotterdam Study, which evaluated the association of reduced HRV and mortality during a 3- to 6-year (mean 4 years) follow-up of 2,088 men and 3,184 women aged 55 years and over.[61] The HRV (SDNN) was calculated from computer-measured RR intervals of the standard 10-s ECGs. Comparing the lowest quartile of SDNN with the third quartile, the relative risk of cardiac mortality was

1.8 (1.0, 3.2) and of all-cause mortality 2.3 (1.0, 1.8). A surprising observation was that the relative risk of cardiac mortality was even higher, 2.3 (1.3, 4.0), when comparing the highest quartile of SDNN with the third quartile, than that for the lowest quartile. The authors concluded that both increased and decreased HRV evaluated from the 10-s ECG recording is associated with a significantly increased risk of cardiac mortality in older men and women.

4A.5.2 Differing Risk of Adverse Events in Studies with Differing Design

Results from three reports from studies with differing design are listed in Table 4A.7.

4A.5.2.1 ARIC Reports

The first report used HRV data from a random subsample ($n = 900$) of ARIC participants who

TABLE 4A.7 Differing risk of adverse events in reports from two ARIC studies and a survey from a healthy older Finnish cohort.

	ARIC[62]	ARIC[63]	Turku Health Survey[64]
Record length	2 min	2 min	24 h
Sample evaluated	A random sample of 900 men and women without CHD 395 subjects with incident CHD and 140 with CVD death	11,654/14,075 ARIC participants; CHD-free at baseline; 11% diabetics	325 men and women, after exclusion of 22 with arrhythmias or recording artifacts (initial random sample 480; participation rate 72%)
Age at baseline	45–65 years at baseline in 1987–1989	45–65 years at baseline in 1987–1989	≥65 years
Follow-up	Through 1993	Through end of 1996; mean follow-up 8 years	10 years
Relative risk RR (95% CI)	CVD mortality SDNN 1.98 (1.06, 3.70) pNN50 3.44 (1.69, 7.02) All-cause mortality SDNN: 1.50 (1.02, 2.21) pNN50: 2.35 (1.57, 3.50)	CHD mortality Nonsignificant for all HRV variables in nondiabetic and diabetic groups Incident CHD, nondiabetics Nonsignificant for all HRV variables Incident CHD, diabetics HF: 1.55 (1.13, 2.13) LF: 1.47 (1.07, 2.02) SDNN: 1.49 (1.07, 2.07)	Cardiac mortality SDNN <120 ms: 1.14 (0.83, 1.59) Slope β < −1.5: 2.05 (1.40, 2.99) All-cause mortality SDNN <120 ms: 1.16 (0.95, 1.77) Slope β < −1.5: 1.74 (1.42, 2.13)
Comments	Adjusted for age, sex, race, diabetes, hypertension, smoking and seven other demographic and clinical variables; not adjusted for heart rate	Adjusted for age, sex, race, fasting glucose, hypertension, smoking, heart rate, and four other clinical and demographic variables	Adjusted for age, sex, and clinical variables that had a significant univariate association with the endpoint; cutpoints of variables optimized for risk. Relative risk was 2.84 (1.71, 4.70) for cerebrovascular mortality

HF high frequency power, *LF* low frequency power, *SDNN* standard deviation of RR intervals of normally conducted QRS complexes of sinus node origin (NN intervals), *pNN50* proportion of successive forward differences of NN intervals >50 ms; *Slope* β power-law regression slope.

were CHD-free at the baseline and "cases."[62] The "cases" were 395 participants with incident CHD and 140 CVD deaths between the time of the baseline sampling (1987–1989) through 1993. The HRV data set was divided into tertiles by each time-domain HRV variable (SDNN, RMSSD, SDSD, and pNN50). Poisson regression for the case-cohort design was used to compute relative risk of various endpoints (all-cause, CVD and cancer mortality, and incident CHD). With the middle tertile as the reference group, the risk of CVD mortality and all-cause mortality was high for all of the time-domain HRV variables, ranging from approximately two to well over three for CVD mortality, and from 1.5 to well over two for all-cause mortality. Relative risks were higher for RMSSD, SDSD and pNN50 than for SDNN. Risk data only for SDNN and pNN50 and only for CVD and all-cause mortality are shown in the summary in Table 4A.7. The risk of incident CHD was significant for pNN50 only (not shown).

The results from a later ARIC report from 2002 in Table 4A.7 used data available from 11,654 ARIC participants who had a completed a 2-min HRV recording.[63] The study objective was to perform risk comparison between 1,275 diabetics and the remaining study group of the CHD-free ARIC population. The mean follow-up was 8 years, 3 years longer than that in the first ARIC report in Table 4A.7. None of the frequency-domain and none of the time-domain HRV variables were significantly associated with the risk of CHD mortality in the diabetes-free group, and the risk of non-CHD mortality was significant only for LF variance. (This study reported CHD and non-CHD mortality, whereas the first study reported CVD and all-cause mortality as the fatal endpoints.) The risk of incident CHD was not significant for any of the HRV variables in the non-diabetic group. The results in the diabetic group revealed a nonsignificant association with CHD mortality, and like in the nondiabetic group, the association with non-CHD mortality was significant only for LF variance. In contrast, the risk of incident CHD in diabetics was significant (excess risk of approximately 50%) for both of the frequency-domain variables and for two of the time-domain variables.

The relative risks reported in both ARIC studies were adjusted for a variety of clinical and demographic variables, as noted in Table 4A.7. The first report also reveals that the HR differed considerably between the tertiles of the HRV variables: for instance for SDNN, it was 74 cpm in the lowest tertile, 67 cpm in the middle tertile, and 63 cpm in the highest tertile ($p < 0.001$). In the second study but not in the first study, the adjustment for HR was included among the adjusted covariates. Risk analysis for HR in the first study indicated that with the adjustment for age, race and gender, HR had a significant association with all-cause and CVD mortality. With the adjustment including all other clinical and demographic factors, HR retained a significant association with all-cause mortality (HR 1.82 [1.29, 2.57]). This result again suggests that HR may contain significant independent risk of all-cause mortality. It is unlikely, however, that the difference in the HR adjustment would explain the main differences in the observed risks in these two ARIC reports.

4A.5.2.2 The Turku Health Survey

The risk data in the third report summarized in Table 4A.7 come from an elderly population health survey in the city of Turku, Finland.[64] The study established the power-law regression slope (β) of the log–log plot of the power density function versus frequency as the most powerful single predictor of mortality. The investigators performed a thorough analysis to sort out HRV variables that are truly independent predictors of mortality. The study group was extracted from a health survey population of elderly residents of the city as a random sample of 347 of 480 (participation rate 72%) men and women ≥ 65 years of age. Excluded were 22 subjects with arrhythmias (atrial fibrillation, sick sinus syndrome) or artifacts in the 24-hour Holter recording. Thus, the final sample was 325 subjects. Ten-year mortality follow-up was performed, and the mortality endpoints used for risk analysis were all-cause, cardiac and cerebrovascular mortality. The mortality rate in the study group was high, 53%.

The power-law regression slope $\beta < -1.5$ separated relatively well those who did and did not die. Comparing survivors and those who had died, slope β, lnVLF, lnLF and SDNN differed significantly between the groups (lnULF and lnHF power were not significantly different, neither was the

HR RR interval). The slope β was the best single univariate predictor of mortality. For all-cause mortality, the odds ratio was 7.9 (3.7, 17.0), $p < 0.0001$. Of special interest was the independent predictive value of HRV variables when entered into multivariate risk models. The investigators noted that correlations between VLF, LF values and SDNN were relatively high ($r > 0.7$ for all) but substantially lower between β and SDNN ($r = 0.16$), VLF ($r = 0.37$), or LF ($r = 0.34$). The latter set was selected for stepwise proportional hazards analysis to evaluate independent significant predictors of mortality. With adjustment for age and sex, the power-law slope β and SDNN were both independent predictors of all-cause mortality, cardiac mortality, and the power-law slope also of cerebrovascular mortality. The occurrence of frequent ventricular ectopics ($\geq 10/h$) was also a significant predictor of cardiac mortality (VLF and LF power were not significant predictors of mortality).

As shown in Table 4A.7, when all factors (clinical, laboratory, and Holter variables) that had a

significant association with mortality in univariate analysis were included in the model, the power-law slope β remained the only significant independent predictor of mortality. In addition, the history of chronic heart failure remained a significant predictor of all-cause and cardiac mortality, and the history of CVD a predictor of cerebrovascular mortality. In the final full model, the relative risk for the slope β was 2.05 (1.40, 2.99) ($p = 0.0002$) for cardiac mortality and 1.74 (1.42, 2.13) ($p < 0.001$) for all-cause mortality. The power-law slope appears to be a potentially attractive indicator of excess mortality risk in older segments of the general population. This is evident particularly considering the high prevalence of abnormal findings using the dichotomized slope value.

Regrettably, prevalence data are commonly omitted in risk evaluation reports. Even high relative risks reported may have little meaning from an epidemiological point of view (prevention) if the HRV variable identifies just a small fraction of high risk subjects.

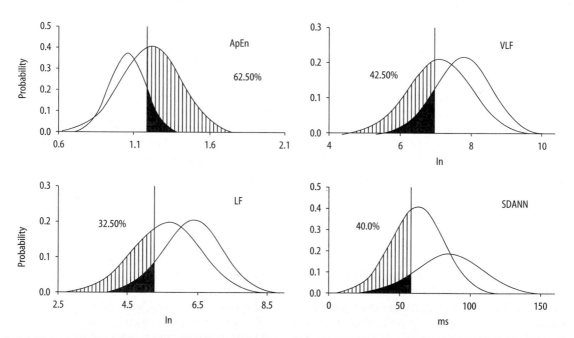

FIGURE 4A.3 Distribution of the values of approximate entropy (*ApEn*), very low frequency power (*lnVLF*), low frequency power (*lnLF*) and SDNN in 40 post-MI patients and age-matched healthy subjects. The vertical line identifies the 90th percentile value of the distribution (probability density function) in healthy subjects. ApEn discriminated over 60% of the MI group compared to approximately 40% by lnVLF and SDNN and slightly over 30% by lnLF power. (Source: Mäkikallio et al.[75] J Am Coll Cardiol 1996;28: 1005–11. Copyright © 1996 The American College of Cardiology Foundation. Reproduced with permission.)

The power-law slope appears to be a potentially unique independent predictor of mortality. This variable should be included in future studies on ECG risk evaluation.

4A.5.2.3 The Zutphen Study

The Zutphen Study in a male cohort evaluated SDNN from the standard 12-lead ECG.[65] The study groups consisted of two cohorts: middle-aged men aged 40–60 years with 25 years of follow-up; and 885 men aged 65–85 years with a 5-year follow-up. The relative risk of total mortality in middle-aged men with SDNN <20 ms compared with men with SDNN 20–39 ms was 2.1 (1.4, 3.0). The trend towards excess risk did not reach a significant level in the older men. Of interest was the observation that noncoronary causes of death contributed substantially to the increased total mortality risk. The association of reduced HRV with CHD mortality and sudden death was less consistent.

4A.5.3 Reduced Heart Rate Variability and Mortality Risk in Survivors of Acute Myocardial Infarction

The interest in HRV reduction as a marker of adverse cardiac events escalated after the 1987 report by Kleiger et al. demonstrated that it was associated with increased mortality after acute MI.[66] The investigators evaluated mortality risk in a 31-month follow-up of 808 survivors of acute MI. Patients with SDNN >100 ms from 24-hour Holter ECG recorded 11 days after the onset of the acute phase had a 5.3-fold excess mortality risk compared to patients with SDNN <50 ms after adjustment for other Holter features and demographic and clinical characteristics including left ventricular ejection fraction.

Time-domain measures such as SDNN and frequency-domain components of HRV have been shown in numerous studies to predict mortality risk when measured in the early post-infarction period. Subgroup analyses from some studies have suggested that it may be possible to distinguish even between subgroups of high risk post-MI patients more likely to experience arrhythmic vs nonarrhythmic death using multiple prediction variables.

Hartikainen et al. investigated associations of HRV, ventricular ectopic complexes, QRS prolongation in signal-averaged ECG and left ventricular ejection fraction with arrhythmic and nonarrhythmic death in 575 survivors of acute MI.[67] There were 47 cardiac deaths (29 arrhythmic, 18 nonarrhythmic) during the follow-up period of up to 2 years. In univariate analysis, all four variables were significantly associated with cardiac death and with the exception of left ventricular ejection fraction, also with arrhythmic death. In multivariate analysis, depressed HRV index, ventricular ectopic complexes ($p < 0.001$) and low ejection fraction ($p < 0.01$) were associated with nonarrhythmic death, and depressed HRV index ($p < 0.001$) and runs of ventricular ectopic complexes ($p < 0.05$) with arrhythmic death. Subcategories of variables in these small subgroups identified patients predominantly at risk of arrhythmic or nonarrhythmic death. Such observations from subgroup analyses need validation in other independent studies.

4A.5.3.1 Frequency-domain HRV Measures and Mortality in Acute MI Survivors

Bigger et al. evaluated mortality risk for 24-hour frequency-domain HRV variables in 331 patients from the Cardiac Arrhythmia Pilot Study (CAPS) who had survived for 1 year after acute MI.[68] None of the patients was on antiarrhythmic drugs at the onset of the follow-up. The investigators used cutpoints for RR variability derived from the Multicenter Post-Infarction Program (MPIP), and they also derived dichotomized cutpoints optimized to produce strongest association with mortality. The average follow-up was 788 days. In univariate analyses, each RR interval variability measure was strongly associated with mortality. The prevalence of RR variability values below the cutpoints was approximately 20%, lower for HF power. For optimized cutpoints, relative risks ranged from 3.4 to 5.6, shown in Table 4A.8. The LF/HF power ratio was a weaker but still significant predictor of mortality (RR 2.5, $p < 0.01$). The univariate relative risks were slightly lower when the original cutpoints were used. However, the prevalence of abnormal RR variability below the cutpoint values was substantially lower for MPIP cutpoints (Table 4A.8).

TABLE 4A.8 Univariate estimates of mortality risk associated with frequency-domain measures of heart rate variability for two sets of thresholds in 331 patients with 24-hour Holter recordings 1 year after acute myocardial infarction.

	ULF	VLF	LF	HF
Optimal cutpoint				
Threshold (ms^2)	<5,000	<600	<120	<35
Prevalence (%)	20.2	22.1	19.3	14.5
Relative risk	3.4	5.6	5.6	3.6
p	<0.001	<0.001	<0.001	<0.001
MPIP cutpoints				
Threshold (ms^2)	<1,600	<180	<35	<20
Prevalence (%)	3.0	5.1	4.2	5.4
Relative risk	5.2	4.1	4.5	2.4
p	<0.01	<0.01	<0.01	ns

MPIP Multicenter Post-Infarction Program, *ULF* ultra low frequency power, *VLF* very low frequency power, *LF* low frequency power, *HF* high frequency power. Source: Bigger et al.[68] J Am Coll Cardiol 1993;21:729–36. © 1993 The American College of Cardiology. Reproduced with permission.

The sample of post-MI patients in the above study had a relatively high prevalence of other post-infarction risk predictors, associated with a significant mortality. Of note was the 30% incidence of congestive heart failure during the first post-infarction year, with a relative risk of 4.2 (p < 0.001), and the 24% prevalence of nonsustained ventricular tachycardia, with a relative risk of 2.7 (p < 0.01). With seven covariates (age, congestive heart failure, left ventricular ejection fraction and New York Heart Association functional class, rales during the coronary care unit stay, and two ventricular arrhythmia variables) used simultaneously with each single RR variability measure in Cox regression model, several RR variability measures were no longer significant predictors of mortality. The variables that still retained a significant, strong association with mortality were VLF power (RR 4.4, p < 0.01) and LF power (RR 3.8, p < 0.01).

Many reports from observational studies on mortality risk in post-MI patients for various HRV measures have been published. Only a few have been validated in larger studies. Some of the other reports by Bigger et al. are examined here in some detail because they come from larger validation studies and provide examples of careful, comprehensive analyses of the diverse aspects of the relationships involved.

Bigger et al. evaluated mortality risk for frequency-domain measures of RR variability (appropriately denoted by the authors as heart period variability [HPV] rather than HRV) in a larger group of MI patients (n = 715) with 24-hour Holter recordings obtained 2 weeks after acute MI.[69] All patients in the study were <70 years old. As in other studies, each frequency-domain RR variability measure had a moderately strong or strong univariate association with all-cause, cardiac, and arrhythmic death. With dichotomized cutpoints selected to maximize the hazards ratio, the prevalence of low RR variation (proportion of patients below cutpoint) ranged from 10 to 15%. Relative risks were strong for each RR variability measure for all-cause, cardiac, and arrhythmic death. For all-cause deaths the unadjusted relative risks were 4.4 for ULF power, 4.3 for VLF power, and 3.3 for LF power (p < 0.001 for all). The relative risk was also strong for total power (4.1, p < 0.001). The relative risk was significant but weaker for HF power (2.5, p < 0.05).

With the adjustment for five known clinical risk factors (age, left ventricular ejection fraction, New York Heart Association functional class, rales during the coronary care unit stay, and arrhythmias detected in 24-hour Holter), total, ULF and VLF power each retained a significant association with mortality, with relative risk ranging from 2.1 to 2.3 (p < 0.05).

In an attempt to identify high risk subgroups using combinations of risk factors and RR variability measures, the performance of the combinations was compared using their sensitivity and specificity for detecting total deaths. Very low frequency power alone had a sensitivity of 30% at a specificity of 92%, and ULF power alone, a sensitivity of 28% at a specificity of 93%. Ultra low frequency power in combination with VLF power had a 20% sensitivity at a specificity of 96%. At the same level of specificity, ejection fraction in combination with either ULF or LF power had a sensitivity for identification of deaths that was similar to the ULF/LF combination. Thus, ULF power <1,600 ms^2 combined with LF power <35 ms^2 in their 24-hour Holter recording 2 weeks after MI identified a 5.7% subgroup of these post-MI patients aged <70 years who had a mortality risk of 48% in 2.5 years.

Bigger et al. also evaluated in the above group of 715 patients the predictive value of short-term (2–15 min) RR variability measures.[27] The investigators again used optimal cutpoints (to provide the greatest difference in mortality rates for variables obtained from 24-hour recordings) and evaluated mortality risk during 2- to 4-year follow-up. The unadjusted relative risks differed relatively little between various mortality endpoints, or between 15-min daytime segments and 24-hour recordings. For all-cause mortality, the relative risk for HF was 2.3, for VLF 2.4, and for LF 3.5 ($p < 0.001$ for all), and they were approximately within the same range for 24-hour recordings.

Baroreflex sensitivity assessment is another clinical test that may enhance the prognostic value of HRV. The Autonomic Tone and Reflexes After Myocardial Infarction investigators reported results from this multicenter prospective study on 1,284 patients with recent MI (<1 month).[70] The primary endpoint was cardiac mortality during 21-month follow-up. Cardiac mortality was 17% for the combination of low SDNN (<70 ms) and reduced baroreceptor sensitivity to intravenous phenylephrine (<3.0 ms per mmHg) compared to 2% when both HRV and baroreceptor sensitivity were well preserved (SDNN >105 ms and baroreceptor sensitivity >6.1 ms per mmHg).

Therapeutic treatment of the acute as well as the post-acute phase of MI has evolved considerably since the early 1980s with thrombolytic therapy, revascularization, angiotensin-converting enzyme inhibitors, and β-blocking therapy. The question coming up frequently is whether the results from HRV studies performed in earlier periods, particularly those before optimal and more widespread use of β-blockers, are still valid.[71]

4A.5.4 The Importance of Advanced Dynamic HRV Analysis

The research group of Huikuri with their collaborators has performed comprehensive evaluations of HRV measures and mortality in survivors of acute MI, including in patients receiving optimal β-blocker medication.[31,72–75] These studies have also pointed out the prognostic importance of more advanced dynamic RR variability measures such as the short-term scaling component.

In the report of Tapanainen,[72] the prognostic significance of SDNN and several spectral and fractal HRV parameters was evaluated in patients from a prospective cardioverter-defibrillator pilot study of three clinical centers involving 697 out of 806 consecutive patients who survived acute MI and who had satisfactory Holter recordings. Both unedited (removing only artifacts) and edited RR interval series (including only sinus complexes) were used for detrended fractal analysis.

Optimal cutpoints for HRV parameters that maximized relative risk for all-cause mortality were used in risk evaluation. In univariate analyses, all RR variability measures were significant predictors of all-cause mortality, with relative risks ranging from 2.37 for SDNN and lnULF power to as high as 5.05 for unedited short-term scaling exponent α1 ($p \leq 0.001$ for all). In multivariate models with adjustment for wall motion abnormalities and other clinical variables, the short-term scaling exponent α1 remained as the most powerful predictor, with relative risk 3.90 (2.03, 7.49, $p < 0.001$). The relative risks for lnULF, lnVLF and lnLF power were all over twofold but statistically nonsignificant ($p < 0.05$ for each). Interestingly, the LF/HF ratio was an almost equally strong multivariate predictor as the short-term scaling exponent α1, with relative risk 3.49 (1.76, 6.90, $p < 0.001$). In previous studies before β-blocker medication was widely used, frequency-domain variables in lower frequency bands were generally reported to be more important mortality risk predictors than LF/HF ratio. Mortality risk associated with the power-law regression slope demonstrated the potential of nonlinear HRV analysis in risk prediction in post-MI patients.

The report by Mäkikallio et al. illuminates the potential value of another HRV measure from nonlinear analysis, the approximate entropy (ApEn).[75] The investigators compared spectral composition and ApEn derived from a group of 40 consecutive Q wave MI patients >1 month after acute MI referred for angiography because of angina pectoris with an age-matched group of healthy subjects. Patients with diabetes or atrial fibrillation were excluded, and cardioactive drugs (except nitroglycerin) withdrawn. Distributions of ApEn, lnVLF, lnLF and SDNN values (probability density functions) of the two groups, reproduced in Figure 4A.3, show that at a comparable level of the threshold in the healthy group (90th percentile), ApEn discriminated 62.5% of the MI patients compared to 42.5% by lnVLF, 40.0% by SDNN and 32.5% by lnLF. The authors concluded that ApEn can detect increased intrinsic randomness or unpredictability of RR interval dynamics in post-MI patients, an abnormality not easily detected by common HRV statistics. It remains to be seen how ApEn will compare with the slope (β) of the power-law regression line as an independent predictor of risk in post-MI patients and other abnormal conditions.

As mentioned at the beginning of this chapter, more details about the interpretation and procedures used in analysis of HRV data are summarized in Chapter 4B.

References

1. Rautaharju PM, Zhou SH, Calhoun HP, Spodick DH. Distribution of sinus heart rates in community-based populations. In: Macfarlane PW, Rautaharju P (eds). Electrocardiology '93. XXth International Congress on Electrocardiology, 1993. Singapore: World Scientific Publishing Co. Pte. Ltd, 1994, pp 265–8.

2. Palatini P. Need for a revision of the normal limits of resting heart rate. Hypertension 1999;33:622–5.

3. Boyett MR, Jewell BR. Analysis of the effects of changes in rate and rhythm upon electrical activity in the heart. Prog Biophys Molec Biol 1980;36: 1–52.

4. Cohen I, Giles WR, Noble D. Cellular basis for the T wave of the electrocardiogram. Nature 1976;262: 657–61.

5. Antzelovitch C, Zygmunt AC, Dumaine R. Electrophysiology and pharmacology of ventricular repolarization. In: Gussak I, Antzelovitch C (eds). Cardiac Repolarization. Bridging Basic and Clinical Science. Totowa, New Jersey: Humana Press, 2003, pp 63–89.

6. Nobel D, Cohen I. The interpretation of the T wave of the electrocardiogram. Cardiovasc Res 1978;12: 13–27.

7. Azbel MY. Universal biological scaling and mortality. Proc Natl Acad Sci USA 1994;91:12453–7.

8. Levin HJ. Rest heart rate and life expectancy. J Am Coll Cardiol 1997;30:1104–6.

9. Medalie JH, Kahn HA, Neufeld HN. Five-year myocardial infarction incidence. II. Associations of single variables to age and birthplace. J Chron Dis 1973;26:329–49.

10. Schroll M, Hangerup LM. Risk factors of myocardial infarction and death in men aged 50 at entry. A ten-year prospective study from the Glostrup Population Studies. Dan Med Bull 1977;24:252–5.

11. Eriksen J, Rodahl K. Resting heart rate in apparently healthy middle-aged men. Eur J Appl Physiol 1979;42:61–9.

12. Dyer AR, Persky V, Stamler J et al. Heart rate as a prognostic factor for coronary heart disease and mortality: findings in three Chicago epidemiological studies. Am J Epidemiol 1980;112:736–49.

13. Kannel WB, Kannel C, Paffenbarger RS, Cupples LA. Heart rate and cardiovascular mortality: The Framingham Study. Am Heart J 1987;113: 1489–94.

14. Gillum RF, Makuc DM, Feldman JJ. Pulse rate, coronary heart disease, and death: the NHANES I Epidemiologic Follow-Up Study. Am Heart J 1991; 121:172–7.

15. Reunanen A, Karjalainen J, Ristola P et al. Heart rate and mortality. J Intern Med 2000;247:231–9.

16. Benetos A, Rudnichi A, Thomas F et al. Influence of heart rate on mortality in a French population: role of age, gender, and blood pressure. Hypertension 1999;33:44–52.

17. Greenland P, Daviglus ML, Dyer AR et al. Resting heart rate is a risk factor for cardiovascular and noncardiovascular mortality: the Chicago Heart Association Detection Project in Industry. Am J Epidemiol 1999;149:853–62.

18. Palatini P, Thijs L, Staessen JA et al. Predictive value of clinic and ambulatory heart rate for mortality in elderly subjects with systolic hypertension. Arch Intern Med 2002;162:2313–21.

19. Fujiura Y, Adachi H, Tsuruta M et al. Heart rate and mortality in a Japanese general population: an 18-year follow-up study. J Clin Epidemiol 2001;54:495–500.

20. Seccareccia F, Pannozzo F, Dima F et al. Heart rate as a predictor of mortality: the MATISS project. Am J Public Health 2001;91:1258–63.

21. Zuanetti G, Mantini L, Hernandez-Bernal F et al. Relevance of heart rate as a prognostic factor in patients with acute myocardial infarction: insights from the GISSI-2 study. Eur Heart J 1998:19(Suppl F):F19-F26.

22. Perski A, Olsson G, Landou C et al. Minimum heart rate and coronary atherosclerosis: independent relations to global severity and rate of progression of angiographic lesions in men with myocardial infarction at a young age. Am Heart J 1992; 123:609–16.

23. Chaitman BR. Abnormal heart rate responses to exercise predict increased long-term mortality

regardless of coronary disease extent: the question why? J Am Coll Cardiol 2003;42:839–41.

24. Cole CR, Blackstone EH, Pashkow F et al. Heart-rate recovery immediately after exercise as a predictor of mortality. N Engl J Med 1999;341: 1351–7.

25. Cole CR, Foody JM, Blackstone EH, Lauer MS. Heart rate recovery after submaximal exercise testing as a predictor of mortality in a cardiovascularly healthy cohort. Ann Intern Med 2000;132:552–5.

26. Vivekananthan DP, Blackstone EH, Pothier CE et al. Heart rate recovery after exercise is a predictor of mortality, independent of the angiographic severity of coronary disease. J Am Coll Cardiol 2003;42:831–8.

27. Bigger JT, Fleiss JL, Rolnitzky LM, Steinman RC. The ability of several short-term measures of RR variability to predict mortality after myocardial infarction. Circulation 1993;88:927–34.

28. Bigger JT Jr, Fleiss JL, Steinman RC et al. Correlations among time and frequency-domain measures of heart period variability two weeks after acute myocardial infarction. Am J Cardiol 1992;69: 891–8.

29. Umetani K, Singer DH, McCraty R, Atkinson M. Twenty-four hour time domain heart rate variability and heart rate: relations to age and gender over nine decades. J Am Coll Cardiol 1998;31:593–601.

30. Tsuji H, Venditti FJ, Manders ES et al. Determinants of heart rate variability. J Am Coll Cardiol 1996;28:1539–46.

31. Pikkujämsä S. Heart rate variability and baroreflex sensitivity in subjects without heart disease. MD thesis, University of Oulu, Finland. Oulu University Library, 1999.

32. Abdel-Rahman AR, Merrill RH, Wooles WR. Gender-related differences in the baroreceptor reflex control of heart rate in normotensive humans. J Appl Physiol 1994;77:606–13.

33. Liao D, Barnes RW, Chambless LE et al. Age, race, and sex differences in autonomic cardiac function measured by spectral analysis of heart rate variability – the ARIC study. Atherosclerosis Risk in Communities. Am J Cardiol 1995;76:906–12.

34. Huikuri HV, Pikkujämsä SM, Airaksinen KEJ et al. Sex-related differences in autonomic modulation of heart rate in middle-aged subjects. Circulation 1996;94:122–5.

35. Huikuri HV, Kessler KM, Terracall E et al. Reproducibility and circadian rhythm of heart rate variability in healthy subjects. Am J Cardiol 1990;65:391–3.

36. Niemelä MJ, Airaksinen KEJ, Huikuri HV. Effect of beta-blockade on heart rate variability in patients with coronary artery disease. J Am Coll Cardiol 1994;23:1370–7.

37. Kamath MV, Fallen E. Diurnal variation of neurocardiac rhythms in acute myocardial infarction. Am J Cardiol 1991;68:155–60.

38. Cook JR, Bigger JT Jr, Kleiger RE et al. Effect of atenolol and diltiazem on heart period variability in normal persons. J Am Coll Cardiol 1991;17: 480–4.

39. Beta-Blocker Heart Attack Research Group. A randomized trial of propranolol in patients with acute myocardial infarction. JAMA 1982;247: 1707–14.

40. Lampert R, Ickovics JR, Viscoli CJ et al. Effects of propranolol on recovery of heart rate variability following acute myocardial infarction and relation to outcome in the Beta-Blocker Heart Attack Trial. Am J Cardiol 2003;91:137–42.

41. Bigger JT, Fleiss SL, Steinman RC et al. RR variability in healthy, middle-aged persons compared with patients with chronic coronary heart disease or recent acute myocardial infarction. Circulation 1995;91:1936–43.

42. Bigger JT Jr, Fleiss JL, Rolnitzky LM. Time course of recovery of heart period variability after myocardial infarction. J Am Coll Cardiol 1991;18:1643–9.

43. Casolo GC, Stroder P, Signorini C et al. Heart rate variability during the acute phase of myocardial infarction. Circulation 1992;85:2073–9.

44. Lombardi F, Sandrone G, Pernpruder S et al. Heart rate variability as an index of sympathovagal interaction after acute myocardial infarction. Am J Cardiol 1987;60:1239–45.

45. Liao D, Evans GW, Chambless LE et al. Population-based study of heart rate variability and prevalent myocardial infarction. The Atherosclerosis Risk in Communities Study. J Electrocardiol 1996;29: 189–98.

46. Malik M, Farrelli T, Camm AJ. Circadian rhythm of heart rate variability after acute myocardial infarction and its influence on the prognostic value of heart rate variability. Am J Cardiol 1990;66: 1049–54.

47. Huikuri HV, Niemelä MJ, Ojala S et al. Circadian rhythm of frequency domain measures of heart rate variability in healthy subjects and patients with coronary artery disease: effects of arousal and upright posture. Circulation 1994;90:121–6.

48. Lombardi F, Sandrone G, Mortara A et al. Circadian variation of spectral indices of heart rate variability after myocardial infarction. Am Heart J 1992;123: 1521–9.

49. Vanoli E, Adamson PB, Ba-Lin et al. Heart rate variability during specific sleep stages. A comparison

of healthy subjects with patients after myocardial infarction. Circulation 1995;91:1918–22.

50. Task Force of the European Society of Cardiology and the North American Society of Pacing and Electrophysiology. Heart rate variability. Standards of measurement, physiological interpretation, and clinical use. Circulation 1996;93:1043–65.

51. Langewitz W, Ruddel H, Schachinger H. Reduced parasympathetic cardiac control in patients with hypertension at rest and under mental stress. Am Heart J 1994;127:122–8.

52. Guzzetti S, Dassi S, Pecis M et al. Altered pattern of circadian neural control of heart period in mild hypertension. J Hypertens 1991;9:831–8.

53. Kienzle MG, Ferguson DW, Birkett CL et al. Clinical hemodynamic and sympathetic neural correlates of heart rate variability in congestive heart failure. Am J Cardiol 1992;69:482–5.

54. Casolo G, Balli E, Taddei T et al. Decreased spontaneous heart rate variability in congestive heart failure. Am J Cardiol 1989;64:1162–7.

55. Saul JP, Arai Y, Berger RD et al. Assessment of autonomic regulation in chronic congestive heart failure by the heart rate spectral analysis. Am J Cardiol 1988;61:1292–9.

56. Binkley PF, Nunziata E, Haas GJ et al. Parasympathetic withdrawal is an integral component of autonomic imbalance in congestive heart failure: demonstration in human subjects and verification in a paced canine model of ventricular failure. J Am Coll Cardiol 1991;18:464–2.

57. Townend JN, West JN, Davies MK et al. Effect of quinapril on blood pressure and heart rate in congestive heart failure. Am J Cardiol 1992;69:1587–90.

58. Tsuji H, Larson MG, Venditti FJ et al. Impact of reduced heart rate variability on risk for cardiac events. Circulation 1996;94:2850–5.

59. Tsuji H, Venditti FJ, Manders ES et al. Reduced heart rate variability and mortality risk in an elderly cohort. The Framingham Study. Circulation 1994; 90:878–83.

60. Liao D, Cai J, Rosamond WD et al. Cardiac autonomic function and incident coronary heart disease: a population-based case-cohort study. The ARIC Study. Am J Epidemiol 1997;145:696–706.

61. de Bruyne MC, Kors JA, Hoes AW et al. Both decreased and increased heart rate variability on the standard 10-second electrocardiogram predict cardiac mortality in the elderly: the Rotterdam Study. Am J Epidemiol 1999;15:1282–8.

62. Dekker JM, Crow RS, Folsom AR et al. Low heart rate variability in a 2-minute rhythm strip predicts risk of coronary heart disease and mortality from several causes: the ARIC Study. Atherosclerosis Risk in Communities. Circulation 2000;102: 1239–44.

63. Liao D, Carnethon M, Evans GW et al. Lower heart rate variability is associated with the development of coronary heart disease in individuals with diabetes: the Atherosclerosis Risk in Communities (ARIC) study. Diabetes 2002;51:3524–31.

64. Huikuri HV, Mäkikallio TH, Airaksinen KEJ et al. Power-law relationship of heart rate variability as a predictor of mortality in the elderly. Circulation 1998;97:2031–6.

65. Dekker JM, Schouten EG, Klootwijk P et al. Heart rate variability from short electrocardiographic recordings predicts mortality from all causes in middle-aged and elderly men. The Zutphen Study. Am J Epidemiol 1997;145:899–908.

66. Kleiger RE, Miller JP, Bigger JT Jr, Moss AJ. Decreased heart rate variability and its association with increased mortality after acute myocardial infarction. Am J Cardiol 1987;59:256–62

67. Hartikainen J, Malik M, Staunton A et al. Distinction between arrhythmic and nonarrhythmic death after acute myocardial infarction based on heart rate variability, signal-averaged electrocardiogram, ventricular arrhythmias and left ventricular ejection fraction. J Am Coll Cardiol 1996;28:296–304.

68. Bigger JT Jr, Fleiss JL et al. Frequency domain measures of heart period variability to assess risk late after myocardial infarction. J Am Coll Cardiol 1993;21:729–36.

69. Bigger JT Jr, Fleiss JL, Steinman RC et al. Frequency domain measures of heart period variability and mortality after myocardial infarction. Circulation 1992;85:164–71.

70. La Rovere M, Bigger J Jr, Marcus F et al. Baroreflex sensitivity and heart rate variability in prediction of total cardiac mortality after myocardial infarction. ATRAMI (Autonomic Tone and Reflexes After Myocardial Infarction) investigators. Lancet 1998; 351:478–84.

71. Zuanetti G, Neilson JMM, Latini R et al. Prognostic significance of heart rate variability in post–myocardial infarction patients in the fibrinolytic era. Circulation 1996;94:432–6.

72. Tapanainen JM, Bloch Thomsen PE, Køber L et al. Fractal analysis of heart rate variability and mortality after an acute myocardial infarction. Am J Cardiol 2002;90:347–52.

73. Tapanainen J. Non-invasive predictors of mortality after acute myocardial infarction. MD Thesis, University of Oulu, Finland, 2003.

74. Tapanainen JM, Still AM, Airaksinen KEJ, Huikuri HV. Prognostic significance of risk stratifiers of mortality, including T wave alternans, after acute myocardial infarction: results of a prospective follow-up study. J Cardiovasc Electrophysiol 2001; 12:645–53.

75. Mäkikallio TH, Seppänen T, Niemelä M et al. Abnormalities in beat to beat complexity of heart rate dynamics in patients with a previous myocardial infarction. J Am Coll Cardiol 1996;28: 1005–11.

4B
Methodological Considerations in Heart Rate Variability Analysis

Heart rate variability (HRV) analysis was introduced in the early 1960s with the advent of special purpose computers suitable for collecting RR interval histograms and producing autocorrelation functions. The initial impetus came from the report of Hon and Lee, who used fetal electrocardiography to demonstrate a reduced HRV in fetal distress.[1] Early reports of Sayers and Hyndman from the Imperial College[2,3] popularized HRV analysis among the medical engineering profession, and ever since the field has been a playground of medical engineers and other professionals interested in time series analysis. RR intervals produce seemingly endless series of point processes in various physiological and clinical conditions, and they provide an ideal realm for statistical modeling.

The report by the Task Force of the European Society of Cardiology and the North American Society of Pacing and Electrophysiology in 1996 is a comprehensive review of HRV analysis methodology, with extensive references and proposals for nonrestrictive standardization.[4] The source signal for HRV analysis is a point process generated from the RR intervals, or NN intervals of normally conducted QRS complexes, excluding ventricular and supraventricular premature and nonpremature ectopic complexes and artifacts. The interval histogram (tachogram) of this point process is sampled at nonequal time intervals. The length of the RR interval preceding sample i (RR_{i-1}) is assigned to sample i. This histogram is constructed by dividing the x axis, the length of the RR interval, into finite class intervals with equal time increments (such as 8 ms) and counting the number of RR intervals falling into each class interval. When normalized with respect to the total number of intervals included in the display, the histogram is an approximation to the probability density function of RR interval distribution. The choice of the time increments, the class interval, depends on the total number of counts of the intervals analyzed and the sampling rate. The minimum increment is determined by the sampling rate. For instance, with the sampling rate of 128 samples per second, which many older Holter scanners used, the minimum increment is closest to 8 ms ($1/128 = 7.81$). The total recording interval and the number of counts has to be high enough to produce a fairly smooth distribution of the counts.

The triangular index (TIN) is the baseline width of the triangular approximation of the normalized NN histogram (Figure 4B.1). If unedited or inadequately edited RR series are used, without removing intervals preceding and following ectopic complexes and artifacts, various extrapolation or more sophisticated algorithms[4] must be used to exclude them.

In spectral analysis, it is preferable to use some interpolation scheme to transform the irregularly sampled point process into a continuous function of time whereby the RR interval function is sampled at equal time intervals. The RR interval histogram is transformed to "instantaneous HR" and spectral analysis is then performed (Figure 4B.2). As pointed out by Taylor and Lipsitz, analysis of HR function and RR interval function may not yield identical results because one is a nonlinear, inverse function of the other.[5] Strictly

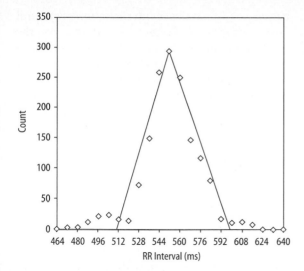

FIGURE 4B.1 Triangular index obtained as a triangular approximation to RR interval histogram normalized to the total count of normally conducted complexes.

speaking, instantaneous HR does not exist but instantaneous RR interval does. It would definitely be preferable to distinguish between HRV and RR variability and use an acronym RRV for the latter. HRV is so deeply ingrained in medical use that any other acronym for it would be ignored.

The Task Force cited above proposed the following definitions, already used by many investigators, for high and low frequency components of HRV in spectral analysis:

- Total power to be determined in the frequency range 0.04–0.4 Hz.
- High frequency (HF) component from 0.15 Hz to 0.4 Hz.
- Low frequency (LF) component from 0.04 Hz to 0.15 Hz.

The omission of frequency components below 0.04 Hz from total power estimation is a rather pragmatic approach but is justifiable if the main goal is to evaluate autonomic system balance.[6] Also, there are a number of problems in the estimation of the spectral components below the LF range and in the interpretation of their physiological mechanisms. The HF and LF power is calculated by integrating the spectral density function in the frequency windows specified. It is noted that the total power is the total variance of the periodic components from 0.04 Hz to 0.4 Hz. Normalized HF and LF components are obtained by expressing them as the fraction of total power in this frequency band.

The LF/HF ratio is generally used as an expression for sympathovagal balance.[7-9] Although at

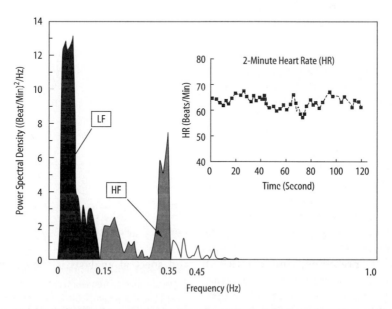

FIGURE 4B.2 Power spectral density function from a 2-min sequence of normally conducted complexes first transformed into an "instantaneous" heart rate function and then sampled at equally spaced time points (constant time increments).

times criticized,[10] it has received prominent attention in medical literature on HRV and risk assessment although in general it is not the best predictor of excess risk of adverse events.

The Task Force suggests that the very low frequency (VLF) below 0.04 Hz be omitted from spectral analysis of short-term recordings in part because it is affected by trend removal algorithms and because of the uncertainty of its origins and physiological background. Very low frequency components have been attributed to oscillations due to thermoregulation or the modulation of the tone of the peripheral arterial system and arterial pressure by the renin–angiotensin–aldosterone system. A 1998 report by Taylor et al. on a series of controlled experimental procedures on healthy young adults revealed that although VLF oscillations are influenced by the renin system, they are primarily under the control of the parasympathetic system: the blockade by atropine decreased VLF variability by 92%.[11]

Spectral analysis of HRV looks deceptively simple. There are numerous considerations, however, that are critical for proper use of these methods and proper understanding of the meaning of the measures obtained, as pointed out by the Task Force report. These include careful editing for validation of the QRS typing, correct identification of ectopic or premature complexes, proper interpolation in case of rejected QRS complexes or rejection of noisy segments of the recording, accurate detection of the fiducial time points derived from the QRS complexes with reliable algorithms and with adequate sampling rate, etc.

Frequency domain methods used for calculating power spectral density are characterized as parametric and nonparametric methods. Whereas parametric methods are based statistically on various probability models, nonparametric methods do not expect any specific statistical models to describe the characteristics of the sequence or the overall distribution.

Heart rate variability can be quantified using measures derived in frequency as well as in time domain. The interpolated RR function of time sampled at equal intervals is used for analysis, and it is readily amenable for both types of analysis. In general, spectral analysis of HF and LF components is preferably performed using stationary short-term recordings such as 5-min segments

because of difficulties in interpretation of spectral measurements of 24-hour recordings. On the other hand, time domain measures are preferable for analysis of long-term records because they are easier to calculate and interpret. However, both types of analyses have been used in a wide variety of situations.

4B.1 Heart Rate Variability −1/f Model

In power spectral analysis, the variance or the power (P) varies with the spectral frequency (F) as a power function, whereby $P = k*F^{\beta}$, or $\ln P = \ln k + \beta * \ln F$, where β is the exponent of the power function or the slope of the graph of ln spectral power against ln frequency (Figure 4B.3). (It is immaterial whether the axes are on ln or log base 10 scale.)

When $\beta = -1$, the variance decreases by a factor of 10 for frequency decrease by a decade, a characteristic of normal HRV and 1/F noise, in contrast to white (random) noise when $\beta = 0$. The more negative (abnormal) the value of α, the larger the fraction of power in the ultra low frequency (ULF) and LF bands of the power density spectrum. When $\beta = -2$ (the power decreasing

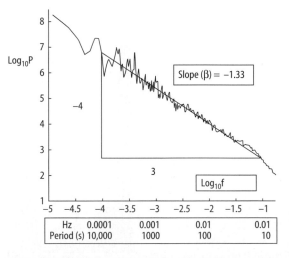

FIGURE 4B.3 Power spectral density function (variance or power [P] versus spectral frequency) on a log–log scale. The slope (negative) of the function is the exponent β of the power spectral density. (Courtesy of Dr Peter P. Domitrovich and Dr Phyllis Stein, Washington University School of Medicine, St Louis, Mo.)

rapidly as an inverse square function of F), the behavior has the characteristics of Brownian motion noise. When $\beta = 0$, all frequencies have equal power densities, representing characteristics of white noise.

Saul et al. investigated these functional relationships in healthy young men and found that the slope of this power relationship to frequency ranged from -0.93 to -1.07, with an average value of -1.02.[12] This 1/f relationship was first reported in 1982 by Kobayashi and Musha.[13] In an extensive 1996 report, Bigger confirmed these observations in a group of 274 healthy middle-aged persons and found the average slope to be -1.06 (SD 0.12).[14] The value of this negative exponent was approximately twice as large, -2.08 (SD 0.22) in 19 patients with heart transplant and it was -1.15 (SD 0.19) in 715 survivors of acute myocardial infarction (MI). These interesting observations reveal a great deal of information relevant to the interpretation of the meaning of spectral analysis data and heart rate variance in general.

A layman's synopsis of the salient features and relationships in spectral analysis of HRV may be summarized as follows:

1. Let V = variance or power in the HR spectrum. V is expressed as the total power in a given frequency band such as HF, LF, VLF and ULF power, or the power/unit frequency (F), which is the value of the spectral density function corresponding to a given value of F.

2. The slope β of lnV versus lnF plot is a parameter that is fundamentally different from the estimates of spectral power in various customary measures of HR power spectrum. The slope reflects the distribution of the power over various frequency bands rather than the magnitude. When $\beta = -1$, the power is inversely proportional to the frequency (or linearly proportional to the cycle length of the frequency of variation).

3. At frequencies corresponding to VLF and ULF bands, the power spectrum has the characteristics of a broad band signal, meaning that no single frequency dominates the power distribution. Total variance increases the wider the band of frequencies included in the observation, i.e. the longer the recording period analyzed.

4. Total power per decade of frequency is constant (for instance comparing power in the decade 10^{-4}–10^{-3} with that in the decade 10^{-3}–10^{-2}) within ULF and VLF regions. The variance of HR with cycle length from 100 (2 min) to 1,000 s (20 min) will be equal to the variance of much slower oscillations with cycle lengths from 1,000 s to 10,000 s (3 h). However, the power density or V/unit F (ms^2/Hz) is ten times higher in the lower frequency decade than that in the higher frequency decade because the higher frequency decade covers ten times more frequencies (higher band width).

5. The steeper the slope β, the more power is distributed in the lower frequency ranges compared to the higher frequency ranges.

6. In heart transplant patients with denervated hearts (unless re-innervation takes place), the exponent approximating $\beta = -2$, the power is inversely proportional approximately to the square of the frequency (or linearly proportional to the square of the cycle length of the variation).

7. In frequency ranges corresponding to LF and HF variations, the lnV versus lnF functional relationship is nonlinear because of the modulation by respiration.

4B.2 Chaotic and Fractal Characteristics of Heart Rate Variability

Nonlinear interacting cardiovascular control systems with long feedback loops acting on the SA node bring another dimension to HRV analysis. Heart rate variability has sudden "bursts" or nonlinear trends, for instance following an ectopic premature complex and other more unpredictable random-looking variations. Diurnal and other very slow periodic variations may appear as slow trends in HRV data. Then there are various kinds of more and less random components in HRV. Application of methodology from chaos theory has enhanced our understanding of the nature of HRV, as succinctly expressed by Bassingthwaighte: "Explaining why we cannot predict exactly is an improvement over not understanding at all".[15]

Chaos is an aperiodic behavior of a given variable of a bounded deterministic system that is unpredictable over a large time scale. Fractile behavior is a special form of chaos. It has "self-similar", scale-invariant structures with intrinsic irregularity characteristics that remain similar when composed by smaller or larger subunits. Fractals do not have a single length scale and the size of fractals cannot be described by ordinary geometric display or terms. The geometric dimension of fractiles is defined by terms like Hausdorff dimension or correlation dimension. Two of the newer nonlinear measures of HRV appear to be of special interest in the assessment of the risk of adverse events associated with HRV: the scaling exponent (α) and the so-called approximate entropy (ApEn).

4B.3 Detrended Fluctuation Analysis and the Scaling Exponent

Detrended fluctuation analysis has the advantage that it is less influenced by nonstationarities than HRV statistics that do not remove local trends in the series. Time series like the RR intervals RR(i) plotted against interval number i are detrended first by generating integrated series I(k) from RR(i) starting from i = 1 to successively increasing values of k: $I(k) = \Sigma[RR(i) - meanRR(i)]$, where the sum is calculated from i = 1 to k with increasing values of k.

The integrated interval series I(k) are divided into boxes of equal length n and each box is detrended by subtracting local trend $I_n(k)$, in order to obtain detrended series D(k) as $D(k) = I(k) - I_n(k)$. The process is repeated for successively increasing numbers of box size n. Subsequently, function F(n) is calculated as a function of box size n: $F(n) = SQR\{(1/N)^*\Sigma[D(k)]^2\}$, where the sum is calculated from k = 1 to N and SQR is square root.

The value of F(n), when plotted against n on a log–log scale, increases with the size parameter n. The slope of the log–log function is the scaling exponent α. The scaling exponent of this function derived from interval series is related to the negative value of the slope of the log–log plot of the power spectral density versus frequency: $\beta = -(2^*\alpha - 1)$.

Thus, when the scaling exponent $\alpha = 1$, $\beta = -1$, for 1/f behavior. Scaling exponent is generally calculated for shorter interval windows with n from 4 to 11 intervals ($\alpha 1$, short-term scaling exponent) and for windows >11 intervals ($\alpha 2$, long-term scaling exponent).

4B.4 Approximate Entropy

Entropy in general is a measure of the order in a system. A highly ordered system is easily predictable, offers no surprises and its information content is low (high entropy). A more disordered system is more complex to encode, its information content is high and the entropy low. As described originally by Pincus in 1991,[16,17] the functional definition of the ApEn is considerably more complex than that for simple time domain HRV parameters, which are mostly based on standard deviations, so the order of the data in the sequence is immaterial. The order of the data in the sequence analyzed is critical for ApEn. There are conditions where these two approaches provide similar information, and there are conditions where the behavior of these two kinds of measures differs.

Approximate entropy is not a magnitude statistic like most HRV variables. It is a measure of regularity or the lack of it. Like power spectral calculations, ApEn is vulnerable when calculated from HR series that are nonstationary, with one or more local trends.[17] Algorithms for ApEn were defined by Pincus,[16,17] and a concise summary can be found in the appendix of the paper by Mäkikallio et al.[18] That paper compares ApEn characteristics of 40 patients with Q wave MI and an age-matched group of 40 healthy subjects. Analysis was performed after carefully editing and removing trends, premature complexes and artifacts. The paper has also an excellent description of the dependence of RR interval data on shuffling the sequence and adding artificial frequency components and noise with quantified characteristics. Key observations are summarized in the following:

1. As expected, Gaussian (white) noise signals produced ApEn values close to 2 (between 1.94 and 2.02), and 1/f-type sequences closer to 1, between 0.8 and 0.85.

2. Shuffling of 1/f-type sequences increased ApEn to >1.9, and shuffling interval sequence data

of MI patients and healthy subjects also substantially increased ApEn values.

3. ApEn values increased when the relative content of VLF power in artificial signals was decreased, and a slight artificial addition of HF power increased ApEn values proportionally.

4. Adding white Gaussian noise to a real RR interval sequence with differing signal to noise ratios had a minor effect of ApEn. Increasing signal to noise ratio by a factor of 2 (from 8 to 16) decreased ApEn <1%.

A variety of aspects of nonlinear and other HRV analysis methods are discussed in the 1996 monograph of Malik and Camm.[19]

References

1. Hon EH, Lee ST. Electronic evaluations of the fetal heart rate patterns preceding fetal death: further observations. Am J Obstet Gynecol 1965:87: 814-26.
2. Sayers BM. Analysis of heart rate variability. Ergonomics 1973;16:17-32.
3. Hyndman B. The role of rhythms in homeostasis. Kybernetik 1974;15:227-36.
4. Task Force of the European Society of Cardiology and the North American Society of Pacing and Electrophysiology. Heart rate variability: standards of measurement, physiological interpretation, and clinical use. Circulation 1996;93:1043-65
5. Taylor JA, Lipsitz LA. Heart rate variability. (Letter to the editor.) Circulation 1997;95:280.
6. Liao D, Cai J, Rosamond WD, Barnes RW, Hutchinson RG, Whitsel EA, Rautaharju P, Heiss G. Cardiac autonomic function and incident coronary heart disease: a population-based case-cohort study. The ARIC Study. Am J Epidemiol 1997;145:696-706.
7. Brovelli M, Baselli G, Cerutti S, Guzzetti S, Liberati D, Lombardi F et al. Computerized analysis for an experimental validation of neurophysiological models of heart rate control. In: Computers in Cardiology. Silver Spring, MD: IEEE Computer Society Press, 1983, pp 205-8.
8. Pomeranz B, Macaulay JB, Caudill MA, Kutz I, Adam D, Gordon D et al. Assessment of autonomic function in humans by heart rate spectral analysis. Am J Physiol 1985;248:H151-3.
9. Pagani M, Lombardi F, Guzzetti S, Rimoldi O, Furlan R, Pizzinelli P et al. Power spectral analysis of heart rate and arterial pressure variabilities as a marker of sympathovagal interaction in man and conscious dog. Circ Res 1986; 58:178-93.
10. Eckberg DL. Sympathovagal balance. A critical appraisal. Circulation 1997;96;3224-32.
11. Taylor JA, Carr DL, Myers CW, Eckberg DL. Mechanisms underlying very-low-frequency RR-interval oscillations in humans. Circulation 1998;98: 547-55.
12. Saul JP, Albrecht P, Berger RD, Cohen RJ. Analysis of long term heart rate variability: methods, 1/f scaling and implications. In: Computers in Cardiology. Silver Spring, MD: IEEE Computer Society Press, 1987, pp 419-22.
13. Kobayashi M, Musha T. 1/f fluctuations of heart beat period. IEEE Trans Biomed Eng 1982;29: 456-7.
14. Bigger JT, Steinman RC, Rolnitzky LM, Fleiss JL, Albrecht P, Cohen RJ. Power law behavior of RR-interval variability in healthy middle-aged persons, patients with recent acute myocardial infarction, and patients with heart transplants. Circulation 1996;93:2142-51.
15. Bassingthwaighte JB. Chaos in cardiac signals. Adv Exp Med Biol 1993;346:207-18.
16. Pincus SM. Approximate entropy as a measure of system complexity. Proc Natl Acad Sci USA 1991; 88:2297-301.
17. Pincus SM, Golberger AL. Physiologic time-series analysis: what does regularity quantify? Am J Physiol 1994;266:H1643-56.
18. Mäkikallio TM, Seppänen T, Niemelä M, Airaksinen KEJ, Tulppo M, Huikuri HV. Abnormalities in beat to beat complexity of heart rate dynamics in patients with a previous myocardial infarction. J Am J Cardiol 1996;28:1005-11.
19. Malik M, Camm AJ (eds). HR Variability. Armonk, New York: Futura, 1996.

5
Supraventricular Dysrhythmias

Synopsis

Significance

Supraventricular dysrhythmias cover a variety of arrhythmic conditions ranging from innocent supraventricular ectopic complexes to re-entrant tachycardias requiring therapeutic action or, at times, more demanding intervention.

Mechanisms

The mechanisms range from abnormal automaticity with ectopic impulse formation to re-entrant circuits involving AV node or atria (atrial fibrillation [AF] and atrial flutter [AFL]). Atrial flutter is an atrial re-entrant arrhythmia where the re-entrant circuit encloses the tricuspid valve ring. Atrial flutter generates flutter waves commonly at approximately 300 cpm. Atrial fibrillation is a high rate atrial tachycardia (>430 cpm) where the atrial excitation pattern is more or less chaotic, with multiple interacting wavelets wandering around zones or islets of refractory tissue in the atria. Sustained AF is the most common chronic arrhythmia that is associated with increased risk of adverse events. The ventricular response rate can be slow, moderate or high depending on the refractory period of the AV node and the strength of the atrial excitation fronts reaching the upper part of the AV node. These factors are amenable to modification by therapeutic action.

Prevalence and Incidence

Atrial flutter is rare below 35 years of age. The prevalence of AFL is known to increase with age and is twice as high in men as in women. The incidence estimate of AFL from a single available large study was approximately 22/100,000 annually. The reported prevalence of AF in community-based populations aged 60 years and older ranges from 2% to 5–6% overall, strongly increasing with age in women but not in men. The reported prevalence ranges from less than 2% for lone AF to over 9% for AF with other comorbid conditions. There is evidence for a significant trend over time in AF prevalence in men (particularly strong for AF associated with myocardial infarction). The prevalence increase over time in women is insignificant. Approximate estimates of annual incidence rate of AF expressed as 1,000 person-years of observation in age group 65–74 range from 10 to less than 20 in men and from 5 to 10 in women, and in age group 75–84 years from 20 to over 40 in men and from 14 to less than 20 in women.

Classification Problems

Atrial fibrillation and AFL are at times difficult to differentiate and many studies have combined these conditions. Asymptomatic episodes remain ordinarily undetected and they will often bias prevalence/incidence estimates.

Associated Conditions and Confounding Factors

For incident AFL, these are: history of congestive heart failure and chronic obstructive pulmonary disease; for AF: age, history of congestive heart failure and valvular disease, enlarged left atrium, abnormal mitral or aortic valve function, treated hypertension, and stroke.

Associated Risk

The relative mortality risk for sole AFL (without AF) from a single study was 1.2 (95% CI 1.2, 2.6; not considerably lower than that for sole AF); it was 1.7 for 6-month and 2.5 for 12-month follow-up periods (not significant for either), and substantially lower than the mortality risk for sole AF for these shorter periods. The reported mortality risk in community-based populations for AF ranges from nonsignificant to an approximately twofold increase, and in persons hospitalized for AF during the first 6 months after hospital discharge a nearly eightfold increase. The risk of stroke associated with AF has been estimated to be nearly threefold in men and over twofold in women. In terms of stroke prevention, ventricular rate control in AF has been found to be as effective as attempts to restore and maintain sinus rhythm. With the exception of re-entrant tachycardias, other supraventricular tachycardias (abnormal automaticity and ectopic complexes) are not considered to be associated with excess risk of adverse events.

Abbreviations and Acronyms

AF – atrial fibrillation
AFFIRM – Atrial Fibrillation Follow-up Investigation of Rhythm Management
AFL – atrial flutter
AFL1 – atrial flutter type 1
AFL2 – atrial flutter type 2
AV – atrioventricular
CHD – coronary heart disease
CHF – congestive heart failure
CHS – Cardiovascular Health Study
COPD – chronic obstructive pulmonary disease

CVD – cardiovascular disease
ESVC – ectopic supraventricular complex
EVC – ectopic ventricular complex
f wave – fibrillatory wave
F wave – flutter wave
LVH – left ventricular hypertrophy
MI – myocardial infarction
RBBB – right bundle branch block
RR – relative risk
SVT – supraventricular tachycardia
WPW – Wolf-Parkinson-White syndrome or ECG pattern

5.1 Introduction

Supraventricular dysrhythmias involve different mechanisms ranging from supraventricular ectopic complexes to atrioventricular (AV) re-entrant tachycardias (Figure 5.1). A commonly used categorization of supraventricular tachycardias (SVT) includes atrial tachycardia, AV junctional re-entrant tachycardia, and sino-atrial (SA) nodal re-entrant tachycardia (shaded categories in Figure 5.1). Atrioventricular nodal junctional

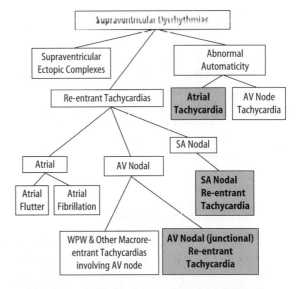

FIGURE 5.1 Categories of supraventricular tachycardias. Most re-entrant tachycardias are usually identified as individual entities. The shaded categories are often collectively grouped under one category called supraventricular tachycardia because their differentiation is difficult from the standard 12-lead ECG.

re-entrant tachycardia is the most common category, accounting for 50–60% of SVT. Atrioventricular nodal rhythm is often classified as a separate entity from other supraventricular dysrhythmias. The relatively rare high rate AV node tachycardia is at times difficult to differentiate from other supraventricular tachycardias if the nodal retrograde P waves are not visible.

The main mechanisms of supraventricular tachycardias include re-entry circuit and abnormal automaticity in an ectopic atrial focus or multifocal firing. In SA node re-entrant tachycardia, the micro re-entrant circuit is thought to involve the structure of the SA node. More familiar categories of re-entrant tachycardias are atrial fibrillation (AF), atrial flutter (AFL), and Wolf-Parkinson-White (WPW) syndrome.

The topics in this chapter will be presented in the following order: AFL, AF, supraventricular ectopic complex, and the primarily non-re-entrant SVT. The criteria for each condition were adapted mainly from the Novacode classification system.[1]

5.2 Atrial Flutter

Atrial flutter and AF are often combined in ECG classification for epidemiological studies because differentiation between them from standard 12-lead ECG is at times difficult. The prevalence of AFL is thought to be relatively low in comparison with the prevalence of AF, and risk evaluation reports for AFL alone are rare in populations outside the hospital. Pathophysiological mechanisms involved are different in AFL and AF, and these conditions also have different implications regarding their clinical management and prognosis.

5.2.1 Criteria for Atrial Flutter

Atrial flutter is characterized by the absence of P waves, the presence of the flutter (F) waves $\geq 100\,\mu V$ peak-to-peak with repetitive regular morphology in leads II, aVF, or V1. Classification criteria for AF are listed in Table 5.1. Ventricular rate in AFL depends on the dominant AV conduction, which is dependent on the functional properties of the AV node. The term "macro re-entrant"

implies the existence of a fairly long pathway where the re-entrant circuit rotates, as indicated by the long cycle interval. Spectral analysis of the flutter wave periodicity has revealed that the cycle length is not constant. It is modulated by the autonomic nervous system through a reflex control mechanism that regulates respiration, and also by the ventricular response rate, which is dependent on the dominant conduction through the AV node.[2] Hemodynamic factors are evidently involved in this variation of the periodicity.

TABLE 5.1 Classification criteria for atrial flutter categories.

Category	Criteria (for a 10-second record)
Atrial flutter/fibrillation (AFL/AF), screening criteria	C1. No P waves are present C2. Flutter waves (F) $\geq 100\,\mu V$ peak-to-peak with repetitive, regular morphology present in II or V1 C3. Fibrillation waves (f) or F waves with irregular cycle intervals or amplitudes in II, III or aVF C4. RR intervals irregular, with fewer than 3 within 40-ms class interval AFL/AF = C1 and (C2 or C3 or C4)
Atrial flutter type 1 (AFL1*)	C1. Five or more RR intervals, each with F waves C2. F ≤ 333 cpm (cycle interval ≥ 180 ms or 4.5 mm at paper speed 25 mm/s) C3. At least partial regularity of RR intervals, with ≥ 3 within 2 class intervals of 20 ms) AFL1 = C1 and C2 and C3
Classic atrial flutter type 1 (AFL1C)	C1. Criteria for AFL1 are met C2. F waves predominant in II or aVF, sawtooth pattern, with a negative initial leading edge notch with respect to baseline from QRS onset AFL1C = C1 and C2
Variant atrial flutter type 1 (AFL1V)	C1. Criteria for AFL1 are met C2. F waves predominant in II or aVF, sawtooth pattern, with a positive initial leading edge notch with respect to baseline from QRS onset AFL1V = C1 and C2
Atrial flutter type 2 (AFL2)	C1. F waves sustained for ≥ 5 RR intervals C2. F ≥ 333 cpm (cycle interval 141–179 ms or 3.6–4.4 mm at paper speed 25 mm/s) AFL2 = C1 and C2

* AFL1 with 1 : 1 AV conduction is coded as supraventricular tachycardia.
Source: Rautaharju et al.[1] *J Electrocardiol* 1998;31:157–87. © 1998. Reproduced with permission from Elsevier.

F waves in atrial flutter type 1 (AFL1) commonly occur at a rate of around 300 cpm. The associated ventricular rate is often approximately 150 cpm because of 1:2 conduction of the F waves through the AV node to the ventricles. The conduction rate is 1:2, 1:3, 1:4 etc, and it often varies, depending on the strength and timing of the F wave front reaching the AV node.

The classic AFL1 F waves are characterized with the initial notch (at the start of the leading edge of the saw tooth) that is negative with respect to the ECG baseline. This indicates counterclockwise rotation of the re-entrant right atrial circuit and craniocaudal propagation in the lateral free anterior wall followed by propagation in the opposite (caudocranial) direction in the septum and the posterior wall. The less common variant type AFL1 has a positive initial notch because of the counterclockwise rotation of the F wave front. The re-entrant circuit is rarely in the left atrium.

Atrial flutter type 2 (AFL2) patterns are less stable. It has more irregular re-entrant circuits than ALF1. At F rate >350 cpm, the F wave morphology tends to become more irregular in amplitude and cycle length, and the partial regularity of the RR intervals is often not present, like in AFL1.

5.2.2 Mechanism of Generation of Atrial Flutter

The conditions in the atria commonly considered necessary for flutter type 1 are: (1) some initiating trigger mechanism; (2) the existence of areas with differing action potential duration, refractory period, and conduction velocity; and (3), some anatomical or functional obstacles (or both) to form the pathway for the re-entrant circuit. The functional obstacle may be formed by fractionated and colliding wave fronts. The functional block may exist between the lateral and posterior walls of the right atrium, extending the obstacle from the tricuspid valve ring upwards toward the superior vena cava. The site of the re-entry is the isthmus between the inferior vena cava, the annulus of the tricuspid valve, or the ostium of the coronary sinus, as has been shown by the ablation techniques used to stop this arrhythmia. Atrial activation mapping data have shown that the re-entrant circuit is in the right atrium, with excitation proceeding in a counterclockwise direction in the anterior–right view of the atrial septum, obliquely from the right side.[a]

Right atrial endocardial mapping has made it possible to document in more detail temporal patterns of right atrial excitation and the re-entrant pathway in the common form of type 1 AFL.[3] From the re-entry site with a slower conduction velocity, a new excitation cycle starts with wave fronts speeding in the general direction from caudal to cranial parts in the septum to the superior vena cava region. There they turn around and the excitation front propagates from a cranial to caudal direction along the crista terminalis and the free lateral right atrial wall to the isthmus. Thus, the flutter circuit may rotate in a path enclosing the tricuspid ring.[4] Immediately after one cycle is completed, the next cycle begins as soon as excitation exits from the isthmus to the lower septum. Conduction velocity in the isthmus was estimated by Shah et al. to be on the average 0.6 m/s compared to approximately 1 m/s in other parts of the right atrium.[5]

Although the counterclockwise motion of re-entrant circuits in the right atrium is the landmark of the classic common form of type 1 AFL, the ECG features of the F waves in body surface ECG leads are determined mainly by the left atrium, as shown by Okumura et al. in their epicardial activation data in dog left atrium.[5] The posteroinferior left atrium was activated early compared with the activation time at the Bachmann's bundle in the cranial area of the left atrium. This activation sequence can be expected when the left atrium (and the septum) is excited dominantly in the caudocranial direction. A positive flutter wave was observed when the Bachmann's bundle area was activated early in comparison with the posteroinferior left atrium,

---

[a] There is some confusion about the terminology regarding what is clockwise and what is counterclockwise rotation of the re-entrant circuit. Some of the investigators displaying activation maps in the posteroanterior view describe a clockwise flutter circuit,[5] where others see a counterclockwise rotation when viewed in the anteroposterior direction.

indicating left atrial excitation dominantly in a craniocaudal direction. A finding not so easily reconciled was that the presence of craniocaudal excitation of the free wall of the right atrium (presumably counterclockwise rotation in frontal view) had no consistent relationship with the F wave polarity in lead II. It is not known whether this observation reflects differences in dog and human ECG in relation to anatomic position of the heart in the chest.

Cheng et al. described a subtype of right atrial flutter called lower loop re-entry.[6] This pattern of atrial flutter can exist in some patients in conjunction with the typical counterclockwise atrial flutter, sharing the isthmus as a common re-entry point and right atrial re-entry pathway involving portions of the posterior right atrium and lower segments of crista terminalis. Thus, the episodes of lower loop re-entry coexisting with typical atrial flutter may result in flutter waves with similar morphologies but with two different cycle lengths. In the report of Cheng et al., the typical counterclockwise flutter wave mean cycle length was 272 ms (221 cpm). The cycle lengths of the lower loop re-entry flutter waves were shorter, ranging from 170 ms (373 cpm) to 250 ms (240 cpm), mean 217 ms (276 cpm). In body surface ECGs the flutter waveforms were similar, with negative initial portion of the flutter waves in inferior leads and positive in V1. However, the positive terminal portion of the flutter wave in inferior leads was absent in lower loop re-entry.

The triggering mechanism initiating AFL is assumed to be the occurrence of critically timed atrial ectopic complexes. Waldo et al. postulated that type 1 AFL does not start spontaneously but that AF is usually the transitory arrhythmia immediately preceding the onset of AFL.[7] Atrial flutter is experimentally induced by atrial pacing, and there is evidence that the initiation is dependent on the pacing site.[8] Slowly conducting isthmus in the pathway may also form a unidirectional or in some atrial activation patterns a bidirectional block. In pacing studies in 46 patients, Suzuki et al. demonstrated that pacing in the coronary sinus area induces a counterclockwise flutter circuit (viewed from front), and pacing from the low lateral right atrium initiates a clockwise clutter circuit.[9]

5.2.3 Prevalence of Atrial Flutter

There are no reliable prevalence data available in general populations with clear separation in the classification of atrial flutter and fibrillation. The age trend in the prevalence of AFL apparently parallels that of AF. The prevalence of AFL is probably approximately one-tenth of that of AF, so that AFL prevalence is likely to be well below 1%, perhaps approaching 1% in old age groups. The prevalence of AFL is approximately twice as high in men as in women.

5.2.4 Incidence of Atrial Flutter

There is a scarcity of epidemiological information available about AFL in general populations. As mentioned, most studies have focused solely on AF or included AFL in the overall AF count. The Marshfield Epidemiological Study Area (MESA) in Central Wisconsin has accumulated unique data on the incidence of AFL and its predisposing factors from the shared medical records of two clinical centers that provide almost all health care in the region covering 58,820 area residents.[10] The report on AFL covered approximately 220,000 person-years of observation, with AFL documentation by approximately 29,000 ECGs and rhythm strips, 1,100 Holter ECG and 500 ambulatory event recordings from area residents. Final selection was done by cardiac electrophysiologists from approximately 2,000 recordings with potential AFL incident cases. Each incident AFL case was matched for age and gender by controls without previously documented atrial arrhythmias chosen randomly from the MESA residents.

During the 4 years of ascertainment, there were 181 new AFL cases diagnosed among 58,820 MESA residents. Nearly all new AFL cases were >50 years of age. It was noted that over one-half (58%) of the incident AFL cases also had at least one episode of AF. The overall incidence of AFL in the general population was 88/100,000 (Figure 5.2). The overall annual incidence of AFL was approximately 22/100,000 (9/100,000 for sole AFL). Adjusted for age, the approximate overall annual incidence of AFL in men was 31/100,000. In women, the incidence was one-half of that in men: 15/100,000. Age-specific AFL incidence increased progressively with age in both men and women.

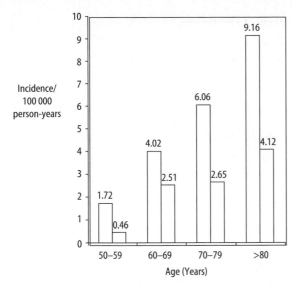

FIGURE 5.2 Incidence of atrial flutter by age in men (*white bars*) and women (*shaded bars*) over an average of 4 years of follow-up in the Marshfield population in central Wisconsin. The annual overall incidence is approximately one-quarter of that indicated, and the incidence of sole AFL without AF approximately one-half of the overall annual incidence. (Source: Granada et al.[10] J Am Coll Cardiol 2000;36:2242–6. Copyright © 2000 The American College of Cardiology Foundation. Reproduced with permission.)

5.2.5 Predisposing Factors for Atrial Flutter

In the Marshfield study population, histories of congestive heart failure (CHF) and chronic obstructive pulmonary disease (COPD) were identified as the two significant factors associated with incidence of AFL. The relative risk was 3.5 (1.7, 7.1; $p = 0.001$) for CHF and 1.9 (1.1, 3.4; $p = 0.02$) for COPD. The investigators calculated population-attributable risk and estimated that 15.8% and 11.6% of AFL cases in the cohort could be attributed to CHF and COPD, respectively.

5.2.6 Actions of Drugs on Atrial Flutter

There is a functional relationship between the refractory period (T), the average conduction velocity (v), and the minimum length of the rotation pathway or pathways. This is because the time it takes for the flutter circuit to travel once around is equal to the refractory period (note that s = wavelength [λ] of the flutter wave): T = s/v, or s = λ = T*v.

Evidently T is the longest refractory period of the atrial fibers in the pathway. The above relationships are modified by actions of certain cardioactive drugs. Acetylcholine shortens the wavelength λ by 30–40% mainly because T shortens. With guanidine, T is prolonged, v shortened, and prolongation of λ is less pronounced. Thus, consideration of λ appears useful in evaluation of antiarrhythmic drug effects.[11]

Ordinarily, the wavelength (the distance the excitation front travels during the duration of the refractory period) is so long in comparison with the size of the atria that a stable re-entrant circuit cannot be established and possible short runs of rapid re-entrant responses terminate spontaneously. A shorter wavelength makes it possible to establish a single stable re-entrant circuit and atrial flutter can be established if a relatively large area with a conduction block is present. With a further shortening of the wavelength either with slower conduction velocity due to depressed conduction or with a shortening of the refractory period, re-entrant circuits and AF can be established more easily even in the presence of small areas with a conduction block.

5.2.7 Atrial Flutter and Mortality Risk

A report from the Marshfield study group in 2002 compared AFL and AF mortality in 577 patients and matched controls during a total of 4,775 person-years of follow-up.[12] For short-term (0–6 months) mortality, the relative risk (RR) in patients with sole AFL was increased but not significantly (RR 1.7 [0.6, 5.3], $p = 0.35$). This contrasts with the relative risk for sole AF at 6 months: sevenfold compared to the controls (RR 7.1 [4.0, 13], $p = 0.0001$). During the 7–12 months follow-up period, the relative risk for AFL alone had increased to 2.5 but it still had not reached a statistically significant level ($p = 0.15$). The number of cases with AFL alone was considerably smaller ($n = 76$) than that with sole AF ($n = 396$). During the entire follow-up, the relative risk for sole AFL was 1.7 (1.2, 2.6, $p = 0.007$), not substantially lower than that for sole AF, which was associated with a relative risk of 2.4 (1.9, 3.1, $p < 0.0001$). These models were adjusted for age, sex, and clinical risk factors (heart failure, COPD, rheumatic heart disease, smoking history, thyroid abnormalities, and diabetes mellitus).

The Marshfield study results suggested that effective treatment of AFL will have an impact at least on short-term mortality. Cardioversion is the initial therapeutic action of choice, or pacing if cardioversion is not successful. Drug therapy is used to reduce the risk of recurrent episodes. The goal of pharmaceutical therapy is to terminate or at least to achieve adequate rate control in AFL. Calcium channel blockers are in general effective. Avoiding class I and III drugs is advisable in the prehospital setting – they may convert the conduction ratio for F waves to 1:1 by improved AV conduction.

5.2.8　Atrial Flutter and Quality of Life

Common complaints in AFL are history of palpitations, fatigue or poor exercise tolerance, dyspnea, and occasionally syncope. The symptoms in AFL are generally dependent on ventricular rate, which may or may not be high, depending on the conduction ratio for F waves. This emphasized the importance of adequate rate control if high ventricular rate is associated with symptoms.

5.3　Atrial Fibrillation

Atrial fibrillation is a high rate atrial tachycardia (>430 cpm) with more or less chaotic patterns of atrial excitation. The proportion of atrial excitatory waves that are conducted to the ventricles is limited by the AV node (its refractory period) and the strength of the atrial excitation fronts reaching the upper part of the AV node. The ventricular response rate may be slow, moderate or high, depending on the above factors. Atrial flutter and AF are often combined in ECG classification for epidemiological studies because differentiation between them from standard 12-lead ECG is occasionally difficult.

5.3.1　Atrial Fibrillation Criteria

The criteria for AF (Table 5.2) are seemingly simpler than those for AFL. As mentioned before,

TABLE 5.2 Criteria for atrial fibrillation.

Category	Criteria
Atrial fibrillation (AF)	C1. Screening criteria for AF or atrial flutter (AFL) (defined in Table 5.2) are met
	C2. Criteria for AFL type 1 and type 2 are not met
	AF = C1 and C2
Atrial flutter/fibrillation (AFL/AF)	Defined in Table 5.1
AFL/AF with possibly dominant AV conduction	C1. Fibrillation waves (f)
	C2. Flutter waves (F) with ≥100 µV peak-to-peak in ≤4 RR intervals
	C3. RR interval differences ≤40 ms (or within two adjacent 20-ms class intervals), indicating possibly dominant AV conduction
	AFL/AF with possibly dominant AV conduction = (C1 or C2) and C3

these two conditions are at times difficult to differentiate. They may both coexist with a transition from one to the other and meeting the criteria for AFL/AF combined.

5.3.2　Mechanism of Atrial Fibrillation

The most plausible mechanism for this high rate re-entrant atrial tachycardia is the existence of multiple re-entrant wavelets with fractionated wave fronts, although more than one mechanism may be involved in special circumstances. The existence of multiple interacting wavelets wandering around zones or islets of refractory tissue in the atria is the basic characteristic of AF.[13,14] A high firing rate shortens atrial action potential duration and the refractory period and the wavelength. The wavelength is the product of the conduction velocity and the refractory period. The shorter the wavelength, the higher the number of simultaneous wavelets possible. Atrial fibrillation occurs at shorter wavelengths that can be induced by rapid stimulation of atrial appendix with simultaneous vagal stimulation or acetylcholine infusion, and it continues spontaneously as long as vagal stimulation or acetylcholine infusion is maintained.

The multiple wave hypothesis of Moe and Abildskov is based on a model that incorporates nonhomogeneous distribution of refractory periods.[14] Self-sustained activity is initiated by a premature firing at sites with short refractory periods. Short wavelength increases the likelihood of simultaneous existence of multiple re-entrant pathways with randomly wandering wavelets coexisting. The wavelets may encounter refractory elements and become extinguished or divide and combine by fusion or collision with neighboring wavelets, changing the direction and magnitude of the wave fronts. Alessie et al. demonstrated that the existence of relatively few wavelets (even three to six) is enough to maintain AF.[15] The question of a rapidly firing focus as an integral element of maintaining AF is open, as is the question whether spontaneously occurring AF has the same initiating mechanism as AF induced in these experiments.

Electrophysiological characteristics of the atria are altered with the induction of AF in goats. Repetitive induction of AF results in progressive shortening of the effective atrial refractory period and prolongation of the duration of transient AF periods, which gradually (within a week) become sustained.[16,17] In addition to the shortening of the effective refractory period after the induction of AF, there is attenuation or a change to an inverse relationship of the normal physiological adaptation to rate changes. Similar alterations have been reported in humans after only several minutes of AF or rapid atrial pacing, suggesting a transient shortening of the atrial wavelength whereby AF may perpetuate itself.[18]

Flecainide, a class 1C antiarrhythmic drug, attenuates the shortening of action potential durations with increasing firing rate, resulting in the increase of the wavelength.[19] Thus, the conditions decreasing the chances of re-entry work in favor of termination of AF. Prolongation of the wavelength by slowing down the conduction velocity in atria may work in two ways. Re-entry may be facilitated because the myocytes have more time to recover from the refractoriness. On the other hand, longer wavelength promotes lengthening of the re-entrant pathway, which, in principle, should decrease the rate of the fibrillatory waves. Premature stimuli associated with longer wavelengths are more likely to induce AFL than AF.[6]

5.3.3 Precursors of Atrial Fibrillation

Rheumatic heart disease with mitral stenosis used to be a common clinical condition precipitating AF. With the reducing prevalence of rheumatic heart disease, other precursors have taken a more prominent role as determinants of AF or as contributing factors in its evolution. Comorbidity includes conditions such as valvular heart disease, cardiomyopathy, myocardial infarction (MI), metabolic and electrolyte abnormalities, left ventricular hypertrophy (LVH), left atrial enlargement, thyrotoxicosis, pneumonia, and other infections. Atrial fibrillation is common after surgery for the repair of Fallot's tetralogy, and the incidence is high in other valvular procedures. It is a complication in 10% to 30% of coronary artery bypass grafts. Atrial fibrillation occurring as an isolated condition has been a subject of debate.

5.4 Prevalence and Incidence of Atrial Fibrillation

5.4.1 Lone Atrial Fibrillation

As noted, AF usually occurs with other comorbid clinical conditions. The prevalence as well as the incidence of isolated or "lone" AF varies, depending on how refined methods and on how strict criteria are used to define coexisting conditions. In an insured population, up to 41% of the subjects with chronic AF were considered free of cardiac disease, at least in part because of the low sensitivity in detecting overt disease in retrospective analysis of life insurance medical examinations.[20]

In the Reykjavik study of 9,067 32- to 64-year-old randomly selected residents, one-third of the prevalent AF was considered as "lone" AF (absence of associated cardiovascular disease [CVD], COPD or thyrotoxicosis).[21]

In the Olmsted County study, cumulative count was established in County residents hospitalized with AF during an observation period from 1950 to 1980 (3,623 patients).[22] In 2.7% the AF was determined to be lone (without overt CVD or other conditions precipitating AF). The report included hospitalized residents 60 years old or younger, with a mean age of 40.9 years.

In a report on the 30-year follow-up of the Framingham study participants, AF was considered to be lone in 32 out of 193 men (16.6%) and in 11 out of 183 women (6.0%) who developed AF (incident AF).[23]

5.4.2 Age and Gender and the Prevalence and Incidence of Atrial Fibrillation

The prevalence of AF depends on the general health of the study population and the prevalence of comorbid conditions. Of primary interest is the prevalence in unselected or randomly selected populations.

5.4.2.1 The Reykjavik Study

In the Reykjavik study, the cross-sectional prevalence was low: 25 out of the 9,067 men and women

had AF (0.28%) in this randomly selected population 32–64 years of age.[21] Atrial fibrillation turned out to be chronic in all 25 subjects, as confirmed in subsequent examinations. The AF prevalence was substantially higher in men than in women, with a male/female prevalence ratio of 2.73.

5.4.2.2 The Busselton Study

In the Busselton study in Western Australia, triennial surveys were performed of a population sample of 1,770 men and women aged 60 years and over at entry in 1966.[24] The last triennial survey was in 1981 and the latest follow-up was done in 1983. At the entry examination, AF was found in 40 subjects (2.3%) (Table 5.3). Incident AF was observed in 47 subjects during the period from the baseline to the last follow-up. The cross-sectional prevalence varied in succes-

TABLE 5.3 Atrial fibrillation and the risk of stroke and all-cause death in three reports from diverse populations.

Items compared	Busselton study[24]			Whitehall study[37]	British Regional Heart study[37]
Report population	Out of 1,770 persons aged >60 years, 87 with AF at baseline or incident AF at any of the five triennial follow-up examinations from 1966 to 1981			63 men with nonrheumatic AF selected from 80 men with AF found in screening of 19,018 London civil servants aged 40–69 years	48 men with nonrheumatic AF selected from 54 men with AF documented from 7,727 patients aged 40–59 years in group practices in 24 towns
Cohort assembly	1966–1968			Between 1967 and 1969	1979–1980
AF Prevalence (%) (all five triennials combined)	Age	Men	Women	–	–
	60–64	1.1	2.3		
	65–69	3.3	2.7		
	70–74	8.6	5.5		
	75+	15.0	8.4		
	2.3% overall				
Follow-up	2–17 years			16–18 years	8 years
Mortality risk or risk of stroke	Mortality risk			Mortality risk	Risk of stroke
	Men		Women	Only 33% of the AF group survived at 15 years, compared with 82% in the main cohort. This gives the mortality ratio 3.7	There was only one stroke in the study group, relative risk 2.3, not significant
	1.96 (1.4, 2.8)		2.35 (1.5, 3.6)		
	CVD mortality				
	Men		Women	Risk of stroke (all)	
	2.2 (1.3, 3.7)		2.3 (1.2, 4.3)	6.9 (3.0, 13.5)	
	Risk of stroke			There were only 9 strokes (8 fatal) in the study group. Age-adjusted rate of fatal stroke 13.8/1,000 person-years	
	Men		Women		
	2.7 (1.1, 6.4)		2.3 (1.2, 4.3)		
Adjustment	Age			Age	Age
Comments	Incidence of new AF by age in any of the triennial intervals ranged between 2 and 24/1,000 persons			Among potential predictors of stroke, significant association only for systolic and diastolic blood pressure	Age-adjusted rate of stroke 3.3/1,000 person-years

sive triennial surveys over 17 years. The prevalence ranged from 5/1,000 to 24/1,000, and was strongly dependent on age, particularly in men. The male/female ratio was less than 0.5 in persons 60–64 years old, and it increased to 1.8 at age 75 years old and older. (These rates differ from those listed in Table 5.3, which represent the cumulative aggregate prevalence by age from all five triennial examinations, and are a mixture of initial prevalence and incident cases.) Similarly, the cumulative incidence in the successive 3-year intervals ranged from 5/1,000 to 15/1,000. (It is not clear whether this is the incidence per 1,000 or the incidence per 1,000 person-years of follow-up.)

5.4.2.3 The Framingham Cohort

The association between age and the incident AF was evaluated in the Framingham cohort.[25] The incidence of AF increased exponentially in men from 6.2 at age 55 to 64 years to 75.9 at age 85 to 94 years, and in women from 3.8 to 62.8, respectively, expressed per 1,000 person-examinations. In a sex-specific multivariable model including clinical conditions associated with the development of AF (CHF, valvular heart disease, MI), for each decade of advancing age the odds ratio of developing AF was 2.1 for men and 2.2 for women. This implies that AF incidence increases as a power function of age with an exponent of approximately 2 for each increment of a decade after the age of 50 years. In a multivariable model adjusting for clinical AF precursor conditions (age, smoking, diabetes, LVH, hypertension, MI, CHF and valvular heart disease), male gender was associated with a 50% higher likelihood of developing AF (odds ratio 1.5 [1.3, 1.8], $p < 0.0001$).

5.4.2.4 The Manitoba Study

A similar increase of AF incidence with age, as in the Framingham study, was reported from the Manitoba follow-up study.[26] The study was initiated in 1948 and it involved 3,983 male air crew recruits with mean age 31 (90% between 20 and 39 years) with the latest follow-up in 1992. The age-specific incidence, which was less than 0.5/1,000 person-years of observation before the

age of 50 years, increased to 2.3 by age 60 years and 16.9/1,000 person-years by age 85 years. The exponent for age estimated from Figure 1 of the Manitoba report (not shown) is nearly 2.

5.4.2.5 The Cardiovascular Health Study

In the 24-hour ambulatory ECG recordings of a subsample of 1,327 participants at the baseline of the Cardiovascular Health Study (CHS), the combined prevalence of AF and AFL (sustained or transient) was 3.3% in men and 2.8% in women.[27] The prevalence of AF and AFL determined from the standard 10-second 12-lead ECG in 5,152 CHS participants at baseline was higher, 6.2% in men and 4.8% in women.[28] Atrial fibrillation was identified: (1) by ECG criteria alone in the standard 12-lead ECG; (2) by questionnaire self-report alone (Did a doctor ever tell you that you have AF? If not sure, answer "Don't know"); or (3), by both procedures. Self-report accounted for only one-half of the AF prevalence in women and slightly less than one-half in men. Evaluation of the anti-arrhythmic medication use indicated that self-reports were likely to be reliable. Although AF prevalence tended to increase with age, the trend was significant in women only ($p < 0.0001$). This contrasts with the age trend for incident AF, as will be noted later.

The CHS investigators also reported the results from an AF incidence study.[29] The results were based on AF incidence data from three sources: (1) ECG at each annual examination; (2) self-report of AF; and (3) discharge diagnosis obtained from every hospitalization reported. Excluding subjects with prevalent AF at the baseline and subjects with electronic pacemakers, 4,844 subjects at risk of new-onset AF were included in the incidence study. There were 304 incident AF cases during the follow-up of an average of 3.28 years duration. Nearly a third (29%) of the total study group was classified as having clinical CVD at the baseline, and 71% were considered CVD-free. The incidence of AF had an increasing trend with age, particularly in men. The annual incidence rate expressed per 100 person-years was 1.8 in men and 1.0 in women in the two youngest age groups combined (65–74 years), and 4.3 in men and 2.2 in women in the two oldest age groups combined (75–84 years).

5.4.3 Time Trends in the Prevalence of Atrial Fibrillation

The Framingham study evaluated secular trends in the prevalence of AF.[30] The test for time trends was performed using the generalized estimation equation method, which adjusts for repeated measurements in the same subjects.[31] The model used included age, sex, and examination number as independent variables. The examination number makes it possible to test for the significance of time trends in the prevalence. The evaluation included persons aged 65–84 years, and the time period covered was 22 years, from 1968 to 1989 (10th and 20th biennial examinations). There was a marginally significant trend in AF prevalence from ECGs in routine biennial clinic examinations in men ($p = 0.08$) but not in women ($p = 0.55$). The report notes that this rate from biennial examinations was only half of that from all sources including hospitalizations.

Comparing AF prevalence by sex at the 10th and 20th examinations from ECGs obtained from private physicians and hospitalizations combined, the age-adjusted rate increased in men from 3.2 to 9.1% ($p = 0.002$) and in women from 2.8 to 4.7% ($p = 0.60$). Thus, the male to female ratio of AF prevalence increased substantially during the study period, from 1.14 to 1.94. There was a rather drastic increase in AF prevalence in men with prior MI, from 4.9 to 17.4%. There was no significant increase in this same category in women. Age-adjusted prevalence of MI did not increase significantly in either sex. This again suggests that prior MI predisposes to propensity to AF in men, perhaps reflecting the association with improved MI survival in men, although AF prevalence increased also in men without prior MI.

The Framingham data confirm AF prevalence in hospital discharge data in the USA between 1982 and 1993, according to the survey data in 1979 and 1992 by the National Center for Health Statistics.[32,33] The Framingham investigators noted that increasing time trend and age trend in AF prevalence may have clinical implications in view of the aging population and the fact that the stroke incidence doubles in successive age decades.

5.4.4 Predictors of Prevalent Atrial Fibrillation

5.4.4.1 The Cardiovascular Health Study

In the CHS population, only age and history of CHF, valvular disease and stroke retained a significant association with AF in a multivariate stepwise selection model that included seven covariates (age, male gender, and five clinical conditions: history of MI, angina, CHF, valvular heart disease, and stroke).[28] In univariate models, six of the other variables suggesting subclinical disease were significantly associated with AF: abnormal left ventricular wall motion, abnormal ejection fraction, evidence of mitral stenosis, aortic regurgitation, enlarged left atrium, and electrocardiographic estimate of left ventricular mass.

5.4.5 Predictors of Incident Atrial Fibrillation

5.4.5.1 The Framingham Cohort

In the 38-year follow-up of 2,090 male and 2,641 female members of the original Framingham cohort, CHF in men and women and valvular disease in women were identified as the strongest predictors of incident AF.[25] After adjusting for age and clinical risk factors for AF, men had a 1.5 times greater likelihood of incident AF than women ($p < 0.001$). For CHF, the odds ratio in a sex-specific multivariable model adjusting for other risk factors was 4.5 for men and 5.9 for women ($p < 0.001$ for both). For valvular disease, the odds ratio was 3.4 ($p < 0.001$) for women and 1.8 ($p < 0.01$) for men. Other overt clinical cardiac diseases with a significant association with incident AF were diabetes mellitus and hypertension in both sexes and MI in men, all with an approximately 50% excess risk of developing AF. It is of interest that the multivariable model remained largely unchanged after excluding subjects with valve disease. Age was also a strong predictor, as expected, with an odds ratio 2.1 in men and 2.2 in women ($p < 0.001$ for both). Adjusting only for age, ECG-LVH was associated with a threefold excess of age-adjusted risk for incident AF in men and a nearly fourfold excess risk in women.

In a separate study in a subgroup of 1,924 participants, echocardiographic measurements were available for evaluation of the risk for incident AF.[34] After adjusting for age, sex, hypertension, coronary artery disease, CHF, diabetes, and valve disease, independent predictors of incident AF were left atrial size, left ventricular wall thickness (septal + posterior wall), and left ventricular fractional shortening (inverse association).

5.4.5.2 The Manitoba Study

Clinically overt cardiac disease conditions with a pronounced association with incident AF in the Manitoba follow-up study[26] were CHF and valvular heart disease, like in the Framingham study. The covariate with the strongest association with incident AF in the multivariable model (including all risk factors significant in univariate analyses) was cardiomyopathy, with a relative risk of 4.07 (1.45–11.45). In contrast with the Framingham study, where the association between ischemic heart disease and incident AF was relatively weak in men, in the Manitoba follow-up study the relative risk of AF was 3.62 (2.59, 5.07) for MI, 2.84 (1.91, 4.21) for angina pectoris, and 2.21 (1.62, 3.00) for isolated ST or T wave abnormalities in the absence of overt ischemic heart disease (Minnesota code categories 4.1.2–4.4 and 5.2–5.4). Ischemic heart disease was present in over one-third of the men who developed AF later. Of the cardiac symptoms, palpitations, supraventricular and ventricular rhythm disturbances each had a significantly increased relative risk for incident AF. These apparent manifestations of subclinical cardiac disease may also reflect possible association with transient AF that escaped documentation until later.

5.4.5.3 The Cardiovascular Health Study

A number of clinical precursors and potential risk factors for new-onset AF were identified in the CHS incidence study.[29] In a stepwise multivariate model including the whole incidence study group, prominent risk factors were valvular heart disease (RR 2.42 [1.62, 3.60]), coronary heart disease (CHD) (RR 1.48 [1.13, 1.95]), left atrial diameter (RR 1.74 [1.44, 2.11]), and diuretic use (RR 1.51 [1.17, 1.97]). Diuretic use most likely reflects hypertension and possibly LVH. Increased risk was also significantly associated with systolic blood pressure (RR 1.11 [1.05,

1.18] for a 10-mmHg increment), glucose (RR [1.03, 1.08] for mmol/l), and age (RR 1.05 [1.03, 1.08]). The association between left atrial size and the incidence of AF showed a progressively increasing relative risk, compared to the group with left atrial diameter ≤3.00 cm. Factors with a significant association with reduced risk of incident AF were β-blocker use (RR 0.61 [0.41, 0.91]), good lung function as reflected by forced expiratory volume in one second (RR 0.75 [0.59, 0.94]), and for unexplained reasons, cholesterol level (RR 0.86 [0.76, 0.98]).

Clinically, prolonged PR interval is known to precede initiation of AF or AFL, and it may be a manifestation of sick sinus syndrome.[35] It is also known that delayed retrograde excitation of the left atrium due to interatrial block with P wave duration exceeding 120 ms predisposes to incident atrial flutter and fibrillation.[36] In CHS, the relative risks identified for various independent predictors of incident AF were similar in magnitude when evaluated in separate multivariate models for participants with and without clinically overt CVD. In a multivariate stepwise model for the group with CVD at baseline, one additional variable entered into the model: first degree AV block, with a relative risk of 2.11 (1.03, 3.35).

5.4.6 Left Atrial Size and the Incidence of Atrial Fibrillation

A strong relationship was found in the CHS between echocardiographic left atrial size and incident AF (Figure 5.3).[29] In a multivariate stepwise model, a 1-cm increment of the left atrial diastolic dimension was associated with a 74% excess in the incidence of AF (RR 1.74 [1.44, 2.11]). This prospective incidence study indicates that left atrial enlargement precedes incident AF, and left atrial enlargement is more likely to be a precipitation factor or a substrate for the initiation of AF rather than a consequence of AF. There has been some controversy about this relationship, which probably relates to the fact that causal relationships are more difficult to evaluate if the study population consists of prevalent rather than prospective incident cases of AF. In the echocardiographic study from Framingham cited above,[34] a

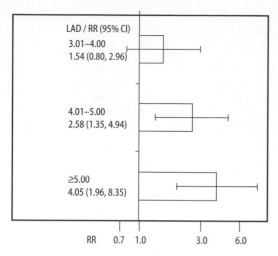

FIGURE 5.3 Association between left atrial dimension (LAD, cm) and the incidence of atrial fibrillation/flutter in the Cardiovascular Health Study. Relative risk (RR, with 95% confidence limits on logarithmic scale) in three subgroups stratified by LAD compared with the reference group with LAD ≤3.00 cm. (Source: Psaty et al.[29] Circulation 1997;96:2455–61. Copyright © 1997 American Heart Association. Reproduced with permission from Lippincott, Williams & Wilkins.)

0.5-cm increment in left atrial size was associated with 39% increased risk of incident nonrheumatic AF, an excess risk comparable to that in the CHS study.

5.5 Atrial Fibrillation and the Risk of Mortality and Stroke

5.5.1 Prevalent Atrial Fibrillation and Mortality Risk

Risk data from various studies on the association of AF with mortality and stroke differ widely. These differences are due to differences in age and other study population characteristics, selection criteria, etc. Among the main reasons for the diversity of the results are the differences in age structure, etiological factors for AF (rheumatic versus nonrheumatic), and the study endpoints. These differences are exemplified by the data from three reports in Table 5.3, and in another set of three reports in Table 5.4.

5.5.1.1 The Busselton Study

In a report from the Busselton study in a Western Australia community, the risk estimates presented were from a study group of 87 men and women aged 60 years and older with AF. There were 40 prevalent AF cases at the baseline of the study and 47 incident AF cases detected from the triennial examinations.[24] The mortality risk (all-cause and CVD) as well as the risk of stroke during a 2- to 17-year follow-up ranged between approximately 2 and 2.7, with no notable differences between men and women (significant for all).

5.5.1.2 The Whitehall and London Civil Servants Studies

In the Whitehall study of 63 men with non-rheumatic AF screened from London civil servants aged 40–69 years, only 33% survived at 15 years, compared with 82% of men in the main cohort.[37] This gives the mortality ratio of 3.7. The risk of stroke was 6.9 (3.0, 13.5). For fatal stroke, the mortality ratio was as high as 14.6. In the British Regional Heart study summarized in the same report as the Whitehall study, there were 48 men aged 40–59 years with nonrheumatic AF selected from group-practice patients. The relative risk of stroke was 2.3 (0.1, 12.7). It should be noted that there was only one stroke in the latter study group. Based on these limited numbers, the age-adjusted rate of stroke was 3.3/1,000 person-years. There were also very few strokes (ten) in the Whitehall study, two of them fatal. The investigators concluded that these lower rates of stroke in nonrheumatic AF may imply a lesser potential benefit from preventive measures.

5.5.1.3 The Reykjavik Study

The first report in the second set of three AF studies (Table 5.4) is from the Reykjavik study.[21] This was a survey of a community population sample of 9,067 men and women aged 32–64 years. The AF prevalence was 0.28% (male/female ratio 2.73). Compared to the age- and sex-matched control group, the 14-year all-cause mortality in this small AF group was higher (32%) than in the control group (20%) but the difference was not significant. The relative risk for CHD mortal-

TABLE 5.4 Atrial fibrillation and mortality risk in a randomly selected community population and in two studies on residents hospitalized for atrial fibrillation from defined geographic areas with a single main provider of health care.

Items compared	Reykjavik[21]	Olmsted[22]	Marshfield[12]
Report population	25 persons (18 men, 7 women) with AF (all considered chronic) from a randomly selected population of 9,067 (age range 32–64 years)	97 patients with lone AF (87% males) out of 3,623 hospitalized AF patients from residents of the county, excluding 97% of AF cases with other comorbid conditions. Age range 10–60 years, mean 44 years	577 patients with AF or AFL from 58,820 residents of the study area that captured nearly all hospitalizations and deaths. Age not indicated
Cohort assembly	1967–1969 and from a second phase 3 years later	1950–1980	Source data collected for 4 years starting July 1, 1991
Prevalence (%)	2.76/1,000; male/female ratio 2.73	Standardized data not reported	Standardized data not reported
Comorbid conditions	Nonsignificant difference from matched control group: hypertensive heart disease (by ECG/X-ray) 20%, ischemic heart disease 20%, chronic obstructive pulmonary disease 8%	None by definition	Not reported
Follow-up (years)	14	Mean 14.8	Up to 7.3, mean 3.6
Comparison group	Age- and sex-matched group of 50 persons	Expected survival in age- and sex-matched sample of white west north central US population in 1970	Control group of 577 (age- and sex-matched?)
Mortality risk (95% CI)	All-cause mortality increase not significant (32 vs 20% in the control group). For CVD mortality (including stroke), relative risk 6.1, from stroke alone 12.3 ($p < 0.05$ for both)	Survival 98 and 94% after 10 and 15 years, respectively, with no significant difference between the AF group and age- and sex-matched control group or between isolated, recurrent or chronic AF	Entire follow-up: RR 2.4 (1.9, 3.1) $p < 0.001$ First 6 months: 7-fold increased risk for ≥13 months, nearly twofold excess risk
Adjustment	–	–	Age, sex, CHF, chronic pulmonary disease, rheumatic heart disease, smoking history, thyroid abnormalities, and diabetes mellitus
Comments	–	AFL apparently excluded. Stroke incidence 5 per >1,400 person years (0.35/100 person-years). Cumulative actuarial incidence 1.2% at the end of the 15th year	–

AF atrial fibrillation, *AFL* atrial flutter, *RR* relative risk.

ity was 6.1 and for stroke mortality 12.3 ($p < 0.05$ for both).

5.5.1.4 The Olmsted County Study

The second report in Table 5.4 presents the prognosis in 97 patients with lone AF (excluding other comorbid conditions). This group was extracted for all patients hospitalized for AF from the 3,623 residents of the Olmsted County in Minnesota where one institution (the Mayo Clinic) serves as the primary care provider for the area.[22] The patients with lone AF were 60 years old or younger, and the mean follow-up period was 14.8 years. The survival rate was not significantly different between the lone AF group and the age- and sex-matched control group. The authors concluded that the risk of stroke in lone AF in patients under the age of 60 years is very low.

5.5.1.5 The Marshfield Study

The third report in Table 5.4 comes from a geographic region in Michigan, the Marshfield study, similar to the Olmsted study.[12] The report included risk data of 577 patients with AF or AFL, captured from all hospitalizations between July 1, 1991 and June 30, 1995. The mean follow-up was 3.6 years (up to 7.3 years). Mortality risk data, comparing the AF group with the control group (apparently matched for age and sex) revealed an over twofold increased risk for the entire follow-up period, and 7.8 (4.1, 15) for the initial 6 months ($p < 0.0001$ for both periods). The excess early mortality risk was largely because of the higher mortality risk for AF than for AFL. The report apparently com-

prised all AF cases and not only nonrheumatic AF.

5.5.2 Incident Atrial Fibrillation and the Risk of Mortality and Stroke

All-cause mortality risk and the risk of stroke associated with incident AF were significantly increased in two reports from the Framingham study and a report from a Canadian long-term study (Table 5.5).

5.5.2.1 The Framingham Reports

The first Framingham report covered a follow-up of 30 years of 303 incident AF cases from 15 bien-

TABLE 5.5 Incident atrial fibrillation and the risk of death and stroke from two Framingham reports and from a Canadian long-term study.

Item compared	Framingham study[38]	Framingham study[40]		Manitoba study[26]
Report population	303 of 5,184 study participants, aged 30–89 years, incident AF occurring with during 15 biennial periods from 1948 to 1978	621 participants, aged 55–94 years, with incident AF or AFL (48% men) occurring during 20 biennial periods from 1948 to 1988		300 men with incident AF during 44-year follow-up; the men, eligible for pilot training, were aged 18–62 years at entry in 1948
Follow-up (years)	30	Up to 40		Up to 44
Incidence/1,000 person-years	Men 5.9, women 3.8. Incidence strongly age-dependent: rate <1 at age <50 years; threefold increase in men and twofold increase in women in each successive decade (2-year incidence of chronic nonrheumatic AF)	–		Age-specific incidence of AF: <0.5 at age <50 years, 2.3 by age 60 years, 16.9 by age 85 years. 5.7 at age >60 years, 9.7 at age >70 years
Comparison group	Participants without AF	Approximately two subjects without AF matched for each AF subject by age, sex, time of incident AF		Remaining 3,683 men of the cohort
Mortality risk or risk of stroke	Overall 2-year rate of strokes 76/1,000 in persons with AF vs 6.2/1,000 in persons without AF (rate ratio 12.3). The proportion of strokes associated with AF 14.7% increasing progressively from 6.7% at age 50–59 years to 36.2% at age 80–89 years	Mortality risk Men 1.5 (1.2, 1.8)	Women 1.9 (1.6, 2.3)	Mortality risk 1.31 (1.08, 1.59) Risk of stroke 2.07 (1.43, 3.01)
Adjustment	–	Age, hypertension, smoking, diabetes, ECG-LVH, MI, CHF, valvular heart failure, and stroke		Significant predictors of AF in multivariable models (ischemic heart disease, valvular disease, CHF, hypertension, cardiomyopathy, palpitations, obesity, other arrhythmias)

AF atrial fibrillation, *CHF* congestive heart failure, *ECG-LVH* left ventricular hypertrophy by ECG criteria, *MI* myocardial infarction.

nial periods.[38] The study group was free of rheumatic heart disease and did not have an AF at the start of each biennial examination. The overall rate of stroke in participants with chronic nonrheumatic AF was 76/1,000 persons, compared with 6.2/1,000 in persons without AF. This gives the rate ratio as high as 12.3. Nearly 15% of all strokes were associated with AF, with the proportion increasing progressively from 7% at age 50–59 years to 36% at age 80–89 years.

A later Framingham report (not shown) summarized the risk of stroke associated with incident nonrheumatic AF in 311 participants after 34 years of follow-up.[39] The study estimated that the risk of stroke was more than tripled in the presence of hypertension, more than doubled in the presence of CHD, more than fourfold in the presence of CHF, and nearly fivefold in the presence of AF. When adjusted for the other comorbid conditions, the relative risk of stroke for AF ranged from 2.6 to 4.0 in the youngest three age groups (50–59 years). In the oldest age group (80–89 years), the relative risk for AF was 4.5, comparing the oldest age group with the youngest ($p < 0.001$).

The second Framingham study report in Table 5.5 covers data from up to 40 years of follow-up of 621 participants aged 55–94 years with incident AF (possibly including AFL).[40] Compared to matched controls without AF selected at the time of the occurrence of the incident AF, the overall mortality risk ratio in men was 1.5 (1.2, 1.8) and in women 1.9 (1.6, 2.3) (adjusted for age, hypertension, smoking, diabetes, and LVH by ECG criteria). In the subgroups without heart disease or CVD events, the mortality risk ratio was 2.4 (1.8, 3.3) in men and 2.2 (1.6, 3.3) in women.

5.5.2.2 The Manitoba Report

The third report in Table 5.5 comes from a 44-year follow-up of the Manitoba study of men who were eligible for a training program for Royal Canadian Air Force personnel in the 1940s, during and after the Second World War until 1948.[26] The all-cause mortality risk for AF compared with the rest of the cohort without AF was 1.31 (1.08, 1.59), the CVD mortality risk 1.41 (1.11, 1.80), and the risk of stroke 2.07 (1.43, 3.01).

5.5.3 Atrial Fibrillation and the Quality of Life

Atrial fibrillation can be asymptomatic and occur only once or twice a lifetime. It can become more chronic, with episodes lasting for hours or weeks and it can become sustained permanently, resistant to drug therapy and difficult to control by radiofrequency ablation. Atrial flutter often goes back spontaneously to a normal sinus rhythm or it can revert into AF. Concerning the apparent beneficial effect of β-blocker use, it is known that asymptomatic episodes of AF are over ten times more common than symptomatic episodes.[41] The apparent reduced risk of incident AF with β-blocker use may in part be due to reduced symptoms and thus reduced likelihood of detection of paroxysmal episodes.

Both AF and AFL often have a significant impact on the quality of life. Subjects with AF in the MONICA-Augsburg survey were significantly more likely to have sleep disturbances and deteriorated self-reported health status than age- and sex-matched controls.[42] Dyspnea and the feeling of general weakness are often related to palpitations and high heart rate, and reduced exercise tolerance is associated with worsening of these symptoms. In type 1 AFL with 1 of 2 conduction ventricular rate is commonly approximately 150 cpm (one-half of the flutter rate), and the ventricular response rate in AF is often 100–150 cpm and very irregular. Chronic AF leading into CHF may be associated with lightheadedness, syncope and cardiac arrest as an outcome.

Van den Berg et al. evaluated autonomic function and symptoms as predictors of the quality of life in 73 patients with frequent paroxysmal AF.[43] The patients had on the average a 3-year history of one paroxysm a week of 2 hours duration. Quality of life assessed by a health survey questionnaire was significantly lower ($p < 0.01$) in patients with paroxysmal AF than in matched controls in four of the eight subscales (physical and emotional role functions, vitality, and general health). Heart rate variability measures of autonomic function (baroreflex sensitivity, total power, response to deep breathing, and heart rate variability response to standing up) were predictive of all of the four subscales in a multivariate model ($p < 0.05$). Interestingly, the frequency of paroxysm was predictive only of physical function. Symptoms, severe respiration in particular, were also significant predictors of low scores at the level of $p < 0.05$. Structural heart disease was not a significant Predictor of quality of life.

The quality of life is a factor to be considered when contemplating intervention for AF.

5.5.4 Intervention for Atrial Fibrillation and Mortality Risk

5.5.4.1 Rate Control versus Rhythm Control

The current conservative medical strategy for control of AF is either rhythm-control therapy (cardioversion followed by drug therapy to maintain sinus rhythm) or rate control (permitting AF to continue and using rate-controlling drugs to alleviate symptoms), with anticoagulant therapy recommended in both approaches. The results from two intervention reports will be considered next (Table 5.6). The first report by the Atrial Fibrillation Follow-up Investigation of Rhythm Management (AFFIRM) investigators is from a controlled randomized multicenter clinical trial involving 4,060 patients considered at high risk of stroke or death.[44] A large fraction (71%) of the patients had a history of hypertension and 38% had coronary artery disease. Two-thirds (65%) of the 3,311 patients with echo evaluation had an enlarged left atrium, and a quarter (26%) had depressed left ventricular function. The 5-year mortality rates, the primary endpoint of the trial, were 23.8 and 21.3% in the rhythm-control and the rate-control group, respectively, with a hazard ratio 1.15 (0.99, 1.34), $p = 0.08$. There were more hospitalizations and adverse drug effects in the rhythm-control group than the rate-control group. Most strokes in both groups occurred after discontinuation of anticoagulant therapy or with a sub-therapeutic level of the drug. The authors concluded that the rhythm-control approach offers no advantage over the rate-control strategy, and in fact may have a potentially higher risk of adverse drug effects.

The second report in Table 5.6, also from 2002, compared rate-control and rhythm-control therapies in 522 patients in whom AF persisted after previous cardioversion.[45] Serial cardioversions were used in the rhythm-control group, otherwise

therapeutic approaches were similar to those in the AFFIRM study. In the rhythm-control group of 266 patients, 39% were in sinus rhythm after a mean of 2.3 years, compared to 10% of the 256 patients in the rate-control group. The primary endpoint (composite death from CVD, heart failure, thromboembolic complications, bleeding with the implantation of a pacemaker, and severe adverse drug effects) was documented in 44 (17.2%) and 60 (22.6%) in the rate-control and the rhythm-control groups, respectively. The authors concluded that the rate control is not inferior to rhythm control, and may be an appropriate therapy in patients with recurrent sustained AF after cardioversion.

5.5.4.2 Circumferential Ablation around Pulmonary Vein Ostium

From the pathophysiological point of view, it still would be a rational goal to restore the normal sinus rhythm in AF patients, to avoid the need for long-term anticoagulation and adverse effects of antiarrhythmic drugs, the risk of thromboembolism, and to achieve improved cardiac function and long-term survival. Atrial fibrillation may substantially reduce cardiac output and cerebral blood flow. Like therapeutic approaches to many cardiac conditions, the strategies for AF control keep changing with the introduction of new drugs and invasive procedures.

The third report in Table 5.6 summarizes new results from an extensive Italian study on circumferential ablation creating conduction block around each pulmonary vein ostium.[46] The ablation group of 589 patients was compared with a group of 582 patients with antiarrhythmic medication for rhythm control throughout the follow-up period. The two groups were obtained from 1,171 referral patients with symptomatic AF. The trial was not strictly randomized for ethical reasons, and the choice of the treatment group was made either by the patient or by the judgment of an electrophysiologist. The Kaplan-Meier plots for survival rates of the two groups were compared, and they were also compared with the life expectancy in the general Italian population of the same age and gender. Hazard ratios were determined from Cox models to estimate treatment effect on all-cause mortality, adverse

TABLE 5.6 Comparative effect of intervention strategies for atrial fibrillation control in three clinical trials.

	AFFIRM study[44]	Dutch AF control study[45]	Italian ablation study[46]
Report population	4,060 patients with AF at high risk of stroke or death, enrolled in a multicenter study; mean age 70 years, 61% males	522 patients with persistent AF or AFL (in 7%) after previous cardioversion, randomly assigned to rate- or rhythm-control groups; mean age 68 years, 63% males	589 referral patients with AF who underwent circumferential pulmonary vein ablation and 582 patients receiving medical treatment for sinus rhythm control (antiarrhythmics and cardioversion, if necessary)
Primary objective	To compare rate and rhythm control in AF for all-cause mortality	To compare rate and rhythm control in AF for a composite endpoint (testing the hypothesis that rate control was not inferior to rhythm control)	To compare ablation with medical treatment of AF for effectiveness for long-term maintenance of sinus rhythm
Comorbid conditions	Hypertension in 71% (predominant diagnosis in 51%), CAD in 38% (predominant diagnosis in 26%)	History of hypertension 49% (proportion higher in rhythm-control group), chronic obstructive lung disease 20%, CHF 50%, CAD 27%, valvular disease 17%, cardiomyopathy 9%	Hypertension 46 and 43% in the ablation group and medical group, respectively; CAD 23 and 22%, respectively; diabetes, cardiomyopathy and chronic lung disease approximately 10, 10 and 5%, respectively, in both groups
Primary endpoint	All-cause mortality	Composite death from CVD, CHF, thromboembolic causes, bleeding, pacemaker implantation, and severe drug side-effects	AF recurrence, all-cause mortality
Follow-up	Mean 3.5 years (maximum 6 years)	2.6 years from the assembly of the cohort between June 1, 1998 and July 1, 2001	Median follow-up 900 days
Comparison group Mortality risk (95% CI) or difference in composite endpoint	Rate-control group HR 1.15 (0.99, 1.34), $p = 0.08$	Rate-control group 17.2%, outcome rate difference 5.4%(−11.0, 0.4), with absolute difference ≤10.0%, confirming the noninferiority of the rate control. With the adjustment for hypertension prevalence difference between the groups, the absolute difference (rate-control group − rhythm-control group) −4.2% (−10.0 to 1.5%)	Medical group HR 0.30 (0.24, 0.37) Maintenance of sinus rhythm (entered as time-dependent covariate into Cox regression) was associated with a significant reduction in mortality, with a hazard ratio HR = 0.24 (0.16, 0.37), and adverse events HR = 0.22 (0.15, 0.31) with both groups combined
Comments	The use of multiple drugs was permitted, and warfarin use was common in both study groups. Also, cross-over between the groups was permitted, and was more common in the rhythm-control group ($p < 0.001$)		Survival for ablated patients not different from that for age- and gender-matched general Italian population

AF atrial fibrillation, *AFL* atrial flutter, *CAD* coronary artery disease, *CHD* coronary heart disease, *CHF* congestive heart failure, *CI* confidence interval, *CVD* cardiovascular disease, *HR* hazard ratio.

events, and recurrence of AF. In addition, the effect of maintaining sinus rhythm was evaluated with the Cox model including a time-dependent variable that was assigned a value of 1 until the first recurrent AF occurred, and 0 thereafter.

At the end of the follow-up, 38 (6%) of the patients in the ablation group and 83 (14%) in the medical group had died. The observed survival probabilities at 1, 2, and 3 years were 98, 95, and 92%, respectively, among the ablation group, and 96, 90, and 80%, respectively, in the medical therapy group ($p < 0.001$). The observed survival of the ablated group was not significantly different from that of the age- and gender-matched Italian population. The reduction in the risk of death in the ablated patients was 54%. Maintaining sinus rhythm was associated with a significantly lower mortality risk in all patients combined from both study groups, with hazard ratio 0.24 (0.16, 0.37). Compared with the medical group, the hazard ratio for all-cause mortality was 0.46 (0.31, 0.68), $p < 0.001$, before entering the sinus rhythm variable and it went to 0.66 (0.44, 0.97), $p = 0.04$, after entering the maintained sinus rhythm variable.

Compared with the medical group, the ablation group was more than twice less likely to have morbid events (recurrent AF or other major morbid events) (hazard ratio 0.45 [0.31, 0.64]). Control of recurrent AF translates to improved quality of life, which was, as expected, similarly and significantly reduced for physical and mental functions in both study groups at the baseline compared to the general Italian population ($p < 0.001$). At 1 year, there was a significantly improving time trend ($p = 0.007$) in the ablation group but not in the medical treatment group. In the ablation group, at 6 months the improving score level had reached the level in the general population.

5.5.5 Radiofrequency Ablation and the Quality of Life

Radiofrequency ablation success rate after the initial leaning curve has been reported as high as 93%, with only an exceptional need for repeated ablation during the initial 9 months following the procedure.[47] The impact on quality of life in patients with severe symptomatic chronic drug-resistant AF or flutter is demonstrated by the influence of a successful intervention by radiofrequency ablation.[48] Twelve of the 23 patients received radiofrequency ablation of the AV junction and were placed on pacemaker therapy, and 11 were placed on pacemaker alone (the control group). Comparing the two groups after 15 days, palpitations decreased by 92 and 37%, respectively ($p = 0.004$), rest dyspnea by 79 and 40% ($p > 0.05$), effort dyspnea by 65 and 30% ($p = 0.03$), and exercise intolerance by 54 and 17% ($p = 0.005$). Similar improvements were observed in the control group patients who underwent ablation therapy at the end of the initial controlled study.

There was also a notable improvement in left ventricular function. In 14 of the patients (64%), the New York Association functional class was 3 or higher before ablation but only in three (14%) after ablation therapy.

5.6 Supraventricular Ectopic Activity

Supraventricular ectopic activity discussed here includes atrial ectopic and junctional complexes conducted retroactively to the atria. Like supraventricular arrhythmias in general, supraventricular ectopic activity has received less attention than ventricular ectopic activity mainly because supraventricular ectopic activity is not considered to be associated with excess mortality or morbidity risk.

5.6.1 Criteria for Ectopic Supraventricular Complexes

The criteria for ectopic supraventricular complex (ESVC), including aberrant ESVC and SVT, are defined in Table 5.7, adapted from the Novacode.[1] These criteria, to some extent arbitrary, were formulated to simplify the manual coding procedure. Conditions 3 and 4 in Table 5.7 imply that the P wave is ectopic. The PR interval of the ectopic complex is not always shorter than the PR of the sinal complexes, for instance when the impulse originates in the left atrium. P waveform or polarity is generally changed if the P wave can be distinguished. Condition 5 assumes that the ectopic atrial complex is conducted to the ventricles. It defines the limits for prematurity and acknowledges the fact that the interval following the ectopic complex is generally prolonged. The requirement of sudden shortening and subsequent prolongation of the RR protects against classification of false ectopic complexes in case of marked sinus arrhythmia. Classification of the complex as ectopic on the basis of condition 5 implies that the ectopic premature impulse may occasionally originate outside the SA node even when the P wave morphology is similar to the sinal P wave.

Active impulse formation in atrial cells anywhere outside the SA node can initiate an excita-

TABLE 5.7 Criteria for nonaberrant and aberrant ectopic supraventricular complex and supraventricular tachycardia classification.

ESVC category	Criteria
Nonaberrant ESVC	C1. Basic rhythm is sinus rhythm
	C2. QRS morphology matches the morphology of the sinal QRS complexes, with QRS duration within 20 ms
	C3. P amplitude differs by more than 100 μV from the sinal P waves of the basic rhythm, or there is a retrograde P wave, or no P wave is discernible
	C4. PR is at least 40 ms shorter than the PR of the sinal complexes
	C5. RR of the premature complex is at least 200 ms shorter than the preceding RR and at least 240 ms longer than the RR following the premature complex
	Nonaberrant ESVC = C1 and C2 and (C4 or C5)
Aberrant ESVC	C1. Basic rhythm is sinus rhythm
	C2. QRS duration is ≥20 longer than that of the normally conducted sinal QRS complexes
	C3. Ectopic P wave precedes QRS complex
	C4. RBBB patterns (RSR2 with R2 > R) in V1, with QRS duration ≤140 ms
	C5. QRS ≤140 ms
	Aberrant ESVC = C1 and C2 and (C3 or [C4 and C5])
SVT*	C1. ≥6 successive ESVC
	C2. Ventricular rate ≥95 cpm
	SVT = C1 and C2

ESVC ectopic supraventricular complex, *RBBB* right bundle branch block, *SVT* supraventricular tachycardia.

* Subcategories of SVT are distinguished on the basis of ventricular rate (fast, ≥130 cpm and slow, <130 cpm).

tion wave front that propagates through the atria reaching also the AV node and the SA node. This temporarily suppresses the SA node. The interval from the ESVC to the following sinal QRS complex is longer than the normal RR interval because of the suppressed state of the SA node. The post-ectopic pause is usually not fully compensatory, as is the case with the ectopic ventricular complex (EVC). Thus, the sum of two RR intervals (the intervals preceding and following ESVC) is shorter than the sum of two RR intervals of the basic sinal rhythm. The exception occurs when the normally timed sinus impulse fires before the wave front from the ectopic atrial impulse reaches it and the fusion of the normal sinal and ectopic wave fronts occurs somewhere near the sinus region. In this case the pause following an ESVC may be fully compensatory.

The coupling interval from the preceding sinal QRS to ESVC tends to be constant as it should if atrial conduction, including the conduction in the suppressed area, remains constant. However, variations in the coupling interval are often observed and this is not so easily explained. Excitation of the ventricles takes place like in normal sinal conduction, except when the ESVC is aberrant. The aberrancy is influenced by the timing of the ESVC in relation to the recovery from the refractory period.

Concerning aberrant ESVC, differentiation from EVC can be difficult. There are some helpful hints. The RR interval of the premature EVC is generally at least 200 ms shorter than the preceding RR and at least 240 ms longer than the RR following the premature complex. An ectopic P wave preceding the widened QRS complex in general rules out an ectopic ventricular complex. However, if there is a P wave with normal morphology appearing with the expected timing, a widened QRS is more likely to indicate a fusion complex, and it is classified as a ventricular rather than an aberrant supraventricular complex. True EVC and a fusion complex in general have QRS duration more than 140 ms. Right bundle branch block (RBBB) pattern in V1 has an increased likelihood of indicating an aberrant complex of supraventricular origin because aberrancy often originates from blocked conduction in the right bundle branch. This is because this branch may still be in the functional refractory state if the ectopic impulse originates high in the AV nodal or junctional area.

A short coupling interval of the widened complex and a long RR interval preceding it promote the likelihood of aberrancy.

5.6.2 The Mechanism of Supraventricular Ectopic Activity

Two basic mechanisms are generally considered as a possible explanation for supraventricular ectopic activity. The first is the so-called focal mechanism, which assumes that because of increased excitability and instability in a focal region, these myocytes temporarily act like pacemaker cells and may reach a threshold level for depolarization. Active impulse formation in atrial myocytes anywhere outside the SA node can initiate an excitation wave front, which propagates through the atria.

The second, so-called re-entry mechanism postulates that there is a zone with depressed conductivity in the vicinity of the focal zone where the ectopic impulse originates. When these myocytes reach depolarized state, the surrounding normal tissue has already recovered from the refractory state of the previous normal excitation cycle, and the re-entry from the ectopic focus initiates a new excitation wave front propagating through the atria. A third mechanism for the generation of supraventricular ectopic activity has occasionally been postulated. This postulate asserts that repetitive firing is caused by triggered activity due to delayed afterdepolarizations.

5.6.3 Symptoms of Recurrent Supraventricular Arrhythmias

Recurrent supraventricular arrhythmias, at times called tachyarrhythmias, are commonly symptomatic, occurring with sensation of palpitations, weakness, and at times with syncopes, often with life-long symptoms. Like AF, paroxysmal SVT is a common condition for which antiarrhythmic drug therapy is applied. However, the success rate has not been entirely satisfactory. In paroxysmal SVT, the re-entry is through the AV node or through a concealed bypass tract (AV nodal re-entrant tachycardia and macro re-entrant tachycardias). In the latter, the accessory pathway is commonly in the left atrial or posteroseptal site, less commonly midseptal, anteroseptal site or in the right atrial free wall.[49]

An early report on a population of 382 patients with electronic pacemakers assessed the conditions prevailing before pacemaker implantation.[50] Over one-half of the patients had had syncopal attacks and tachyarrhythmias (54 and 57%, respectively). Supraventricular tachycardia (or atrial tachycardia) was documented in one-third of the patients before pacemaker implantation. The condition, the sino-atrial syndrome, was the only manifestation of heart disease in 20%. Coronary heart disease as an underlying condition was present in 61%, and 20% of the patients had had a previous MI. It was noted that during an average of 23 months of follow-up, syncopal attacks had

stopped in 48 out of 49 patients and tachyarrhythmias were successfully controlled by combined drug treatment in 43 of 51 patients.

Improved electrophysiological procedures (epicardial mapping) have facilitated accurate locating of the accessory pathway. Surgical procedures have recently been used as a therapeutic action in re-entrant SVT, with up to 98% reported success rate in interrupting accessory pathways and mortality rates within 1–2% even among patients with other organic heart disease.[49] Surgical therapy in other forms of SVT is largely limited to AF and to WPW in cases where catheter ablation has not been successful.

5.6.4 Prevalence of Supraventricular Ectopic Complexes

In the Finnish Social Insurance Institution's Coronary Heart Disease Study,[51] the age-adjusted prevalence of any ESVC in the 12-lead ECG (15-s recording) was 1.2% in men and 1.5% in women in this population sample aged 30–59 years. The prevalence of frequent (>10% of complexes) ESVC was 0.5% in both men and women. There was no obvious age trend in the prevalence in men. In women, the prevalence was low in the younger age groups and increased in a stepwise fashion after the age of 45 years. The prevalence of any ESVC was 0.7% in age group 30–44 years and 2.4% in age group 45–59 years. This probably reflects atrial electrical instability with the lability of the autonomic nervous system's modulating functions or hormonal changes with menopause. Hormonal factors may play a role concerning atrial ectopic activity, also reflected in the observed premenstrual increase in the incidence of spontaneous atrial arrhythmias. Induction of SVT during electrophysiological testing has been reported to be diminished at periods of higher estrogen levels during the menstrual cycle.[52]

In CHS, the prevalence of arrhythmic events in 24-hour ambulatory ECG was evaluated in 1,372 men and women 65 years old and older from four communities.[27] Nearly all men and women (97%) had ESVCs; these were frequent (≥ 15/h) in 18% of the women and in 28% of the men ($p = 0.0001$ for gender difference). Persons with frequent ESVC were significantly older than those without them. The prevalence of ESVC activity (≥ 15 complexes/h or runs ≥ 3 complexes) did not differ by gender but it was strongly associated with advancing age. In a multivariate model, an increment by 7 years in age had an odds ratio for ESVC activity 1.53 (1.20, 1.95) in women and 1.77 (1.39, 2.25) in men. Other factors with a significant independent positive association with ESVC activity were increased left atrial size and, in women, also digitalis use.

5.7 Supraventricular Tachycardia

Paroxysmal SVT should be distinguished from tachycardias associated with WPW syndrome and other re-entrant tachycardias with accessory AV pathways. The impression that accessory AV pathways are the most common mechanisms for paroxysmal SVT comes from earlier reports based on hospital discharge statistics because they included a preferential selection for hospital admission of patients amenable to surgical intervention, a selection bias as pointed out by Orejarena et al.[53]

Clinically, the ESVC rate for defining SVT is ≥ 120 cpm. It is more logical, however, to use the limiting rate at the upper normal limit for heart rate for adults, 95 cpm as in Table 5.7, to avoid gaps in classification hierarchy. Supraventricular tachycardia subcategories of fast (ESVC rate ≥ 130 cpm) and slow (ESVC rate <130 cpm) can then be established. Clinically, SVT is categorized also as transient or persistent.

5.7.1 Prevalence and Incidence of Supraventricular Tachycardia – the Marshfield Study

The estimation of the prevalence of SVT is largely limited to data from clinical centers and referral hospitals. The establishment of prevalence estimates in the general population faces several problems. First of all, the prevalence is fairly low and particularly incidence estimation would require a large sample size. Secondly, in paroxysmal SVT, these transient events occur infrequently and the probability of their detection from short-term ECG recordings like the standard 10-s ECG is low.

The Marshfield study from 1998 is presumably the first population-based investigation of parox-

ysmal SVT.[53] Because of the lack of reliable SVT and incidence data from other population-based studies, the results from the Marshfield study are reported here in some detail. Using a unique data pool covering health care reports of approximately 50,000 area residents, the study identified 2,223 potential paroxysmal SVT cases using four ICD-9-CM codes. The review of the ECGs and clinical records of a subsample of 600 patients confirmed only 31 cases of SVT, illustrating the difficulty of extracting true paroxysmal SVT using the ICD codes.

Screening for potential SVT cases in the data base was done using ICD-9-CM codes for paroxysmal SVT and, in addition, three other codes (anomalous AV excitation, other cardiac arrhythmias and cardiac arrhythmia, unspecified). Estimation of the "verifiable fraction" of true paroxysmal SVT cases from the potential prevalence cases from these four categories was done by using a random sample of 600 cases. This process yielded 31 true prevalent cases among the 600 potential cases, i.e. the verifiable fraction was 0.052. The incidence was established by reviewing the records of all area residents with a new potential paroxysmal SVT classification in the same four ICD classification categories as was used for prevalence estimation. This yielded 1,163 potential incidence cases. A review of all records in this group yielded 33 confirmed incident cases, i.e. the verifiable fraction was 0.028. It was also noted that 61% of verifiable incident cases would have been missed if the screening had been limited solely to paroxysmal SVT codes.

The investigators estimated that the crude proportion of the area residents who had received a paroxysmal SVT diagnosis over the 12-year period preceding July 1, 1991 was 2.25/1,000. It was 1.65 in persons less than 65 years old and 6.16 in persons 65 years old and older. The overall incidence of paroxysmal SVT was 35 per 100,000 person-years (95% confidence interval 23–47), estimated retroactively, apparently over the whole 12-year observation period. Thus, it is difficult to get an idea of the annual SVT incidence because of the unknown observation period in each case, or even the average observation period. The incidence per 100,000 person-years was 13 (range 0–27) before the age of 20 years; it was 27 (13–40) in age group 20–64 years, and increased to 122 (60–184) in persons 65 years old and older. The increaseed incidence in older age groups in men was largely related to the common association of paroxysmal SVT with CVD in older men. The increased incidence in postmenopausal women may be associated with hormonal factors. Plasma concentration of ovarian hormones has been reported to correlate with the occurrence of episodes of paroxysmal SVT,[52,54] suggesting that estrogen may protect against initiation of paroxysmal SVT.

The group of 33 new paroxysmal SVT cases in the Marshfield survey was examined in detail. The mean age at the time when SVT was first documented was 57 years, with a wide range (infancy to 90 years). Of the incident cases, 70% were women. The relative risk of incident SVT in women compared to men was 2.0 (1.0, 4.2), and the relative risk for persons ≥65 years compared to persons <65 years old was 5.3 (2.7, 10.5). Cardiovascular disease was present in 20 (61%) of the 33 persons with incident SVT; it occurred in 90% of the men and 48% of the women in this group (the sex difference was only marginally significant [$p = 0.0495$] because of the small number of incident cases). The CVD category here included persons with hypertension, which was present in nearly one-half of the incident cases (15/33). It was noted that ECG evidence of WPW (delta wave and short PR) was observed in only one of the 33 incident cases. Isolated incident SVT in the absence of CVD was defined as lone SVT. Lone SVT was present in 13 of the 33 incident cases – 12 of these 13 were women. The onset of symptoms in lone paroxysmal SVT took place in general earlier in life than SVT in persons with CVD, both in men and in women, and the average ventricular rate of the first documented episode of SVT was higher in persons with lone SVT than in persons with SVT associated with CVD, 186 cpm versus 155 cpm.

In six patients in whom electrophysiological studies were performed, AV nodal re-entry tachycardia was found in five. The subject with WPW syndrome had an AV re-entrant tachycardia termed orthodromic (early antegrade excitation of the ventricles through the bypass tract and re-entry path to the atria through the AV node).

Adjusting for age and gender in the US population according to the 1990 US census as the standard, the adjusted SVT prevalence was 2.29 per 1,000 persons, and the incidence 36 per 100,000 persons. Assuming that the rates can be extrapolated to the entire US population, the investigators estimated that there would be 570,000 persons with paroxysmal SVT in the USA, with nearly 89,000 incident cases per year. Of the nearly 89,000 incident cases, an estimated 35,000 would probably be lone SVT, and approximately 54,000 associated with CVD.

5.7.2 Prevalence and Incidence of Supraventricular Tachycardias in other Studies

In the Manitoba prospective 40-year follow-up study of a group of 3,983 initially healthy men,[55] the reported SVT incidence was 1 per 6,000 person-years, or 17 per 100,000 person-years. This incidence in men between ages 30–80 years included narrow QRS tachycardia, excluding overt WPW, and the incidence was determined for cases before clinical or ECG manifestations of ischemic heart disease. Interestingly, in the Manitoba follow-up study, hypertension did not increase the risk of developing SVT, and 27% of the incident SVT cases subsequently developed AF documented by ECG.

In the CHS population, the prevalence of short SVT runs (≥three successive complexes) in 24-h ambulatory ECG was high, 50% in women and 48% in men.[27]

In a series of 88 successive orthotopic transplantations, SVT occurred at least once in 11 recipients and atrial tachycardia in three recipients.[56] Supraventricular tachycardia is also common after coronary artery bypass surgery.[57] In a series of 800 consecutive patients, 186 (23%) developed postoperative supraventricular arrhythmias. These arrhythmias did not contribute to any of the six deaths during the 30-day postoperative period. In multivariate logistic regression analysis, age of 65 years or more, history of atrial arrhythmia or preoperative premature atrial complexes, and left ventricular end-diastolic pressure 20 mmHg or more were identified as having an independent association with the incidence of postoperative supraventricular arrhythmia. Sinus rhythm was restored by treatment with beta-adrenergic blocking agents or digoxin (or combined therapy) in 82% of patients with supraventricular arrhythmia; the conversion was spontaneous in 6%, and 10% required electrical cardioversion.

References

1. Rautaharju PM, Park LP, Chaitman BR et al. The Novacode criteria for classification of ECG abnormalities and their clinically significant progression and regression. J Electrocardiol 1998; 31:157–87.

2. Stambler BS, Ellenbogen KA. Elucidating the mechanisms of atrial flutter cycle length variability using power spectral analysis techniques. Circulation 1996;94:2515–25.

3. Shah DC, Jaïs P, Haïssaguerre M et al. Three-dimensional mapping of the common atrial flutter circuit in the right atrium. Circulation 1997; 96:3904–12.

4. Cosio FG, Goicolea A, López-Gil M et al. Atrial endocardial mapping in the rare form of atrial flutter. Am J Cardiol 1990;66:715–20.

5. Okumura K, Plumb VJ, Pagé PL et al. Atrial activation sequence during atrial flutter in the canine pericarditis model and its effects on the polarity of the flutter wave in the electrocardiogram. J Am Coll Cardiol 1991;17:509–18.

6. Cheng J, Cabeen WR, Scheinman MM. Right atrial flutter due to lower loop reentry. Mechanism and anatomic substrates. Circulation 1999;99:1700–5.

7. Waldo AL, Cooper TB. Spontaneous onset of type 1 flutter in patients. J Am Coll Cardiol 1996; 28:707–12.

8. Olgin JE, Kalman JM et al. Mechanism of initiation of atrial flutter in humans: site of unidirectional block and direction of rotation. J Am Coll Cardiol 1997;29:376–84.

9. Suzuki F, Toshida N, Nawata H et al. Coronary sinus pacing initiates counterclockwise atrial flutter while pacing from the low lateral right atrium initiates clockwise atrial flutter. Analysis of episodes of direct initiation of atrial flutter. J Electrocardiol 1998;31:345–61.

10. Granada, J, Uribe W, Chyou PH et al. Incidence and predictors of atrial flutter in the general population. J Am Coll Cardiol 2000;36:2242–6.

11. Rensma PL, Allessie MA, Lammers WJEP et al. The length of the excitation wave as an index for the susceptibility to re-entrant atrial arrhythmias. Circ Res 1988;62:395–410.

12. Vidaillet H, Granada JF, Chyou PH et al. A population-based study of mortality among patients with atrial fibrillation or flutter. Am J Med 2002; 113:365–70.

13. Moe GK, Abildskov JA. Atrial fibrillation as a self sustaining arrhythmia independent of focal discharge. Am Heart J 1959;58:59–70.

14. Moe GK, Rheinboldt WC, Abildskov JA. A computer model of atrial fibrillation. Am Heart J 1964:67200–20.

15. Alessie MA, Lammers WJEP, Bonke FIM, Hollen J. Experimental evaluation of Moe's multiple wavelet hypothesis of atrial fibrillation. In: Zipes DP, Jalife J (eds). Cardiac Arrhythmias. New York: Grune & Stratton, 1985, pp 265–76.

16. Wijffels MC, Kirchhof CJ, Dorland R, Allessie MA. Atrial fibrillation begets atrial fibrillation. A study in awake chronically instrumented goats. Circulation 1995;92:1954–68.

17. Wijffels MC, Kirchhof CJ, Dorland R et al. Electrical modeling due to atrial fibrillation in chronically instrumented conscious goats: roles of neurohormonal changes, ischemia, atrial stretch, and high rate of electrical activation. Circulation 1997; 96:3710–20.

18. Daoud EG, Bogun F, Goyal R et al. Effect of atrial fibrillation on atrial refractoriness in humans. Circulation 1996;94:1600–6.

19. O'Hara G, Villemaire C, Talajic M, Nattel S. Effects of flecainide on the rate dependence of atrial refractoriness, atrial repolarization and atrioventricular node conduction in anesthetized dogs. J Am Coll Cardiol 1992;19:1335–42.

20. Gajewski J, Singer RB. Mortality in an injured population with atrial fibrillation. JAMA 1981; 245:1540–4.

21. Onundarson PT, Thorgeirsson G, Jonmundsson E et al. Chronic atrial fibrillation – epidemiologic features and 14 year follow-up: a case control study. Eur Heart J 1987;8:521–7.

22. Kopecky SL, Gersh BJ, McGoon MD et al. The natural history of lone atrial fibrillation. A population-based study over three decades. N Engl J Med 1987;317:669–74.

23. Brand FN, Abbott RD, Kannel WB, Wolf PA. Characteristics and prognosis of lone atrial fibrillation. 30-year follow-up in the Framingham Study. JAMA 1985;254:3449–53.

24. Lake FR, Cullen KJ, de Klerk NH et al. Atrial fibrillation and mortality in an elderly population. Aust N Z Med 1989;19:321–6.

25. Benjamin EJ, Levy D, Vaziri SM et al. Independent risk factors for atrial fibrillation in a population-based cohort. The Framingham Study. JAMA 1994;271:840–4.

26. Krahn AD, Manfreda J, Tate RB et al. The natural history of atrial fibrillation: incidence, risk factors, and prognosis in the Manitoba Follow-up Study. Am J Med 1995;98:476–84.

27. Manolio TA, Furberg CD, Rautaharju PM et al. Cardiac arrhythmias on a 24-hour ambulatory electrocardiography in older women and men. The Cardiovascular Health Study. J Am Coll Cardiol 1994;23:916–25.

28. Furberg CD, Psaty BM, Manolio TA et al. Prevalence of atrial fibrillation in elderly subjects (the Cardiovascular Health Study). Am J Cardiol 1994;74:236–41.

29. Psaty BM, Manolio TA, Kuller LH et al. Incidence of and risk factors for atrial fibrillation in older adults. Circulation 1997;96:2455–61.

30. Wolf PA, Benjamin EJ, Belanger AJ et al. Secular trends in the prevalence of atrial fibrillation: The Framingham Study. Am Heart J 1996;131: 790–5.

31. Liang KY, Zeger SL. Longitudinal data analysis using generalized linear models. Biometrica 1988;73:13–22.

32. Haupt BJ, Graves EJ. Detailed diagnoses and procedures for patients discharged from short-stay hospitals, United States, 1979. Department of Health and Human Services publication no. (PHS) 82–1974–1. Hyattsville, Maryland: National Center for Health Statistics, 1982.

33. Graves EJ. Detailed diagnoses and procedures, National Hospital Discharge Survey. Vital Health Statistics (13). Hyattsville, Maryland: National Center for Health Statistics (118), 1994.

34. Vaziri SM, Larson MG, Benjamin EJ, Levy D. Echocardiographic predictors of nonrheumatic atrial fibrillation. The Framingham Heart Study. Circulation 1994;89:724–30.

35. Chang EK. Principles of Cardiac Arrhythmias, 2nd edn. Baltimore/London: Williams &Wilkins, 1980, p 160.

36. Bayes de Luna A, de Ribot RF. Electrocardiographic and vectorcardiographic study of interatrial conduction disturbances with left atrial retrograde activation. J Electrocardiol 1985;18:1–14.

37. Flegel KM, Shipley MJ, Rose G. Risk of stroke in nonrheumatic atrial fibrillation. Lancet 1987; 1:526–9.

38. Wolf PA, Abbott RD, Kannel WB. Atrial fibrillation: a major contributor to stroke in the elderly. Arch Intern Med 1987;147:1561–4.

39. Wolf PA, Abbott RD, Kannel WB. Atrial fibrillation as an independent risk factor for stroke: the Framingham Study. Stroke 1991;22:983–8.

40. Benjamin EJ, Wolf PA, D'Agostino RB et al. Impact of atrial fibrillation on the risk of death. The Framingham Study. Circulation 1998; 98:946–52.

41. Page RL, Wilkinson WE, Clair WK et al. Asymptomatic arrhythmias in patients with symptomatic paroxysmal atrial fibrillation and paroxysmal supraventricular tachycardia. Circulation 1994; 89:224–7.

42. Gehring J, Perz S, Stieber J et al. Cardiovascular risk factors, ECG abnormalities and quality of life in subjects with atrial fibrillation. Sozial-Präventivmedizin 1996;41:185–93.

43. van den Berg MP, Hassink RJ, Tuinenburg AE et al. Quality of life in patients with paroxysmal atrial fibrillation and its predictors: importance of the autonomic nervous system. Eur Heart J 2001;22: 247–53.

44. Atrial Fibrillation Follow-up Investigation of Rhythm Management (AFFIRM) Investigators. A comparison of rate control and rhythm control in patients with atrial fibrillation. N Engl J Med 2002;347:1825–33.

45. Van Gelder IC, Hagens VE, Bosker HA et al. Rate Control versus Electrical Cardioversion for Persistent Atrial Fibrillation Study Group. A comparison of rate control and rhythm control in patients with recurrent persistent atrial fibrillation. N Engl J Med 2002;347:1834–40.

46. Pappone C, Rosanio S, Augello G et al. Mortality, morbidity, and quality of life after circumferential pulmonary vein ablation for atrial fibrillation: outcomes from a controlled nonrandomized long-term study. J Am Coll Cardiol 2003;42: 185–97.

47. Sathe S, Vohra J, Chan W. Radiofrequency catheter ablation for paroxysmal supraventricular tachycardia: a report of 135 procedures. Aust N Z J Med 1993;23:317–24.

48. Brignole M, Gianfranchi L, Menozzi C et al. Influence of atrioventricular junction radiofrequency ablation in patients with chronic atrial fibrillation and flutter on quality of life and cardiac performance. Am J Cardiol 1994;74:242–6.

49. Prystowsky EN, Packer D. Nonpharmacologic treatment of supraventricular tachycardia. Am J Cardiol 1988;62:74L-77L.

50. Härtel G, Talvensaari T. Treatment of sinoatrial syndrome with permanent cardiac pacing in 90 patients. Acta Med Scand 1975;198:341–7.

51. Reunanen A, Aromaa A, Pyörälä K et al. The Social Insurance Institution's Coronary Heart Disease Study. Acta Med Scand 1983;Suppl 673:1–120.

52. Myerburg RJ, Cox MM, Interian A Jr et al. Cycling of inducibility of paroxysmal supraventricular tachycardia in women and its implications for timing of electrophysiologic procedures. Am J Cardiol 1999;83:1049–54.

53. Orejarena LA, Vidaillet H Jr, DeStefano F et al. Paroxysmal supraventricular tachycardia in the general population. J Am Coll Cardiol 1998; 31:150–7.

54. Rosano GM, Leonardo F, Sarrel PM et al. Cyclical variation in paroxysmal supraventricular tachycardia in women. Lancet 1996;347:786–8.

55. Mathewson FAC, Manfreda J, Tate RB, Cuddy TE. The University of Manitoba Follow-up Study – an investigation of cardiovascular disease with 35 years of follow-up. Can J Cardiol 1987;40:149–55.

56. Pavri BB, O'Nunain SS, Newell JB et al. Prevalence and prognostic significance of atrial arrhythmias after orthotopic cardiac transplantation. J Am Coll Cardiol 1995;25:1673–80.

57. Hashimoto K, Ilstrup DM, Schaff HV. Influence of clinical and hemodynamic variables on risk of supraventricular tachycardia after coronary bypass. J Thoracic Cardiovasc Surgery 1991;101:56–65.

6A
Ectopic Ventricular Activity

Synopsis

Significance

Increased ectopic ventricular complex (EVC) activity has been conceptually considered as one of the possible triggering mechanisms associated with an increased risk of malignant ventricular arrhythmias.

Mechanism

Ectopic ventricular complex is an excitation/repolarization cycle originating in the ventricles outside the normally conducted excitation from the ventricular conduction system and the Purkinje network. Multiple contributing factors have been postulated, including injury currents, slow or blocked conduction in injured or ischemic zones, afterdepolarizations, triggered automatic activity, and circus movement with re-entry.

Risk Factors

These include older age, higher ventricular rate, decreased forced vital capacity, clinical signs of coronary heart disease (CHD), decreased ejection fraction, height, moderately prolonged QT in women, and hypertension in some but not in all reports.

Prevalence

The prevalence of EVC depends heavily on the ECG recording length and the demographic and clinical characteristics of the population, particularly age and the presence or absence of organic heart disease. The prevalence of any EVC in a 10-s record in community-dwelling adult populations is approximately 3%, with no clear gender difference. The prevalence of one or more EVCs in a 2-min record in adults without evidence of organic heart disease is approximately 5–6%, and it increases approximately twofold from age 45 to 65 years. In longer-term recordings, approximately one-third of ostensibly CHD-free adults have at least one EVC/h, with strong age dependence. The prevalence of frequent EVC (>30 EVC/h) in CHD-free adult populations is approximately 7%.

Classification Problems

Spontaneous variability of EVC activity is large; its assessment is an elaborate undertaking.

Associated Risk

Risk evaluation results vary, depending on study group characteristics, recording length, EVC frequency, and the length of the follow-up. Frequent (≥ 30/h) EVC activity has been associated in population studies with an approximately twofold excess age-adjusted risk of all-cause mortality in CHD-free men, with a lower or nonsignificant mortality risk in similar female groups. Independent mortality risk for EVC in survivors of acute myocardial infarction is over twofold.

Effectiveness of Intervention

There is no evidence that suppression of EVC activity by antiarrhythmic drugs will reduce the mortality risk.

Abbreviations and Acronyms

ARIC – Atherosclerosis Risk in Communities Study

BHAT – Beta-Blocker Heart Attack Trial

CAD – coronary artery disease

CAST – Cardiac Arrhythmia Suppression Trial

CHD – coronary heart disease

CHS – Cardiovascular Health Study

cpm – cycles per minute (refers to heart rate)

EVC – ectopic ventricular complex

ISIS – First International Study of Infarct Survival trial

LBBB – left bundle branch block

LVH – left ventricular hypertrophy

MI – myocardial infarction

MIAMI – Metoprolol in Acute Myocardial Infarction

MILIS – Multicenter Investigation of the Limitation of Infarct Size

MRFIT – Multiple Risk Factor Intervention Trial

NHANES – National Health and Nutrition Examination Survey

RBBB – right bundle branch block

VT – ventricular tachycardia

WPW – Wolf-Parkinson-White syndrome or ECG pattern

6A.1 Introduction

This chapter covers ectopic ventricular complexes (EVC), EVC pairs or couplets, and EVC runs or ventricular tachycardias (VT). Ectopic ventricular complexes can be unifocal, with uniform morphology, or multifocal or polymorphic. A run is characterized by its rate and the number of successive EVCs in it. When longer recording periods are evaluated, the run is defined as transient if the number of EVCs in it is less than a constant (for instance 30), and longer episodes are called sustained runs.

6A.1.1 Criteria for Ectopic Ventricular Complexes

Key criteria of EVC are summarized in Table 6A.1. An EVC has a QRS duration of 120 ms or more, or at least 20 ms longer than the QRS duration of

TABLE 6A.1 Criteria for various categories of ectopic ventricular complexes.

Categories	Criteria
Ectopic ventricular complex (EVC)	C1. QRS ≥120 ms or 20 ms longer than normally conducted sinal QRS
	C2. Criteria for aberrant SVEC are not met
	EVC = C1 and C2
QRS fusion complexes	EVC precedes sinal P wave occurring with normal timing in the P wave train. Counted as EVC
EVC doublet	Two EVCs in succession within one R-R interval. (Three EVCs in succession is coded as transient ventricular tachycardia)
Coalescent EVC	EVC overlaps with the ST-T complex of the preceding QRS-T complex
Polymorphic EVC (PEVC)	C1. QRS amplitude differences of EVCs ≥50%
	C2. QRS duration differences of EVCs ≥20%
	PEVC = C1 and C2
Ventricular bigeminy (VBG)	C1. EVC follows every sinal QRS-T complex
	C2. Coupling intervals differ ≤100 ms
	VBG = C1 and C2
Ventricular trigeminy	EVC after every two sinal QRS-T complexes

normally conducted sinal QRS. In the presence of sustained bundle branch blocks or Wolf-Parkinson-White (WPW) pattern, EVC is identified by the prematurity, compensatory pause, and a distinct change in the waveform. A wide QRS complex with an ectopic or premature P wave preceding QRS is classified as an ectopic supraventricular complex with aberrant conduction. A QRS with no P wave preceding and with duration ≤140 ms and RSR2 patterns in V1 is classified as an ectopic supraventricular complex with aberrant conduction. A wide QRS complex preceded by a nonectopic P wave with a normal timing is considered to be a fusion complex, and is counted as an ectopic ventricular complex.

6A.1.2 Mechanisms of Ectopic Ventricular Complex Activity

Multiple contributing factors have been postulated, including injury currents, slow or blocked conduction in injured or ischemic zones, after-depolarizations, triggered automatic activity, circus movement, and re-entry.[1] Normal cells in the ischemic border zone may repolarize earlier than the ischemic zone cells because of slow conduction and delayed excitation in the ischemic zone, and injury current from injured zone cells may re-excite the normal border zone cells thus eliciting an EVC.[2–4]

Unifocal EVCs have a uniform waveform and, in general, a fixed coupling interval from the preceding QRS. The coupling interval is constant because the conduction time from the onset of ventricular excitation to the ischemic zone where the EVC is triggered is constant. If conditions were stationary from one excitation cycle to the next, one would think that a unifocal EVC with a constant coupling interval follows every normally conducted QRS as is the case in ventricular bigeminy. The occurrence of an EVC mainly as an occasional single event suggests that, in general, there is a block in the entrance or exit region of the ischemic zone. Another possibility is that afterdepolarizations from enough ischemic myocytes have to be present so that when summated, current of adequate strength is generated to initiate a premature excitation.

The waveform of unifocal as well as multifocal EVC depends on the site of the focus. Ectopic ventricular complexes arising from the right side of the ventricles resemble the pattern of a left bundle branch block (LBBB), and those arising from the left side that of a right bundle branch block (RBBB). The EVC induces secondary repolarization abnormalities, with discordant T waves (polarity opposite to the main QRS deflection). Normal synchronization with minimal dispersion of the endocardial onset of excitation from the terminations of the Purkinje fibers is lost, and repolarization tends to follow the same sequence as excitation, particularly in EVCs arising from the right ventricle and septum. There may be alterations in the degree of discordance if there are primary repolarization abnormalities such as takes place in ischemic myocardium.

There is, in general, a full compensatory pause following an EVC (the sum of the RR intervals preceding and following EVC is equal to the sum of two regularly conducted sinal RR intervals), although there may be some variations in case of a sinus arrhythmia. The EVC is usually premature, and the sinus node fires at its expected timing although the P wave may be masked by a slightly premature EVC. The normally conducted QRS following EVC is initiated by the next sinus node firing, and it thus comes one normal PP interval after the hidden P wave (2 PP or RR intervals after the P-QRS complex preceding the EVC). If a retrograde excitation from the EVC arrives at the SA node before its normal firing time, the SA node will be "reset". In this case, the pause is longer than fully compensatory. The retrograde excitation from the ectopic focus usually collides with the excitation initiated by the sinus node in the atria or the AV node (atrial fusion complexes). In this situation the P waves are usually not visible because they are masked by the EVCs.

6A.1.3　Risk Factors for Ectopic Ventricular Complex Activity

Among the risk factors for EVC are older age, higher ventricular rate, decreased forced vital capacity, clinical signs of coronary heart disease (CHD), decreased ejection fraction, height, moderately prolonged QT in women, and hypertension (in some but not in all reports).

6A.1.4　Spontaneous Variability of Ectopic Ventricular Complex Activity

The observed prevalence of EVC depends largely on the study population and the method of assessment, primarily the record length. Chapter 6B indicates that it takes a "true" hourly rate of 360 EVCs or higher (as estimated from a 24-h Holter recording) so that a single EVC could be detected with a 63% likelihood in a 10-s routine ECG recording. Similarly, it takes an average "true" hourly rate of 30 EVCs so that at least a single EVC can be found in a 2-min monitoring period.

Several reports have documented that individual variability increases with time interval between the recordings used for evaluation of the variability. This limits the possibility of detecting the efficacy of antiarrhythmic therapy, particularly the long-term efficacy, in an individual patient. It should also be noted that the spontaneous variability is greater in patients with coronary artery disease (CAD) than in those without CAD, and that the variability is higher in patients with more severe level EVC activity (frequent EVC runs).[5]

Toivonen used linear regression analysis comparing EVC frequency in 24-h ambulatory ECG recorded at short intervals (2–14 days) and long intervals (6–12 months) in 20 patients with frequent EVCs.[6] This investigator used the method introduced by Sami et al. to establish a 95% confidence interval for spontaneous EVC variability.[7] The 95% confidence interval estimate for the spontaneously decreased EVC frequency indicated that the decrease had to be 60% from the initial value of 60 EVC/h or more to be used for a significant decrease for records after the shorter time interval. These findings are reasonably consistent with the report of Sami et al. Other studies on short time interval variability have reported equally high or higher reductions required to reach statistical significance. For the longer time interval in Toivonen's study, the lower confidence limit for required EVC reduction reached 100%. The required reduction of EVC pairs or runs occurring with a frequency of two or more events/h in the initial recording was 78% for the short interval. For the longer interval, not even 100% reduction in pairs or runs was significant. This result indicates that the establishment of the long-term efficacy of antiarrhythmic drugs in reducing EVC frequency is possible only when comparing the mean changes in the treatment and control groups, or possibly by designing a drug withdrawal test. The confidence limits for spontaneous EVC activity and the suggested limits for significant reductions in the above reports may have been underestimates because of methodological problems (Chapter 6B).

6A.1.5 Fractile Dimensions of Ectopic Ventricular Complex Activity

Fractile dimension is a special application of deterministic chaos theory. Fractile dimension D is determined by ranking the intervals between successive EVCs from the shortest to the longest, for instance with class intervals from 1 to 10 min (or at a higher time resolution) and plotting the cumulative sum of the EVC counts from each class interval against the ordered interval on a log-log scale (the EVC count in this relationship is the probability density that the interval between EVC pairs is log I or shorter than log I). Fractile dimension is then obtained as the slope of the regression of this relationship. The value of D can vary between 0 and 1. If the cumulative EVC count

increases uniformly over all class intervals, then the slope of the regression or D approaches unity, indicating that the EVC occurrence tends to be random with a uniform rather than clustered distribution over time. Lower values of D, for instance ≤ 0.93 indicate the presence of clustering. Thus, fractile dimension is inversely related to the degree of clustering. In the Cardiac Arrhythmia Suppression Trial (CAST) population, a more refined "high resolution fractal D" (evaluated with a higher time resolution of EVC occurrence) was predictive of arrhythmic death.[8] Fractile dimension was greater in those without arrhythmic events than in those who died, and the difference was manifest in the subgroup randomized into the active treatment group.

6A.1.6 Sympathetic Tone and Clustering of Ectopic Ventricular Complexes

Stein et al. have produced evidence that transient increases in cardiac sympathetic tone immediately preceding EVCs increase the likelihood of reduced fractile dimension in patients with inducible sustained unifocal ventricular tachycardia and frequent (200 or more) EVCs.[9] These investigators inferred the presence of these physiological determinants of EVC clustering by combining the evaluation of the fractile dimension with RR interval variability measures and trends in heart rate during short periods (1–10 min) preceding EVCs. Increased sympathetic tone was considered to occur when the heart rate increased and RR interval variability increased or remained unchanged. Sympathetic tone increase was classified as indeterminate when the increase in heart rate coincided with a decreased heart rate variability (i.e. a decrease in parasympathetic tone). Evidence for increased sympathetic tone preceding clustering was present in 14 of the 30 patients and an indeterminate change in sympathetic tone in a further ten patients. These interesting results also indicate that the clustering tendency in VT patients is different from diurnal variation in EVC frequency because it takes place over much shorter intervals preceding EVCs.

Huikuri et al. evaluated changes in heart rate variability before the onset of sustained and non-sustained (self-terminating) VT episodes in 18 patients with CAD.[10] They found that the ratio of

TABLE 6A.2 Lown's grading of the severity level of ventricular ectopic complexes.

Grade	Definition
0	No ventricular arrhythmias
1	<2 EVCs/min or <30 EVCs/h
3	Multiform EVCs
4A	EVC couplets
4B	≥3 consecutive EVCs
5	Early cycle EVC with R-on-T phenomenon

the low frequency and high frequency variation increased substantially before the onset of VT episodes, suggesting an increased sympathetic tone (or possibly vagal withdrawal?). Interestingly, all frequency-domain measures of heart rate variability were significantly lower before sustained than before nonsustained VT.

6A.1.7 Severity Levels of Ectopic Ventricular Complexes

The occurrence of occasional unifocal EVC in the standard 12-lead ECG is generally considered clinically not significant. As already noted, even a single EVC in a 10-s record means that the average hourly EVC rate may be fairly high. Concerning ambulatory ECG findings, it is generally assumed that the likelihood of the association with clinical disease increases with the frequency of EVCs and from unifocal to multifocal, paired or EVC runs or VT and early EVC (R on T). This Lown grading (Table 6A.2) of the severity of ventricular arrhythmias[11] is in common use, although the validity of this grading in relation to the risk of sudden death can be questioned.[12,13] The Lown grading system is based on the assumption that more complex EVC patterns such as the R-on-T phenomenon warrant a more severe grade and that EVC frequency warrants only a low severity level, both assumptions shown to be invalid in the evaluation of the prognostic significance.[13]

6A.2 Ectopic Ventricular Complex Prevalence

6A.2.1 Community-dwelling Populations

Data from reports with varying ECG recording length will be presented here, starting with EVC

prevalence estimates from studies that have used shorter recording (2 min or shorter), followed by studies that have used longer recording periods (1 or 24 h).

6A.2.1.1 The Finnish Social Insurance Institution Study

In the Finnish Social Insurance Institution study in four geographical areas in Finland and comprising 5,738 men and 5,224 women aged 30–59 years, EVC activity was evaluated from standard 12-lead ECGs recorded with a four-channel electrocardiograph.[14] The record length was apparently 15 s. The age-adjusted prevalence of any EVCs was 2.2% in men and 2.8% in women. The age-adjusted prevalence of frequent EVCs (>10% of all QRS complexes in the record) was 1.0% in men and 1.4% in women. The report demonstrated the age-dependence of the prevalence of EVC in men and in women. The overall EVC prevalence did not differ significantly by gender. However, in age group 45–49 years the prevalence of any EVC in women was well over twice as high as in men, 3.5% versus 1.3%, possibly reflecting the lability of the cardiovascular system in premenopausal women.

6A.2.1.2 The ARIC Study

A cross-sectional analysis of 2-min ECG recordings from the Atherosclerosis Risk in Communities (ARIC) study, representing a probability sample of adults aged from 45 to 64 years in four US communities, revealed that EVC prevalence is dependent on age, ventricular rate, gender, ethnicity, educational level, and the presence of organic heart disease.[15] One of the four ARIC communities was sampled exclusively from the African–American population. The overall prevalence of any EVC among participants without evidence of organic heart disease was 6.9% in men and 4.7% in women. The prevalence increased from age 45 to age 65 years approximately twofold in women and threefold in men. The summary of the results from a stepwise backwards regression model to select independent predictors with a significant association with EVC (Table 6A.3) indicated that the presence of CHD was associated with an odds ratio of 2.55 for the presence of

TABLE 6A.3 Odds ratios for the presence of ectopic ventricular complexes in 2-min ECGs for significant independent predictors of primary interest.

Variable	Odds ratio
Organic heart disease*	2.55 (2.37, 2.73)
Male gender	1.44 (1.31, 1.58)
Age (5-year increment)	1.34 (1.28, 1.41)
Hypertension[†]	1.23 (1.09, 1.38)
Magnesium <1.5 mg/dl	1.28 (1.13, 1.43)

* Defined as coronary heart disease (myocardial infarction by ECG, or history of coronary angioplasty or coronary revascularization surgery), or digitalis or antiarrhythmic medication use.

[†] Diastolic pressure ≥90 mmHg, systolic pressure ≥140 mmHg, or self-reported use of antihypertensive medication.

Source: Simpson et al.[15] Am Heart J 2002;143:535–40. © 2002. Reproduced with permission from Elsevier.

EVC. The excess risk of EVC was 44% in men, increased by 34% for a 5-year increment in age, and by 23% in men with CHD. Among other interesting associations with prevalent EVC was a 16% increase in odds ratio with a 5-cpm increase in heart rate, and a 28% increase with low magnesium level (<1.5 mg/dl). Lower educational attainment was also associated with increased likelihood for EVC, generally associated with other markers of cardiovascular health, possibly in part because of lifestyle differences. With an additional analysis including nine potential predictors, only bundle branch block, body mass index, and β-blocker use were retained as significant independent predictors.

6A.2.1.3 The MRFIT Study

In the Multiple Risk Factor Intervention Trial (MRFIT), 10,880 men aged 35–57 years, ostensibly healthy but considered at high risk for future CHD, were screened for the prevalence of EVCs using a 2-min recording of lead I ECG.[16] The prevalence of EVCs in these middle-aged men was 5.0%. A strong association was found between the presence of EVCs and systolic blood pressure, and between systolic blood pressure and age. There was no significant association between EVC and cigarette smoking.

Prevalence odds ratios were also significant for a number of characteristics of interest in relation to subclinical or clinical disease. The overall EVC prevalence among participants with organic heart disease (CHD, on digitalis or on antiarrhythmic medication) was 22.0% in men and 12.3% in women. The factors that in multivariate analysis (a logistic regression model) had a significant association with the presence of EVC included hypertension and organic heart disease, low magnesium, male gender, ethnicity African–American), and lower educational attainment (less than high school). An increase of the ventricular rate by 5 cpm increased the likelihood of EVC by 16%, and a 5-year increment in age by 34%.

The association of hypertension with EVC prevalence is probably mediated through increased sympathetic tone, increased likelihood of left ventricular hypertrophy (LVH), and increased left ventricular mass. Some echocardiographic studies have also reported that African–Americans are more likely to develop eccentric hypertrophy than Euro-American Americans, although there may not be any significant difference in echocardiographic LV mass.[17]

6A.2.1.4 The Framingham Study

The prevalence of frequent or complex ectopic ventricular activity in 1-h ambulatory ECG records was evaluated in the Framingham Heart Study population in 1971.[18] The population used in the analysis included the survivors of the original Framingham cohort in the 16th biennial examination, the offspring and their spouses. There were 2,425 men (mean age 51.3 years) and 3,064 women (mean age 53.8 years) in the sample with no clinical evidence of CHD. The age-adjusted prevalence of at least one EVC in a 1-h recording of these ostensibly CHD-free persons was 33% in men and 32% in women. The prevalence of frequent (>30/h) EVCs was 7% in both men and women. The combined age-adjusted prevalence of frequent and complex EVCs (multiform, EVC pairs, VT and R-on-T pattern) was 12% in both men and women.

The prevalence rates were considerably higher in the subgroup with clinical manifestations of CHD: 58% in 392 men and 49% in 242 women for ≥1 EVC/h, 17% in men and 19% in women for >30 EVCs/h, and 33% in men and 26% in women for frequent and complex EVCs combined. There was a strong age-dependence of EVC prevalence. In the CHD-free subgroup, the prevalence of frequent and complex EVCs combined was 4.4% in men less than 60 years old, 17.7 in men 60–69 years old, and 34.1% in men over 70 years old. In women, it was 6.0, 14.0 and 24.6% in these age groups, respectively. In the subgroups with clinical evidence of CHD, the prevalence rates in the three age groups of men were 27.8, 39.1 and 51.3%, respectively, and in women with CHD, 11.5, 29.8 and 35.6%, respectively.

6A.2.1.5 Clinically Healthy Women

Early ambulatory ECG studies on ostensibly healthy populations were performed on young healthy volunteers, clinically healthy patients from general practice, or in hospital populations. Romhilt et al. evaluated ectopic activity in 24-h ambulatory ECG in a group of 101 women aged 20–59 years selected at random from the employers of a company.[19] Initial random selection was done to obtain a sample of 40 in each decade from 20 to 49 years and 80 in the decade 50–59 years. Excluded were women with a history of any cardiovascular or pulmonary disease, high blood pressure or the use of antihypertensive medication, or any abnormalities in the 12-lead resting ECG or chest x-ray. Thirty-four of the women (28%) had EVCs in their 24-h recording but the average frequency was less than 1 EVC/h in 24 of them. Only one of the women had an average hourly rate of over ten EVCs. Like in other studies, EVC prevalence (any EVC/24h) increased with age, from 4% in the youngest age group to 67% in the age group 50–59 years. Of interest is the finding that the EVC prevalence was twice as high among women taking medication than among those not on medication (48% versus 24%). The higher EVC prevalence was observed in these healthy women if taking maintenance thyroid medication and in young women if taking oral contraceptives. A higher EVC prevalence was not observed in older women on hormone replacement therapy or in women on other medications.

6A.2.1.6 Cardiovascular Health Study

Like the Framingham study, several other studies have shown that EVC prevalence increases with age. In the Cardiovascular Health Study (CHS) population consisting of men and women 65 years

and older, EVC prevalence (any EVC in 24-h Holter) was 76.0% in women and 88.7% in men.[20] The prevalence of frequent EVCs (mean ≥15 EVCs/h) was 13.7% in women and 24.0% in men. Total prevalence of ventricular arrhythmias was 15.6% in women and 28.5% in men. Thus, ventricular arrhythmias evaluated in detailed analyses consisted almost entirely of EVCs.

In multivariate analyses using logistic regression models, a small subset came out with an independent association with ventricular arrhythmias. These significant covariates were considerably different in men and women. In women, the covariates with a significant association with ventricular arrhythmias were prolonged QT and diuretic use. Prolonged QT (QTI >110%) had an odds ratio (OR) 1.77 (1.10, 2.85), and diuretic use had an OR 1.84 (1.17, 2.88). In men, the covariates with a significant independent association with ventricular arrhythmias were abnormal echocardiographic ejection fraction, forced vital capacity, and standing height. Abnormal ejection fraction had an OR 2.05 (1.25, 3.37). Odds ratios for forced vital capacity and height were derived for interquartile range increments. The OR for a 1.1-liter increment in forced vital capacity was 0.63 (0.47, 0.85) and for an increment of 14 cm in height 2.15 (1.38, 3.33).

Several questions arise from these results in older men and women. No significant independent association was found between increased EVC activity and hypertension although it was strongly associated with other likely correlates of hypertension: both echocardiographic and electrocardiographic LV mass and abnormal LV ejection fraction in men, and diuretic use in women.

The results in these older men and women in the CHS differ from those of the ARIC, which reported a significant association between EVC and hypertension in middle-aged men and women. In CHS women, but not in men, even a moderate QT prolongation was associated with an increased likelihood of ventricular arrhythmias, predominantly frequent EVCs. In another CHS study,[21] hypertension and several clinical and subclinical markers of hypertension had a significant independent association with QT prolongation, including electrocardiographic LV mass, QRS duration, and diuretic use. After adjustment for these factors, women were more than three times more likely to have QT prolongation than men. Some of these confounding factors may be involved in masking the independent association between hypertension and increased EVC activity in older men and women. Increased EVC activity has been reported also in healthy elderly populations in other smaller studies.[22,23]

6A.2.2 Ectopic Ventricular Complex Prevalence in Post-myocardial Infarction Patients

The Beta-Blocker Heart Attack Trial (BHAT) was a placebo-controlled clinical trial that enrolled 3,837 male and female survivors of an acute MI, aged 30–69 years.[24] The trial was designed to test the efficacy of propranolol in improving survival. Of the whole study group, 3,290 patients had a 24-h Holter recording made before randomization, and 1,640 of the patients were assigned to the placebo group. Baseline characteristics in the placebo group showed that 13% had an average of ≥10 EVCs/h, one-third had multiform EVCs, and approximately 20% had EVC pairs or VT runs. Three factors were significantly associated with EVC activity in a multivariate linear regression model that included 11 independent variables, including patient's age, history of a MI prior to the qualifying MI and the presence of congestive heart failure during hospitalization for the qualifying acute MI. The site of the MI, presence of Q waves, serum potassium, and heart rate had no association with EVC activity.

6A.2.3 Ectopic Ventricular Complex Prevalence Trends with Time after Acute Phase of Myocardial Infarction

In the BHAT study population, there was a substantial increase in the EVC prevalence from the initial monitoring period 5–21 days after the acute phase in another 24-h Holter monitoring period performed approximately 6 weeks later.[25] A report from an electrophysiological study by Kuch at al. documented that the inducibility of sustained ventricular arrhythmia is considerably higher 24 days than 5 days after the acute phase of MI.[26]

6A.2.4 Diurnal Variation and Ectopic Ventricular Complex Prevalence

Forty per cent of the post-MI patients enrolled in the CAST trial had significant circadian variation in the occurrence of EVCs, with a peak during the morning hours between 6:00 and 10:00 a.m.[27] The presence of circadian variation was associated with higher age, higher overall frequency of EVCs, history of cardiac arrest, more frequent episodes of VT and slow runs. The CAST patients had clinical evidence of impaired cardiac function, with ejection fraction ≤45%. Excluded were patients with VT runs ≥15 complexes at rate ≥120 cpm. The presence of circadian variation in EVC frequency was not a significant predictor of sudden arrhythmic death.

6A.3 Prognostic Implications of Ectopic Ventricular Complex Activity

6A.3.1 Community-based Populations

Mortality risk evaluation results associated with EVC in representative data from community-based populations are summarized in Table 6A.4.

6A.3.1.1 Finland's Social Insurance Institution's Study

In the Finland's Social Insurance Institution's study, men 40–59 years old with frequent EVCs had a 3.8-fold higher CHD mortality rate than men with no EVCs.[14] The Finnish report also observed that occasional (<10%) EVCs appeared to increase the mortality risk. The number of women with increased EVC activity who died was too small to evaluate relative risk for EVCs. The CHD mortality in middle-aged Finnish men has been the highest in the world so that the men in this study can be considered to represent a high CHD-risk population.

6A.3.1.2 The Framingham Study

In the Framingham study, the presence of frequent or complex EVC activity (Lown grade ≥2) in men without CHD was significantly associated

TABLE 6A.4 Mortality risk for ectopic ventricular complexes in community-based populations.

	Finnish Social Insurance Institution survey from four geographical areas in Finland (1966–72)[14]	Survivors of a CHD-free subgroup of the Framingham original cohort at 12th biennial and the offspring study combined (1971)[18]	Framingham original cohort at 16th biennial and the offspring study at 2nd examination combined (1979–84)[29]
Study group	5,738 men and 5,224 women, ages 30–59; 15- to 20-s ECG; 5-year follow-up	2,727 men (mean age 51 years) and 3,306 women (mean age 54 years)	617 subjects free of apparent CHD and with echo-LVH estimate and Holter ECG recording available
ECG length	15–20 s	1 h	1 h
Follow-up (years)	5	4–6	5.7 for the original cohort, 4.5 for the offspring group
Prevalence	Age-adjusted prevalence: of frequent, EVC (>10%) Men 2.9% Women 2.8%	Age-adjusted prevalence of complex of frequent (>30/h) EVC: 12% in CHD-free men and in women; prevalence 33 and 26% in men and women with CHD, respectively	Prevalence of Lown grade ≥ 2 EVC: Men 28% Women 17%
Mortality risk	Men aged 40–59 years, CHD mortality: RR = 3.8. Mortality rate in women too low for risk evaluation	CHD-free men, all-cause mortality: RR = 2.30 (1.65, 3.20) Men, CHD death or MI: RR = 2.12 (1.33, 3.38). No significant associations in men with CHD or in women with or without CHD	For grade ≥ 2 EVC, mortality ratio: men 3.0, women 2.1. HR ratio for all-cause mortality (age and gender adjusted): HR = 1.80 (1.13, 2.87); with an adjustment for 8 clinical covariates: HR = 1.62 (0.98, 2.68)

CHD coronary heart disease, *EVC* ectopic ventricular complex, *HR* hazard ratio, *RR* relative risk.

with all-cause mortality and also with CHD death or MI.[18] The relative risk, after adjusting for age and a variety of other known CHD risk factors, was 2.30 (1.65, 3.20) for all-cause mortality and 2.12 (1.33, 3.38) for MI and CHD death as combined outcome measures (Table 6A.4). There was no significant association with either of these outcome measures in men with CHD or in women with or without CHD.

Both echocardiographic and ECG estimates of left ventricular mass were strongly associated with increased EVC activity in 24-h ambulatory ECG in the CHS population,[20] and also in 2-min ECGs in the ARIC study.[28] This observation would suggest that EVC activity in subjects with LVH is associated with excess mortality risk. Another Framingham study examined the mortality risk of ventricular arrhythmias in a subgroup of the Framingham population with echocardiographic LVH (Table 6A.4).[29] The study population consisted of the survivors of the original Framingham cohort in their 16th biennial examination and the Framingham offspring study in their second biennial examination. The mean follow-up period was 5.7 years for the original cohort and 4.5 years for

the offspring group. The prevalence of frequent or complex EVC in 1-h Holter ECG was high, 27% in men and 17% in women. The mortality ratio for these subjects with complex EVC activity and echo LVH was 3.0 in men and 2.1 in women. The mortality risk adjusted for age in the pooled group of men and women was 1.80 (1.13, 2.87). The trend toward excess risk prevailed when adjusted for several other risk factors, but the significance level dropped from $p = 0.013$ to $p = 0.058$. No significant excess risk was present for MI or CHD mortality.

6A.3.2 Ectopic Ventricular Complex Activity, Mortality, and Clinical Trials

The evidence for the association of EVCs with clinical disease and mortality in survivors of acute MI comes from analyses of ambulatory 24-h recordings in retrospective as well as in prospective studies.[24,30–34] Summary data from two clinical trials mentioned before, the BHAT and CAST, are presented in Table 6A.5. The BHAT results will be examined first in some detail.

TABLE 6A.5 Mortality risk of ectopic ventricular complexes in survivors of acute myocardial infarction in two clinical trials.

	Beta-Blocker Heart Attack Trial (BHAT)[12]	Cardiac Arrhythmia Suppression Trial (CAST)[38]
Study group considered	1,640 patients of the placebo group	1,727 patients (725 in placebo, 730 in encainide or flecainide, 272 in moricizine group), with ≥ 6 EVC/h* and with ejection fraction ≤ 0.55
ECG length	24-h Holter ECG	24-h Holter ECG
Follow-up	Average 25 months	10 months
Prevalence (%)	≥ 10 EVC/h 12.9% Multiform EVC 32.8% ≥ 10 EVC/h or (VT or EVC pairs) 25.5%	Mean EVC rate 133/h.[†] Nonsustained VT with rate ≥ 120/h in 22% and with rate <120/h in 22%
Mortality risk	Risk of all-cause mortality for ≥ 10 EVC/h: OR = 2.23 (multiple logistic regression model with 15 other risk factors)	Encainide or flecainide therapy 7.7% versus 3.0% in placebo group; RR 2.5 (1.6, 4.5)[‡]

EVC ectopic ventricular complex, *RR* relative risk.

* Amenable to pronounced reduction of EVC rate or the number of runs by drugs in pretrial titration phase.

[†] Evaluated in 1,498 patients with 24-h Holter ECG.

[‡] Placebo group mortality lower than expected due to selection of patients more easily amenable to EVC suppression and had less extensive CHD than patients not randomized.

6A.3.2.1 The BHAT Study

The BHAT study evaluated the mortality risk for ventricular ectopic activity in 1,640 survivors of acute MI assigned to the placebo group of the study.[12] The risk for total mortality adjusted for 15 other risk factors increased by 3% for each increment by 10 EVC in the mean hourly rate. Mean hourly rate ≥ 10 was associated with an over twofold increase in the total mortality risk (odds ratio 2.23), and it was not significantly higher for atherosclerotic sudden death than for atherosclerotic nonsudden death (odds ratios 1.81 and 2.25, respectively). The total mortality risk for mean hourly EVC rate of 10 or more was in fact higher than the odds ratio for total mortality for more complex forms or combinations of EVC activity. For instance, for the presence of multiform EVCs, the odds ratio for total mortality was 1.67, and it was higher for sudden atherosclerotic death than for nonsudden atherosclerotic death (odds ratios 2.43 and 1.21, respectively). Mean hourly EVC rate of 10 or more had 26% sensitivity for predicting total mortality at a specificity of 87%. These sensitivity and specificity levels were equally high for sudden and nonsudden atherosclerotic mortality as for total mortality (Table 6A.5).

The BHAT results indicated that EVC activity in survivors of acute MI is an independent predictor of mortality and not merely a marker of clinical disease and cardiac injury. When stratified into subgroups according to the presence of one or more clinical disease markers (history of an MI prior to the qualifying study entry, acute MI, ST depression in the resting ECG or cardiac enlargement defined by cardiothoracic ratio >0.5), the presence of ectopic count 10 or more increased the all-cause mortality risk in all subgroups. However, the relative risk of total mortality for the presence of ≥ 10 EVCs/h was highest (3.86) in the largest subgroup with none of these clinical characteristics.

In the BHAT population, the mortality risk associated with ectopic ventricular activity persisted when only patients with Q wave infarction were considered. The results from another study on survivors of acute MI had brought up the possibility that the excess risk associated with ectopic activity was significantly increased only in patients with non-Q wave MI.[35] The BHAT results also indicated that the treatment with propranolol did not alter the relation between ventricular ectopic activity and mortality: the risk decreased equally in patients with EVCs assigned to the propranolol treatment group and the placebo group.[36]

6A.3.2.2 The CAST Study

The clinical significance of detecting EVC activity is diminished by the fact that various attempts at suppression of EVCs have not been successful in reducing mortality more than in control groups. The CAST study was designed as a carefully conducted randomized clinical trial to test the hypothesis that EVC suppression by antiarrhythmic drugs encainide, flecainide or moricizine will reduce the risk of arrhythmic death in survivors of acute MI.[38] A pilot study in 500 patients had indicated the feasibility of the design and the choice of the drugs, and the main trial was initiated in 1987. The eligibility criteria of this highly select group of patients included: (1) ≥ 6 EVCs/h; (2) ejection fraction ≤ 0.55 if <90 days and ≤ 0.44 if ≥ 90 days post-MI; (3) achieving $\geq 80\%$ reduction in EVC rate and $\geq 90\%$ reduction in runs of nonsustained VT. The mean EVC rate at baseline was 133/h. Nonsustained VT with rate $\geq 120/h$ was present in 22% and with rate >120/h in another 22%.

One year after the active phase and a mean follow-up time of 10 months, the arm of the trial involving encainide and flecainide was stopped when preliminary analyses indicated a 3.6-fold excess risk of arrhythmic death and nonfatal cardiac arrest in encainide and flecainide groups compared with the placebo. The moricizine arm was continued with modifications of the protocol (selection including more severe EVC activity) as CAST II. This trial was also discontinued prematurely because of an excess mortality rate by the drug during the initial 2 weeks of exposure, and little chance of showing long-term benefit.[38] It is instructive to note that the data base from over 3,000 patients with encainide or flecainide before CAST indicated no such serious proarrhythmic effect of these drugs, as was revealed in a well-designed controlled clinical trial.

6A.3.2.3 The MIAMI and ISIS Trials

Large clinical trials to evaluate the efficacy of β-blocker therapy in prevention of ventricular fibrillation, the Metoprolol in Acute Myocardial Infarction (MIAMI) trial[39] and the First International Study of Infarct Survival (ISIS) trial,[40] did not confirm the earlier reports of reduced incidence of ventricular fibrillation.[41,42] The negative findings in these two studies have been thought to be because of concomitant other antiarrhythmic drug administration.[43]

Although post-MI patients with increased ventricular ectopic activity are at an increased risk of total mortality and sudden arrhythmic death, clinical trial evidence indicates that attempts at EVC suppression with currently available antiarrhythmic drugs are not warranted. The availability of implantable cardioverter defibrillators with improved design and reliability may change the

situation. Also, the prospects of using EVC activity analysis for the assessment of long-term efficacy of antiarrhythmic drugs remain uncertain because of large long-term spontaneous variability.

6A.3.2.4 The MILIS Report

Mortality rates as high as in BHAT have been reported in post-MI patients with reduced LV ejection fraction and EVC rate $\geq 10/h$ by the Multicenter Investigation of the Limitation of Infarct Size (MILIS) investigators[33] and by the Multicenter Post-Infarction Research Group.[34] The incidence of sustained monomorphic VT in the early phase of acute MI (during the first 48 h) is less than 2%. It has been related to the presence of more extensive myocardial damage, and identified as an independent predictor of early mortality, with an odds ratio as high as 5.0.[36]

References

1. Cranefied PF, Aronson RS. Cardiac Arrhythmias: The Role of Triggered Activity and Other Mechanisms. Mount Kisco, New York: Futura Publishing Company, 1988, p. 420.
2. Janse MJ, van Capelle FJ, Morsink H et al. Flow of "injury" current and patterns of excitation during early ventricular arrhythmias in acute regional myocardial ischemia in isolated porcine and canine hearts. Evidence for two different arrhythmogenic mechanisms. Circulation Res 1980;47:151–65.
3. Janse MJ, Kleber AG. Electrophysiological changes and ventricular arrhythmias in the early phase of regional myocardial ischemia. Circulation Res 1981;49:1069–81.
4. Janse MJ, van Capelle FJ. Electrotonic interactions across an inexcitable region as a cause of ectopic activity in acute myocardial ischemia. A study in porcine and canine hearts and computer models. Circulation Res 1982;50:527–37.
5. Pratt CM, Slymen DJ, Wierman AM et al. Analysis of the spontaneous variability of ventricular arrhythmias: consecutive ambulatory electrocardiographic recording of ventricular tachycardia. Am J Cardiol 1985;56:67–72.
6. Toivonen L. Spontaneous variability in the frequency of ventricular premature complexes over prolonged intervals and implications for antiarrhythmic treatment. Am J Cardiol 1987;60: 608–12.

7. Sami M, Kraemer H, Harrison DC et al. A new method for evaluating antiarrhythmic drug efficacy. Circulation 1980;62:1172–9.

8. Anderson JL, Karagounis LA, Stein KM et al. Predictive value for future arrhythmic events of fractal dimension, a measure of time clustering of ventricular premature complexes, after myocardial infarction. J Am Coll Cardiol 1997;30:226–32.

9. Stein KM, Karagounis LA, Anderson JL et al. Fractal clustering of ventricular ectopy correlates with sympathetic tone preceding ectopic beats. Circulation 1995;91:722–7.

10. Huikuri HV, Valkama JO, Airaksinen KE et al. Frequency domain measures of heart rate variability before the onset of nonsustained and sustained ventricular tachycardia in patients with coronary artery disease. Circulation 1993;87:1220–8.

11. Lown B, Wolf M. Approaches to sudden death from coronary heart disease. Circulation 1971;44:130–42.

12. Kostis JB, Byington R, Friedman LM et al. Prognostic significance of ventricular ectopic activity in survivors of acute myocardial infarction. J Am Coll Cardiol 1987;10:231–42.

13. Bigger JT, Feld FM. Analysis of prognostic significance of ventricular arrhythmias after myocardial infarction. Shortcomings of Lown grading system. Br Heart J 1981;45:717–24.

14. Reunanen A, Aromaa A, Pyörälä K et al. The Social Insurance Institution's Heart Disease Study. Baseline data and 5-year mortality experience. Acta Med Scand 1983;673(Suppl):1–109.

15. Simpson RJ, Cascio WE, Schreiner PJ et al. Prevalence of premature ventricular contractions in a population of African American and white men and women: the Atherosclerosis in Communities (ARIC) study. Am Heart J 2002;143:535–40.

16. Crow RS, Princas RJ, Dias V et al. Ventricular premature beats in a population sample. Frequency and associations with coronary risk characteristics. Circulation 1975;52(Suppl III):211–5.

17. Koren MJ, Mensah GA, Blake J et al. Comparison of left ventricular mass and geometry in black and white patients with essential hypertension. Am J Hypertens 1993;6:815–23.

18. Bikkina M, Larson MG, Levy D. Prognostic implications of asymptomatic ventricular arrhythmias: the Framingham Study. Ann Intern Med 1992;117:990–6.

19. Romhilt DW, Chaffin C, Sung CC, Irby EC. Arrhythmias on ambulatory electrocardiographic monitoring in women without apparent heart disease. Am J Cardiol 1984;54:582–6.

20. Manolio TA, Furberg CD, Rautaharju PM et al. Cardiac arrhythmias on 24-h ambulatory electrocardiography on older women and men: the Cardiovascular Health Study. J Am Coll Cardiol 1994;23:916–25.

21. Rautaharju PM, Manolio TA, Psaty BM et al. Correlates of QT prolongation in older adults (the Cardiovascular Health Study). Am J Cardiol 1994;73:999–1002.

22. Camm AJ, Evans KE, Ward DE, Martin A. The rhythm of the heart in active elderly subjects. Am Heart J 1980;99:598–603.

23. Fleg JL, Kennedy HL. Cardiac arrhythmias in a healthy elderly population. Chest 1982;81:302–7.

24. Byington RP. Beta-blocker Heart Attack Trial: design, methods, and baseline results. Beta-blocker Heart Attack Trial research group. Control Clin Trials 1984;5:382–437.

25. Lichstein E, Morganroth J, Harris R, Hubble E. Effect of propranolol on ventricular arrhythmia. The Beta-blocker Heart Attack Trial experience. Circulation 1983;67:5–10.

26. Kuch KH, Costard A, Schluter M, Kunze KP. Significance of timing programmed electrical stimulation after acute myocardial infarction. J Am Coll Cardiol 1986;8:1279–88.

27. Goldstein S, Zoble RG, Akiyama T et al. Relation of circadian ventricular ectopic activity to cardiac mortality. CAST investigators. Am J Cardiol 1996;78:881–5.

28. Simpson RJ Jr, Cascio WE, Crow RS et al. Association of ventricular premature complexes with electrocardiographic-estimated left ventricular mass in a population of African-American and white men and women (the Atherosclerosis Risk in Communities study). Am J Cardiol 2001;87:49–53.

29. Bikkina M, Larson MG, Levy D. Asymptomatic ventricular arrhythmias and mortality risk in subjects with left ventricular hypertrophy. J Am Coll Cardiol 1993;22:1111–6.

30. Kotler MN, Tabatznik B, Mower MM, Tominaga S. Prognostic significance of ventricular ectopic beats with respect to sudden death in the late postinfarction period. Circulation 1973;47:959–66.

31. Ruberman W, Weinblatt E, Goldberg J et al. Ventricular premature beats and mortality after myocardial infarction. N Engl J Med 1977;297:750–7.

32. Moss AJ, Davis HT, DeCamilla J, Bayer LW. Ventricular ectopic beats and their relation to sudden and nonsudden death after myocardial infarction. Circulation 1979;60:998–1003.

33. Mukharji J, Rude RE, Poole WK et al. Risk factors for sudden death after acute myocardial infarction: two-year follow-up. Am J Cardiol 1984;54:31–6.

34. Bigger JT Jr, Fleiss JL, Kleiger R et al. The relationship among ventricular arrhythmias, left ventricular dysfunction, and mortality in the two years after myocardial infarction. Circulation 1984; 69:250–7.

35. Maisel AS, Scott N, Gilpin E et al. Complex ventricular arrhythmias in patients with Q wave versus non-Q wave myocardial infarction. Circulation 1985;72:963–70.

36. Kostis JB, Wilson AC, Sanders MR, Buyington RP. Prognostic significance of ventricular ectopic activity in survivors of acute myocardial infarction who receive propranolol. Am J Cardiol 1988;61:975–8.

37. Denes P, Gillis AM, Pawitan Y et al. Prevalence, characteristics and significance of ventricular premature complexes and ventricular tachycardia detected by 24-hour continuous electrocardiographic recording in the Cardiac Arrhythmia Suppression Trial. CAST investigators. Am J Cardiol 1991;68:887–96.

38. The Cardiac Arrhythmia Suppression Trial (CAST) investigators. Preliminary report: effect of encainide and flecainide on mortality in a randomized trial of arrhythmia suppression after myocardial infarction. N Engl J Med 1989;321:406–12.

39. Hjalmarson A. Metoprolol in Acute Myocardial Infarction (MIAMI). Am J Cardiol 1985;56: 1G–46G.

40. Randomised trial of intravenous atenolol among 16027 cases of suspected acute myocardial infarction: ISIS-1. First International Study of Infarct Survival Collaborative Group. Lancet 1986;2: 57–66.

41. Norris RM, Barnaby PF, Brown MA, Geary GG, Clarke ED, Logan RL, Sharpe DN. Prevention of ventricular fibrillation during acute myocardial infarction by intravenous propranolol. Lancet 1984;2:883–6.

42. Ryden L, Ariniego R, Arnman K et al. A double-blind trial of metoprolol in acute myocardial infarction. Effects on ventricular tachyarrhythmias. N Engl J Med 1983;308:614–8.

43. Olsson G, Rehnquist N. Treatment of ventricular arrhythmias in the coronary patient: what sort of patient? For which rhythm disorder? With what procedure? Am J Cardiol 1989;64:57J–60J.

6B
Record Length, Spontaneous Variability and Suppression of Ectopic Ventricular Complex Activity by Drugs

The first part of this chapter covers the dependence of the observed ectopic ventricular complex (EVC) prevalence on the recording length and the second part considers the influence of spontaneous variability of EVC on the ability to detect a drug effect on EVC suppression efforts.

6B.1 Dependence of Ectopic Ventricular Complex Prevalence on Record Length

The record length of the standard 12-lead ECG varies in general from 10 s when three or more leads are recorded simultaneously to 30 s for single channel recorders, assuming that each lead or lead group is recorded for at least 2.5 s. Recording length can be longer if a separate rhythm strip is recorded.

Let us assume that the occurrence of occasional EVCs is a random process. Assume that the average true frequency would thus be one EVC in a 10-s ECG if the recording was repeated many times or a longer recording period was analyzed. If the recording of the standard 10-s ECG was repeated once, what is the likelihood that there would be no EVCs present? It can be assumed that the EVC occurrence is a Poisson process. With a mean frequency $\mu = 1\,EVC/10\,s$, the probability that there would be no EVC in the record is $Po = e^{-1} = 0.37$, or 37%. Thus, the probability that there would be one or more EVCs in a 10-s record is 63%. It will take a fairly high true hourly EVC rate, 360 EVC/h, in a 24-h Holter recording to have on average one EVC in a 10-s recording, and even then, there is only a 63% chance that it will be detected as one event in a 10-s routine ECG recording. This suggests that the presence of even one EVC in the standard 10-s ECG indicates a fairly high rate.

By similar considerations of the properties of a Poisson process, it can be expected that there is a 63% chance of having one or more EVCs in a 2-min ECG recording if the true average rate is 30 EVCs/h, as shown for instance by the reported repeatability test data from the Multiple Risk Factor Intervention Trial (MRFIT). (This does not mean that if the Holter recording of those who had no EVCs is repeated the next day, one-half would have EVCs – because the prior probability of having 30 EVCs/h or more is low in ostensibly healthy populations, and individuals who have no EVCs in the first Holter are very unlikely to have an average EVC rate of 30 the next day!)

The absence of any EVCs in a 2-min monitoring period indicates that the likelihood of a high EVC rate (360 EVCs/h or more) or complex EVC activity in 24-h Holter is relatively low, which has clinical implications. Individual variability regarding the presence or absence of EVC in short recordings of individuals with frequent EVCs is large, which limits the utility of short monitoring periods for EVC suppression studies. However, even these shorter monitoring periods may provide an adequate estimate of EVC prevalence in comparing contrasting populations and for the assessment of association of EVC with clinical and subclinical disease and other risk factors. In patients with organic cardiac disease, the occurrence of EVCs may not be a random stochastic process with a uniform distribution of the intervals between successive EVCs. There may be diurnal variation and there may be clustering of EVCs in the sequence of their occurrence in time.

6B.2 Spontaneous EVC Variability and Detection of Suppression Effect by Drugs

Suppose we wish to determine when the protective or possible proarrhythmic effect of antiarrhythmic therapy exceeds the limits of spontaneous variability of EVC activity. This will require estimation of the confidence limits of spontaneous variability over a given time interval. Logarithmic transform is usually performed on EVC frequency counts in order to reduce the skew and induce a more normal distribution with equal variances. The frequency counts (for instance average hourly frequency) may be represented by $C1 = \ln (F1 + k)$ and $C2 = \ln (F2 + k)$, where $C1$ is for instance the log EVC count in the control (placebo) period and $C2$ is the log count during the therapeutic intervention period. (It is immaterial whether natural or base 10 log transformation is used.) Commonly, investigators have assigned the value 1 for the constant k.[1-4] $C2 - C1$ has to exceed the 95% confidence limits for the spontaneous variability to indicate a significant difference at the 5% level for a two-sided test. Let $D = 2*SD$, where SD is the standard deviation of the spontaneous variability. Various models have been introduced to determine D. The 95% confidence interval is:

$$C2 - C1 = \ln (F2 + k) - \ln (F1 + k)$$
$$= \ln [(F2 + k)/(F1 + k)] = D, \quad [6B.1]$$

so that the count ratio $(F2 + k)/(F1 + k) = e^D$. The mean values of these count ratios (called variability ratios by Schmidt et al.) do not differ significantly from 0.[5]

Morganroth et al. introduced expressions for per cent reduction in EVC count and its 95% confidence interval.[1] Significant per cent reduction indicating that the count ratio is less than the lower confidence limit becomes:

$$100 * [(1 - (F2 + k)/(F1 + k)] > 100 * (1 - e^{-D})$$
$$[6B.2]$$

or

$$100 * (F1 - F2)/(F1 + k) > 100 * (1 - e^{-D}).$$
$$[6B.3]$$

Equation 6B.3 gives the reduction as an unsigned value. A significant per cent increase in the count ratio is:

$$100 * \{[(F2 + k)/(F1 + k)] - 1\} > 100 * (e^D - 1),$$
$$[6B.4]$$

or

$$100 * (F2 - F1)/(F1 + k) > 100 * (e^D - 1).$$
$$[6B.5]$$

The choice of the value for the constant k can be important. Schmidt et al. have pointed out that using the value $k = 1$ results in an underestimate percentile spontaneous variability and thus in an underestimate of the reduction required to become significant if the frequency count (F1 in Equation 6B.3) is low, as is often the case for EVC pairs or runs.[2] It is noted that the expression on the left side of Equation 6B.3 differs from the exact per cent reduction by a factor $(F1 + k)/F1$ because

$$(F1 - F1)/F1 = (F2 - F1)/(F1 + k)$$
$$* (F1 + k)/F1 \qquad [6B.6]$$

Thus, if the EVC activity level is low, the true per cent reduction required can be obtained by multiplying the term on the left side of Equation 6B.3 by this correction factor.

As mentioned above, the values for D differ for singular EVCs, EVC pairs and runs. Schmidt et al. evaluated over what ranges of k the distributions of the variability ratios for different time intervals were normal (Kolmogorov–Smirnov test). They ended up choosing $k = 0.01$, which was the smallest constant consistent with normal distribution for all types of EVC activity.

Schmidt et al. have also introduced a model for establishing the confidence limits for three-dimensional distribution of the variability ratios of singular EVCs, pairs and runs.[5,6] The per cent reductions required with the three-dimensional model were 28% for singular EVCs, 72% for EVC pairs and 88% for runs for control periods up to

1 week, compared with the per cent reductions of 83, 90 and 95%, respectively, for the one-dimensional model. A progressive increase was documented to require longer control periods.

References

1. Morganroth J, Michelson EL, Horowitz LN et al. Limitations of routine long-term electrocardiographic monitoring to assess ventricular ectopic frequency. Circulation 1978;58:408–14.
2. Pratt CM, Slymen DJ, Wierman AM et al. Analysis of the spontaneous variability of ventricular arrhythmias: Consecutive ambulatory electrocardiographic recording of ventricular tachycardia. Am J Cardiol 1985;56:67–72.
3. Toivonen L. Spontaneous variability in the frequency of ventricular premature complexes over prolonged intervals and implications for antiarrhythmic treatment. Am J Cardiol 1987;60:608–12.
4. Sami M, Kraemer H, Harrison DC et al. A new method for evaluating antiarrhythmic drug efficacy. Circulation 1980;62:1172–9.
5. Schmidt G, Ulm K, Barthel P et al. Spontaneous variability of simple and complex ventricular premature contractions during long time intervals in patients with severe organic heart disease. Circulation 1988;78:296–301.
6. Schmidt G, Morfill GE, Barthel P et al. Variability of ventricular premature complexes and mortality risk. Pacing Clin Electrophysiol 1996;19:976–80.

7A
Left Ventricular Hypertrophy

Synopsis

Significance

Electrocardiographic left ventricular hypertrophy (ECG-LVH) was for a long time one of the primary cardiographic epidemiological diagnostic tools, and it was also clinically important for LVH classification in patients with hypertension, acquired valvular heart disease and congenital valvular defects. The clinical significance of ECG-LVH has diminished with advances in cardiac imaging technology. The epidemiological significance of ECG-LVH is primarily in the realm of risk evaluation.

Mechanism

The R and S wave amplitudes in LVH are increased because the net (uncancelled) excitation wave front is stronger in the hypertrophied left ventricular wall and because of the closer proximity of the enlarged heart to the chest wall (increased solid angle), particularly if cardiac remodeling involves dilatation. The excitation time of the left ventricular wall is moderately increased with increased wall thickness. Structural alterations with increased wall stress, ischemic changes and fibrosis associated with coronary problems are common in advanced LVH, and they account for the repolarization abnormalities.

Risk Factors

Risk factors include functional states resulting in overload and increased wall stress of the left ventricle, most commonly hypertension, less fre-quently genetic and acquired valvular defects; obesity, functional and structural adaptation to myocardial infarction.

Population Prevalence

Apparent LVH prevalence varies widely in community-based populations. Profound ethnic and gender differences have been reported in ECG-LVH prevalence. A higher prevalence has been found in African–American and other black populations than in white men and women. The reported prevalence also varies widely depending on the ECG-LVH criteria used.

Classification Problems

Stratification by gender and race is a necessity. A critical assessment reveals that inappropriate sensitivity/specificity combinations in currently used ECG-LVH criteria produce highly distorted LVH prevalence data and distorted ethnic differences in LVH prevalence. The traditional Sokolow-Lyon voltage and the Minnesota Code high QRS amplitude criteria are prone to confounding by extra-cardiac factors. Cornell voltage criteria are less vulnerable to these confounding factors. QRS amplitude criteria combined with repolarization abnormalities are highly specific and associated with a higher risk of cardiovascular disease (CVD) mortality but they have a low prevalence and a low sensitivity. Assessment of ECG-LVH is more useful in clinical applications when LVH prevalence is higher and other LVH-assertion methods such as echocardiography are available.

Confounding Factors

Confounding factors include: extracardiac factors influencing ECG, such as body weight, obesity, breast tissue, pulmonary conditions (lung resistivity), chest size and shape in relation to cardiac size; QRS axis; antihypertensive therapy; coronary heart disease (CHD) with associated remodeling (compensatory hypertrophy) and ventricular conduction problems. Intracardiac factors are: intracavitary blood and cavity size; cardiac structural alterations such as scar tissue and fibrosis.

Population Trends, Risk Evaluation, Intervention Studies

Profound observed trends over time towards decreasing ECG-LVH prevalence may, to some extent, reflect improved efficiency in hypertension control. However, the role of confounding factors such as increased prevalence of obesity has not been critically assessed. From pharmacological agents used in hypertension control, angiotensin-converting enzyme (ACE) inhibitors (and calcium channel blockers) seem most effective and β-blockers least effective in reducing echocardiographic left ventricular mass. Echocardiographic evidence in high risk hypertensive patients with diabetes has failed to demonstrate improved risk with LV mass reduction with ACE inhibitors. One recent study has reported that reduction of ECG-LVH with therapeutic intervention will reduce the risk of CVD mortality.

Abbreviations and Acronyms

ACE – angiotensin-converting enzyme
BIRNH – the Belgian Inter-University Research on Nutrition and Health study
BMI – body mass index
BSA – body surface area
CAD – coronary artery disease
CARDIA – Coronary Artery Risk Development in Young Adults study
CHD – coronary heart disease
CHF – congestive heart failure
CHS – Chicago Heart Study
CVD – cardiovascular disease
Echo-LVH – echocardiographic left ventricular hypertrophy
ECG-LVH – electrocardiographic left ventricular hypertrophy
HDFP – Hypertension Detection and Follow-up Program
HOPE – Heart Outcomes Prevention Evaluation
LIFE – Losartan Intervention For Endpoint reduction in hypertension study
LVH – left ventricular hypertrophy
LVM – left ventricular mass
LVMI – left ventricular mass index
MC – Minnesota Code
MI – myocardial infarction
MRFIT – Multiple Risk Factor Intervention Trial
NHANES – National Health and Nutrition Examination Survey
PIUMA – Progretto Ipertensione Umbria Monitoraggio Ambulatoriale study
RACE – Ramipril Cardioprotective Evaluation
RIFLE – Risk Factors and Life Expectancy study
TOMHS – Treatment of Mild Hypertension Study
Units (most commonly used):
μV – microvolts
mV – millivolts
$\mu V.s$ – microvolt.seconds
m^2 – meters squared
g/m^2 – grams/meters squared

7A.1 Introduction

Evaluation of left ventricular hypertrophy (LVH) has been one of the most prominent topics in clinical and epidemiological electrocardiography. The literature on this topic is voluminous. Electrocardiographic criteria for LVH are in general simple and easily measured also visually even in high volume applications. The prognostic implications of electrocardiographic LVH (ECG-LVH) in hypertensive patients and other conditions have added to the attractiveness of ECG-LVH in epidemiological applications. Electrocardiographic LVH was for a long time the most important factor among the risk categories of the Framingham prognostic score until it was removed in 1985,[1] apparently reflecting its diminishing role over time as a risk predictor. The well-documented rather low classification accuracy of LVH criteria has not dampened the popularity of their application, although echocardiographic and other imaging modalities (tomography, nuclear magnetic resonance imaging) have diminished the role of ECG-LVH in clinical practice.

Various issues involving ECG-LVH will be presented in detail in this chapter because this topic has received and continues to receive so much attention in epidemiological and clinical research. Broad epidemiological and clinical aspects of ECG-LVH have been reviewed in previous communications.[2–5]

A variety of ECG criteria have been introduced for LVH since the early years of electrocardiography. The focal point of the LVH-related publications of the pioneers was on relative left and right ventricular preponderance, with criteria based on the R and S wave amplitudes in the three bipolar limb leads available those days. A notable example is the "preponderance index", $(RI - RIII) + (SI - SIII)$, introduced by Lewis in 1914,[6] with 1.79 mV as a criterion for LVH. Autopsy documentation as ECG-independent evidence was commonly used. The article by Sir Thomas Lewis in his journal *Heart* had 36 pages, 18 tables with detailed autopsy documentation of ventricular weights and ECG comparisons in 118 cases. Equally impressive is the 1922 article by George Hermann and Frank Wilson: 56 pages with detailed ECG and autopsy documentation of 59 cases.[7] The availability of the chest leads of Wilson after the mid 1940s expanded the scope of LVH studies.

In 1949, Sokolow and Lyon introduced their well-known LVH criterion.[8] Patients with clinical disorders capable of producing left ventricular strain who had QRS-STT abnormalities were selected to the LVH group, suggesting a selection bias by present-day standards. In spite of the selection criteria and selection bias, the sensitivity of these LVH criteria was low, with only 48 out of 147 LVH patients (33%) having LVH by these new ECG criteria. It is perplexing that the Sokolow–Lyon LVH criteria have been and continue to be the most widely used in electrocardiography ever since their inception.

With the improvement in echocardiographic LVH (Echo-LVH) imaging technology, echocardiography has replaced autopsy as the "gold standard" for evaluation of classification accuracy of ECG-LVH criteria. Echocardiographic methodology has its own problems, including technical problems in obtaining satisfactory quality for estimation of left ventricular mass (LVM), particularly in older subjects, intra- and inter-reader variability, and the uncertainty about the appropriate method of "indexing" Echo-LVM to body size.

7A.1.1 ECG-LVH Criteria

Some of the commonly used LVH criteria are listed in Table 7A.1. These include the Sokolow–

TABLE 7A.1 Commonly used ECG criteria for left ventricular hypertrophy.

Criteria	Variables	Criteria sets and limits
Sokolow–Lyon (SL)[8]	RV5 + SV1	1. SL >3,500 µV (men and women)
Minnesota Code MC 3.1[9]	R amplitudes in I, II, III, aVL, aVF, V5	2A. R(I, II, III or AVF) >2,000 µV OR RaVL >1,200 µV OR RV5 >2,600 µV
		2B. 2A and (MC 4.1–4.3 or 5.1–5.3)
Minnesota Code MC 3.1 + 3.3[9]	MC3.1 variables plus RI, SL	3A. MC 3.1 OR SL >3,500 µV OR RI >1,500 µV (men and women)
		3B. 3A and (MC 4.1–4.3 or 5.1–5.3)
Cornell voltage (CV)[10]	RaVL + SV3	4. CV >2,800 µV in men, >2,000 µV in women
Cornell product (CP)[11]	CV • QRSdur	5. CP >240 µV.s (men and women)
Estes score ≥5 (ES5)[12]	Variables above and P'V1	6A. RV5/6 ≥3,000 µV OR (R or S in any limb lead ≥3,000 µV) OR LV strain AND QRS >90 ms (men and women)
Estes score ≥4 (ES4)	RV5, RV6, R and R in limb leads, QRSdur, LV strain*	6B. ES4 AND P'V1 >4 mV.s (men and women)
Framingham	SL, RI, SIII, RaVL, SV1–V2, SL, LV strain	7A. Borderline: SL criteria, or RI >1,100 µV or (RaVL or SV1 or SV2 or (RI + SIII)) ≥2,500 µV
		7B. Definite: Borderline criteria + LV strain

LV left ventricle.

* LV strain refers to downsloping ST segment with negative T wave.

Lyon voltage,[8] the high amplitude R wave criteria of the Minnesota Code (MC),[9] the Cornell voltage,[10] the Cornell product,[11] the Romhilt–Estes score,[12] and the Perugia score.[13] The maximum R in V5 or V6 is often used for Sokolow–Lyon criteria. RV6 larger than RV5 usually reflects misplacement of the lateral lead electrodes too far anteriorly.

The MC is a hierarchic scheme for LVH coding whereby MC 3.3 is coded if MC 3.1 is not present. Code 3.1 or 3.3 is at times combined with repolarization abnormalities (MC 4.1–4.3 and 5.1–5.3) for a more strict set of LVH criteria. The Romhilt–Estes point score is more involved than that shown in Table 7A.1. It includes, for instance, terminal P wave area in V1 and QRS duration as covariates. High amplitude R waves and left ventricular strain account for 3 points each. Recognizing that QRS duration is usually 90 ms or more in subjects with LVH, the simplified logic combination listed in Table 7A.1 for the score ≥4 points can be considered adequate (set 7). The Perugia score uses a combination of variables, including the Cornell voltage and Romhilt–Estes score. Some variations of the Sokolow–Lyon voltage and other amplitude and LV strain criteria have been used in various Framingham reports, shown in Table 7A.1. In 1993, Norman et al. introduced a gender-specific ECG model for improved LVH detection by adjusting the Cornell voltage for age and body mass index (BMI).[14]

7A.1.2 Multivariate ECG Models Estimating Left Ventricular Mass as a Continuous Variable

Numerous problems in attempts to use ECG-LVH as an epidemiological tool, to be discussed later, suggest that it may be more logical to use LVM as a continuous variable for comparison of contrasting populations and, in particular, for evaluation of left ventricular involvement as an end organ in hypertension. These models can be adapted also for predicting LVH using dichotomous or higher discretization levels for the estimated LVM. Several models have been developed for this purpose (Table 7A.2). The first two models[15,16] predict Echo-LVM indexed to body surface area (BSA). The log regression model of Casale et al. validated with autopsy findings predicts LVH adjusted for gender.[17] The last, a race- and gender-specific model, predicts Echo-LVM on a continuous scale.[18]

7A.1.3 Mechanism of ECG-LVH

The primary direct determinant of ECG amplitudes used in LVH criteria is the increased solid angle at various body surface points extended by the propagating ventricular excitation front at various instants of QRS. The body surface potential is directly proportional to the area of the

TABLE 7A.2 Electrocardiographic models predicting echocardiographic left ventricular hypertrophy, left ventricular mass, or left ventricular mass index.

Model	Group	Equation
Wolf et al.[15]	Men	$LVMI = 0.00160 * RaVL + 0.00089 * SV1 + 0.00638 * TnegV6 - 3.0314$
	Women	$LVMI = 0.00210 * RaVL - 0.00877 * SI + 0.01047 * TnegV6 - 1.500$
Rautaharju et al.[16]	White and black men	$LVMI = 0.010 * RV5 + 0.020 * SV1 + 0.028 * SIII + 0.182 * TnegV6 - 0.148 * TposaVR + 1.049 * QRSdur - 36.4$
	White women	$LVMI (g/m^2) = 0.018 * RV5 + 0.053 * SV1 - 0.112 * SI + 0.108 * TposV1 + 0.170 * TnegaVF - 0.094 * TposV6 + 88.5$
	Black women	$LVMI = 0.022 * RaVL + 0.018 * (RV6 + SV2) - 0.014 * RV2 - 0.069 * SV5 + 0.199 * InegaVL + 0.746 * QRSdur - 22.3$
Casale et al.[17]	Men and women	$LVH = EXP < -1.55$, where $EXP = (-0.092 * CV - 0.306 * TV1 - 0.212 * QRS - 0.278 * PtermV1 - 0.559 * Gender + 4.558)$; amplitudes are in mm, QRS duration in seconds $* 100$, PtermV1 area is in mm.s and sex $= 1$ for male, 0 for female
Rautaharju et al.[18]	White men	$LVM = 0.026 * CV + 1.25 * Wt + 34.4$
	Black men	$LVM = 0.024 * CV + 1.18 * Wt + 34.8$
	White women	$LVM = 0.020 * CV + 1.12 * Wt + 36.2$
	Black women	$LVM = 0.023 * CV + 0.87 * Wt + 37.6$

LVM (g) left ventricular mass, *LVMI* (g/m²) left ventricular mass index, *Wt* (kg) body weight; ECG amplitudes are in μV and QRS duration is in ms in all models except for Casale et al. as noted.

excitation front (the solid angle subtended by it) and inversely proportional to the square of the distance from the cardiac source to the recording point. The net uncancelled source potential can be expected to be increased with the increased thickness of the left ventricular wall. Alternatively, solid angle subtended by the excitation front area on the epicardial surface can be used computationally to estimate body surface potentials and ECG amplitudes. Intracardiac factors (cavity blood), intracardiac and extracardiac inhomogeneities (cardiac muscle fibers, lungs, subcutaneous tissue) modify body surface potentials.

There is a wide discrepancy between the ECG-LVH and Echo-LVH, as will be discussed later in this chapter. Whereas Echo-LVH reflects anatomical LVM, ECG-LVH reflects electrical events in living, excitable cardiac tissue.

7A.1.4 Risk Factors for ECG-LVH

Risk factors for ECG-LVH are related to functional states resulting in overload and increased wall stress and thickness of the left ventricle, most commonly sustained hypertension. Compensatory hypertrophy is an adaptation process during the recovery from an acute myocardial infarction (MI). This compensates to some extent the surface potential loss occurring with the loss of excitable muscle tissue. Congenital and acquired valvular defects are still an important etiological factor for LVH. Obesity is often reported to be a risk factor for LVH. Substantial differences exist in the obesity effect between ECG-LVH and Echo-LVH. Concerning ECG-LVH, pronounced racial differences have been reported. Extracardiac factors (subcutaneous fat, resistivity, and distance effects) confound these relationships. Indexing issues complicate the evaluation of the role of the obesity as a risk factor for Echo-LVH.

7A.2 Differences in Prevalence of ECG-LVH in Diverse Populations

The prevalence of LVH by MC 3.1–3.3 criteria based on high amplitude QRS waves varies profoundly in different study populations. Ashley et al. summarized the results from their survey of reported LVH prevalence by MC 3.1 criterion (the second set in Table 7A.1), including many early studies in various community-based populations.[2] In females, the median value of the prevalence stayed below 2% up to the age group 40–49 years and then increased approximately in steps of 2% per decade, reaching approximately 8% in age group 60–69 years and approximately 13% in age group 70 and older. The reported prevalence in young males was substantially higher, with median values ranging from approximately 6 to 9%. Also surprising was the wide interquartile range of the reported values in males, from a low of approximately 2% to a high of 24%. The reported LVH prevalence by MC 3.1 criterion in male populations decreased from extreme high values of the younger males to a median value below 4% in age group 40–49 years. After this, LVH prevalence increased progressively with age in men, as in women, with median values slightly higher in men than in women except at age group ≥70 years.

7A.2.1 Prevalence of ECG-LVH in Community-based Populations

7A.2.1.1 The 1969 Report from the Framingham Study

The Framingham study used descriptive clinical criteria for definite and possible LVH.[19] Although the criteria were not specified in detail, possible LVH category apparently consisted mainly of increased R wave amplitude without repolarization abnormalities. Possible LVH prevalence in men (average of seven successive biennial examinations) had a relatively modest increase with age, from approximately 2% in age groups below 50 years to a peak level of 5% in age group 60–64 years. Definite LVH prevalence by criteria including repolarization abnormalities was not much different in middle-aged and older men than by QRS voltage criteria alone. The prevalence of LVH increased from approximately 1% in middle-aged men to 5% in age group 65–69 years and to 7% in age group 70–74 years. A parallel LVH prevalence increase with age was reported for women, although at a slightly lower prevalence level than in men.

The prevalence levels with QRS voltage criteria alone from the Framingham study are lower than from other populations. For instance, the LVH prevalence by MC 3.1–3.3 criteria in men from the Multiple Risk Factor Intervention Trial (MRFIT; aged 40–59 years) was 11%.[20] In hypertensive men of the study, the prevalence by category 3.1–3.3 criteria was 19%, decreasing to below 3% when repolarization abnormalities (MC 4.1–4.3 or 5.1–5.3) were included in the criteria.

7A.2.1.2 The Seven Countries Study

Left ventricular hypertrophy data from 17 male cohorts aged 40–59 years extracted from the Seven Countries study again show the wide range of LVH prevalence by MC 3.1 criteria in various male populations (Table 7A.3).[21] Electrocardiograms in that international collaborative study were

TABLE 7A.3 Prevalence (%) of electrocardiographic left ventricular hypertrophy by Minnesota Code (MC) high amplitude R wave criterion alone and in combination with ST abnormalities in male cohorts aged 40–59 years in the Seven Countries Study.

Cohort	Population size	High amplitude R waves (MC 3.1)	Combined with ST changes (MC 3.1 + 4.1–4.4)
Crete, Greece	686	5.1	0.3
Corfu, Greece	529	7.6	1.0
Velika Krsna*	510	12.2	1.2
Dalmatia*	669	2.8	0.2
Slavonia*	694	11.4	0.7
West Finland	857	16.2	1.2
Karelia, Finland	814	17.9	1.5
Crevalcore, Italy	993	5.5	1.3
Montegiorgio, Italy	717	3.6	0.4
Railwaymen, Rome, Italy	766	3.4	0.1
Zutphen, Netherlands	877	4.3	0.9
Tanushimaru, Japan	504	7.5	2.0
Ushibuka, Japan	484	14.7	1.5
Switchmen, USA	835	1.6	0.2
Sedentary clerks, USA	847	3.4	0.5
Nonsedentary clerks, USA	155	6.5	0.7
Executives, USA	250	1.2	0.4
Total/weighted mean	11,184	7.4	0.8

* Serbian village Velika Krsna, Croatian villages of Dalmatia on Adriatic coast and Slavonia of former Yugoslavia. Source: Keys et al.[21] Acta Med Scand 1966;460(Suppl):1–392.

recorded following standardized procedures and were coded centrally. The highest prevalence by MC 3.1 was reported in two rural populations of men from West Finland and from Karelia in the eastern part of the country, 16.2 and 17.9%, respectively. At the low end were seven study groups with less than 5% prevalence, with the lowest prevalence among Minneapolis businessmen (1.2%) and US switchmen from the Railroad study (1.6%).Table 7A.3 also reveals that with LVH criteria combining high amplitude R waves with even a mild degree of ST depression (including MC 4.3 or 4.4), LVH prevalence dropped to 2% or less in all of the 17 study groups, and in 11 out of 17 groups it decreased to less than 1%.

Does the wide range of the reported LVH prevalence by the MC high amplitude R wave criteria in the Finnish cohorts truly reflect population differences in LVH? Finnish populations were previously found to have a high prevalence of ECG-LVH, in all likelihood because of physiological adaptation to a high level of occupational physical activity, at least among younger age groups.[22] The prevalence of LVH by high amplitude R wave criteria was also reported to be high among lumberjacks in Finland,[23] and in another population study among Finnish firemen.[24]

The ECGs used in these older studies contained analog circuits for internal calibration that were rarely checked for accuracy with external calibrators. The calibration pulse was visually adjusted for the nominal standard scaling at 10 mm/mV, with the goal to retain an overall gain accuracy within at least ±10%. An examination of the cumulative frequency distribution of the Sokolow–Lyon voltage in these populations revealed that two ECGs, both within the limits of 10% correct gain, may produce a nearly threefold difference in the apparent LVH prevalence.[4]

Wide variations in reported LVH prevalence in various populations are also pronounced by comparing LVH prevalence in the same population according to different LVH criteria. For instance, in the 1998 report from an Italian study on patients referred to hypertension clinics,[25] ECG-LVH prevalence was compared according to seven of the criteria listed in Table 7A.1. The prevalence of LVH ranged from 3.9% according to the Framingham criteria to 17.8% according to the Perugia score.

7A.2.2 Age Trends and Ethnic Differences in ECG-LVH Prevalence

7A.2.2.1 The US National Health Surveys

Computer-ECG software suitable for quantitative analysis of the rest and exercise ECGs for epidemiological surveys was developed at the Central ECG Laboratory at Dalhousie University (later known as the Epidemiological Cardiology Research [EPICARE] Center) in the context of the Seven Countries study in the late 1960s. Electrocardiographic acquisition technology and computer-ECG software development had reached performance level meeting the rigorous requirements for quantitative studies by the time of the start of MRFIT[20,26] and the second US National Health and Nutrition Survey (NHANES 2). NHANES 2 was conducted during 1976–1980 and NHANES 3 during 1988–1994. Electrocardiograms from both of these surveys were processed by the Dalhousie ECG program[27,28] and classified according to the MC criteria.

In NHANES 2 white men (Figure 7A.1), ECG-LVH by the MC 3.1–3.3 criteria decreased from

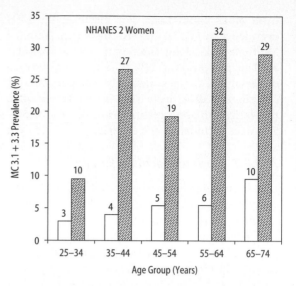

FIGURE 7A.2 Prevalence of LVH according to Minnesota Code 3.1+3.3 criteria by age in NHANES 2 white women (*open bars*) and African–American women (*patterned bars*). Like in men in Figure 7A.1, LVH prevalence is substantially higher in African–American than in white women. An increasing age trend is noted, more consistent in white than in African–American women.

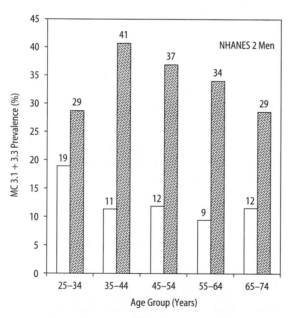

FIGURE 7A.1 Prevalence of LVH according to Minnesota Code 3.1+3.3 criteria by age in NHANES 2 white men (*open bars*) and African–American men (*patterned bars*). The prevalence is substantially higher in African–American than in white men. There is no indication for an increasing age trend in men as in some earlier studies.

age 25–34 years to age 35–44 years and remained relatively unchanged thereafter. In NHANES 2 African–American men, MC 3.1–3.3 prevalence first increased from age 25–34 years to 35–44 years, then declined with age gradually. A slowly increasing age trend was present in white women. In NHANES 2 African–American women, the increase occurred between the first two age groups and there was no systematic trend thereafter (Figure 7A.2).

In NHANES 3 white men, the ECG-LVH prevalence by the MC 3.1–3.3 criteria was approximately 10% in age groups 35–44 and 45–54 years, and there was a small increase to 13% in age groups 55–64 and 65–74 years (Figure 7A.3). No increasing age trend was seen in NHANES 3 African–American men. In NHANES 3, an increasing age trend in MC 3.1–3.3 prevalence was present both in white and African–American women (Figure 7A.4).

There was a drastically higher ECG-LVH prevalence by MC 3.1–3.3 criteria in African–American than in white American men (Table 7A.4) and in

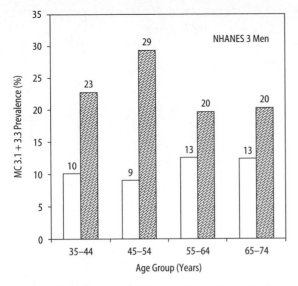

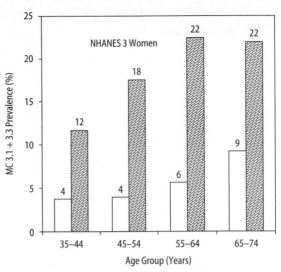

FIGURE 7A.3 Prevalence of LVH according to Minnesota Code 3.1+3.3 criteria by age in NHANES 3 white men (*open bars*) and African–American men (*patterned bars*). As in Figure 7A.1 from NHANES 2 data, the prevalence is substantially higher in African–American than in white men. No prominent age trend like that reported in earlier studies is noted.

FIGURE 7A.4 Prevalence of LVH (Minnesota Code 3.1+3.3) by age in NHANES 3 white women (*open bars*) and African–American women (*patterned bars*). As in Figure 7A.2 from NHANES 2 data, the prevalence is substantially higher in African–American than in white women. An increasing prevalence trend with age is seen both in white and African–American women.

African–American than in white women (Table 7A.5). The ethnic difference was consistent in both of these national health surveys.

7A.2.2.2 The Copenhagen City Heart Study

The Copenhagen City Heart Study[29] provides a representative example of age trends in ECG-LVH

according to the MC 3.1–3.3 high QRS amplitude criteria (Figure 7A.5). That cross-sectional survey was conducted from 1976 to 1978. Combined MC 3.1–3.3 prevalence data of 6,505 men and 7,713 women extracted from the 1981 report again demonstrated a drop in the prevalence in young adult men until age 40–49 years, with little subsequent variation with age. In women, a steady increase in

TABLE 7A.4 Prevalence of left ventricular hypertrophy with Minnesota Code (*MC*) criteria by age in white and African–American men in NHANES 2 and NHANES 3.

Survey	Age group	White men			African–American men		
		n	MC 3.1	MC 3.1–1.3*	n	MC 3.1	MC 3.1–3.3*
NHANES 2	25–34	759	10.8	19.0	115	19.1	28.7
	35–44	557	7.0	11.5	59	25.4	40.7
	45–54	532	7.7	11.8	57	24.6	36.8
	55–64	899	6.6	9.5	109	22.9	33.9
	65–74	864	9.0	11.6	98	21.4	28.6
	35–54	1,089	7.3	11.7	116	25.0	38.8
	55–74	1,763	7.8	10.5	207	22.2	31.4
NHANES 3	35–44	404	4.5	9.4	215	10.2	22.8
	45–54	625	2.6	4.2	218	9.2	29.4
	55–64	689	4.5	6.4	222	12.6	19.8
	65–74	1,371	4.7	6.9	328	12.5	20.4
	35–54	1,029	3.3	6.2	433	9.7	26.1
	55–74	2,060	4.7	6.7	550	12.5	20.2

* Criteria 3A as defined in Table 7A.1.

TABLE 7A.5 Prevalence of left ventricular hypertrophy by Minnesota Code (*MC*) criteria by age in white and African–American women in NHANES 2 and NHANES 3.

Survey	Age group	White women			African–American women		
		n	MC 3.1	MC 3.1–3.3*	*n*	MC 3.1	MC 3.1–3.3*
NHANES2	25–34	849	0.9	2.9	126	1.6	9.5
	35–44	621	0.8	4.0	90	7.8	26.7
	45–54	553	1.1	5.4	88	11.4	19.3
	55–64	985	3.9	5.7	114	18.4	31.6
	65–74	1,015	6.9	9.7	113	15.0	29.2
	35–54	1,174	0.9	4.7	178	9.6	23.0
	55–74	2,000	5.4	7.7	227	16.7	30.4
NHANES 3	35–44	443	1.4	3.6	258	3.9	11.6
	45–54	675	2.1	3.9	274	8.4	17.5
	55–64	669	2.5	5.7	277	10.1	22.4
	65–74	1,389	7.0	9.2	323	14.6	22.0
	35–54	1,118	1.8	3.8	532	6.2	14.7
	55–74	2,058	5.5	8.1	600	12.5	22.2

* Criteria 3A as defined in Table 7A.1.

ECG-LVH prevalence by the MC 3.1–3.3 criteria was seen after age 40–49 years.

7A.2.2.3 Other Studies

Ethnic differences in ECG-LVH prevalence have been reported from several populations with

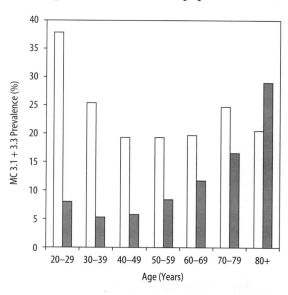

FIGURE 7A.5 Prevalence of LVH (Minnesota Code 3.1+3.3) by age in men (*white bars*) and women (*gray bars*) in the Copenhagen City Heart Study. Consistent with other reports, the high prevalence in young males decreases to a minimum at age 40–49 years. The profound increase in prevalence seen in women from age 40 years is not present in men. (Source: Östör et al.[29] Eur Heart J 1981;2:317–28. Copyright © 1981 European Society of Cardiology. Reproduced with permission.)

varying ECG-LVH criteria.[30-36] The prevalence of ECG-LVH in African–Americans compared to whites was nearly threefold in the Evans County study,[30-32] and over fourfold in the Charleston study.[35] In order to increase the specificity of the LVH criteria, the Chicago area Heart Study defined LVH by MC 3.1 criteria combined with repolarization abnormalities (MC 4.1–4.3 or MC 5.1–5.3).[34] Although the inclusion of repolarization abnormalities in LVH criteria considerably reduces the prevalence, the ethnic differences comparing African–Americans with white Americans were pronounced: 1.6 versus 0.3%, 1.4 versus 0.3%, and 3.5 versus 1.2% in age groups 20–34, 35–49, and 50–64 years, respectively. High ECG-LVH prevalence was also found in civil servants in Nigeria.[36] In that study, ECG-LVH prevalence by MC 3.1–3.3 criteria was 36.3% in men and 16.9% in women.

7A.2.3 The Effect of LVH Criteria used on Age Trends in ECG-LVH Prevalence

Evaluation of ethnic differences in ECG patterns has revealed striking differences in US populations in age trends between the ECG-LVH prevalence by the Cornell voltage and the Sokolow–Lyon voltage criteria.[37] Prevalence of ECG-LVH by the Cornell voltage criterion increased with age in men (Figure 7A.6) and in women (Figure 7A.7). The graphs demonstrate the similarity of the

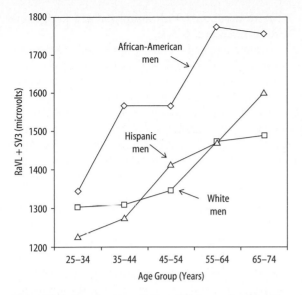

FIGURE 7A.6 Cornell voltage (RaVL + SV3) by age in white, Hispanic, and African–American men. Note consistent increasing trend with age in all three ethnic groups and the substantially higher mean values in African–American compared to white and Hispanic men. (Source: Rautaharju et al.[37] J Electrocardiol 1994; 27(Suppl):20–30. Copyright © 1994. Reproduced with permission from Elsevier.)

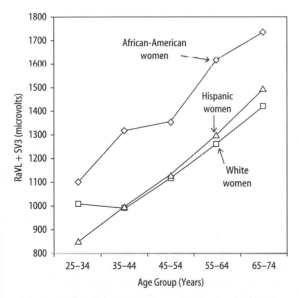

FIGURE 7A.7 Cornell voltage (RaVL + SV3) by age in white, Hispanic, and African–American women. Note consistent increasing trend with age in all three ethnic groups and the substantially higher mean values in African–American compared to white and Hispanic women. (Source: Rautaharju et al.[37] J Electrocardiol 1994;27(Suppl):20–30. Copyright © 1994. Reproduced with permission from Elsevier.)

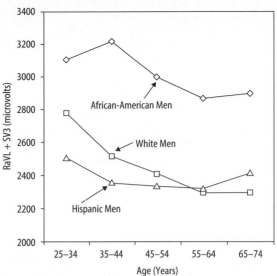

FIGURE 7A.8 Sokolow–Lyon voltage (RV5 + SV7) by age in white, Hispanic, and African–American men. Note the opposite, decreasing age trend in Sokolow–Lyon voltage in all three ethnic groups in comparison to the systematic increase in Cornell voltage with age in Figure 7A.6. The mean values of the Sokolow–Lyon voltage in African–American men are substantially higher compared to white and Hispanic men. (Source: Rautaharju et al.[37] J Electrocardiol 1994;27(Suppl):20–30. Copyright © 1994. Reproduced with permission from Elsevier.)

Cornell voltage between Hispanic and white men and women, and again the drastically higher voltages in African–American men and women compared to the other two ethnic groups in all age groups. The age trend patterns in the ECG-LVH prevalence by the Sokolow–Lyon voltage criteria differed drastically from those by the Cornell voltage criteria in all three ethnic groups in men (Figure 7A.8) and also in women, except in African–American women (Figure 7A.9).

7A.2.4 Echocardiographic versus ECG-LVH – Ethnic Differences

Echocardiographic data, although limited, do not lend support for radical ethnic differences in LVM as would be expected if the ECG prevalence estimates were true. It has become evident that standard ECG criteria overestimate ethnic differences in LVH prevalence.[38] A good example is the report by the Veterans Affairs Cooperative Study Group

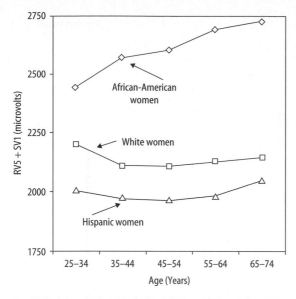

FIGURE 7A.9 Sokolow–Lyon voltage (RV5 + SV1) by age in white, Hispanic, and African–American women. Increasing age trend in Sokolow–Lyon voltage is present only in African–American women, and their mean values are substantially higher compared to white and Hispanic women. (Source: Rautaharju et al.[37] J Electrocardiol 1994;27(Suppl):20–30. Copyright © 1994. Reproduced with permission from Elsevier.)

on Antihypertensive Agents: although there was a threefold ethnic difference in ECG-LVH (31 vs 10%, $p < 0.001$), Echo-LVM indexed either to standing body height or to BSA did not differ significantly by race.[39] Electrocardiographic criteria were not specified but judging from the prevalence, Sokolow–Lyon or similar amplitude criteria were apparently used. Septal and posterior wall thickness and the relative wall thickness ([ratio of posterior wall thickness * 2] to left ventricular diastolic cavity size) were all significantly greater in African–American than in white men. These findings suggest that left ventricular cavity size (a factor influencing ECG amplitudes due to the Brody effect) was not increased in African–American compared to white men.

The Treatment of Mild Hypertension Study (TOMHS)[40] found slightly greater septal and relative wall thickness in African–American than in white study participants ($p < 0.05$). Overall, Echo-LVH (left ventricular mass index LVMI $\geq 134\,g/m^2$ for men and $\geq 110\,g/m^2$ for women) was present in 13% of men and 20% of women, and ECG-LVH was reported to be "virtually absent" by MC 3.1

criteria combined with abnormal repolarization (MC 4.1–4.3 or 5.1–5.3).

In subgroups of the CHS population of men and women 65 years old and older, there was no notable difference in the Echo-LVM between white and African–American men or women.[41]

The Coronary Artery Risk Development in Young Adults (CARDIA) study evaluated associations between Echo-LVM and demographic and coronary heart disease (CHD) risk factors among young adults aged 23–35 years.[42] In a multivariate model, LVM remained independently and positively associated with body weight. After adjustment for a variety of demographic and CHD risk factors including body fatness, height and blood pressure, LVM was 11 g higher in African–American men than in white men (167 ± 43 vs $156 \pm 50\,g$, respectively), and 5 g higher in African–American women than in white women (142 ± 49 vs $137 \pm 43\,g$, respectively).

7A.2.5 Prevalence of ECG-LVH in Hypertensive Cohorts

The Hypertension Detection and Follow-up Program (HDFP) report from 1985 contained ECG-LVH prevalence data in this cohort of 10,940 hypertensive men and women.[43] The study group was selected for a 5-year intervention and follow-up if their diastolic blood pressure (fifth phase) at the second screening visit was 90 mmHg or above. The prevalence of ECG-LVH by the MC 3.1–1.3 criteria was 6.8% in white men, 22.0% in black men, 4.4% in white women, and 12.3% in African–American women, again demonstrating the profoundly higher prevalence in African–American compared to white men and women. The corresponding percentages for ECG-LVH by MC 3.1–3.3 and (4.1–4.3 or 5.1–5.3) criteria were 2.7 and 8.6%, for white and African–American men, respectively, and 1.7 and 7.7% for white and African–American women, respectively.

Prevalence data for LVH have been reported in numerous other studies. However, comparative evaluation of these reported ECG-LVH data in contrasting populations is of relatively little value because of the formidable problems in achieving adequate reliability in LVH prevalence estimates by ECG criteria, as will be discussed later.

7A.2.6 Time Trends in ECG-LVH Prevalence

7A.2.6.1 NHANES Data

In the three successive US National Health Surveys, there have been some striking changes over time in ECG-LVH prevalence according to MC high QRS criteria. There has been a consistent decreasing trend over time in older white and African–American men (Figure 7A.10). Among younger African–American men the prevalence increased between NHANES 1 and NHANES 2, followed by a decline from NHANES 2 to NHANES 3. There has been a consistent decreasing trend over time in African–American women (Figure 7A.11). In older women there was a large decrease in LVH prevalence from NHANES 1 to NHANES 2, with no subsequent difference between NHANES 2 and NHANES 3.

The LVH prevalence by MC 3.1–3.3 criteria from NHANES 1 is included here to evaluate long-term trends in the prevalence of the MC high R wave amplitude criteria for LVH. NHANES 1 was conducted between 1971 and 1975. Electrocardiographic acquisition technology, amplifier design

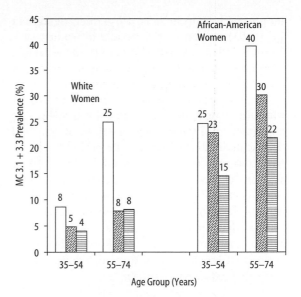

FIGURE 7A.11 Prevalence of LVH (Minnesota Code 3.1+3.3) by age in white women (*left*) and African–American women (*right*) in three successive national health surveys: NHANES 1 (*open bars*), NHANES 2 (*bars with diagonal rectangles*), and NHANES 3 (*bars with horizontal stripes*). A consistent decreasing trend over time is seen in African–American women. Note the large decrease in LVH prevalence in older white women from NHANES 1 to NHANES 2, with no subsequent difference between NHANES 2 and NHANES 3.

and FM magnetic tape recording technology was still in the development phase, and ECG data from the survey should be considered with caution. It was still possible to rescue a substantial fraction of the ECGs from the survey for later computer analysis.[16] As mentioned before, ECG acquisition technology and computer-ECG software development had improved to the level equal to the present-day standards by the time of NHANES 2 and 3.

7A.2.6.2 The Framingham Study

Mosterd et al. reported in 1999 that the population prevalence of ECG-LVH by the Framingham voltage criteria combined with abnormal repolarization has declined from 1950 to 1989 from 4.5 to 2.5% in men and from 3.6 to 1.1% in women in the combined original and offspring cohorts.[44] The decline in the age-adjusted ECG-LVH prevalence was 23% per decade in men and 41% in women ($p < 0.01$ for both). In that same 40-year period, the mean age-adjusted Cornell voltage

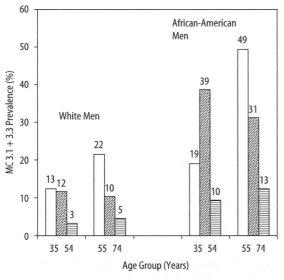

FIGURE 7A.10 Prevalence of LVH (Minnesota Code 3.1+3.3) by age in white men (*left*) and African–American men (*right*) in three successive national health surveys: NHANES 1 (*open bars*), NHANES 2 (*bars with diagonal rectangles*), and NHANES 3 (*bars with horizontal stripes*). A consistent decreasing trend over time is evident in older white and African–American men. Among younger African–American men the prevalence increases between NHANES 1 and NHANES 2, followed by a decline from NHANES 2 to NHANES 3.

amplitude had declined $80\,\mu V$ per decade in men ($p = 0.03$) and $60\,\mu V$ per decade in women ($p = 0.06$). This ECG-LVH decline paralleled the decline in hypertension approximately to one-half in men and nearly to one-quarter in women (defined as systolic blood pressure over 160 mmHg or diastolic blood pressure over 100 mmHg). As expected, antihypertensive medication use had drastically increased during the period, from 2.3 to 24.6% among men and from 5.7 to 27.7% in women. The availability of more effective antihypertensive regimens has unquestionably contributed to the success of hypertension intervention.

The declining trend in ECG-LVH in the Framingham predominantly white population is confirmed by the trends from the three sets of NHANES data, as was shown.

FIGURE 7A.12 Differing influence of demographic factors on the LVH prevalence odds ratio by the Cornell voltage (*CV*) and Sokolow–Lyon based Minnesota Code (*MC*) criteria.

7A.3 Other Determinants of ECG-LVH

7A.3.1 Overweight, ECG-LVH, and Echocardiographic LVH

7A.3.1.1 ECG-LVH and Overweight – NHANES 2 and the Hispanic Health and Nutrition Examination Surveys

The effects of race, age, and obesity on ECG-LVH by the MC 3.1–3.3 and the Cornell voltage criteria from a multivariate model were reported using the data from NHANES 2 and the Hispanic Health and Nutrition Examination Survey.[37] The data demonstrated that the association of demographic extracardiac factors with the two sets of ECG-LVH criteria differed but that the associations with each were relatively uniform in the three ethnic groups. The exception was the overweight status, which had a significant positive association with RaVL and ECG-LVH by the Cornell voltage only in Hispanics, with an odds ratio 1.88 (1.30, 2.72). The association of overweight with ECG-LVH by the MC criteria was inverse in all ethnic groups. Figure 7A.12 summarizes the results in pooled ethnic groups.

The prominent association of ECG-LVH with African–American race by both sets of criteria is evident. The association with age is pronounced for the Cornell voltage and of borderline significance for the MC criteria. The negative associa-

tion between QRS axis and ECG-LVH by the Cornell voltage criteria reflects pronounced horizontal shift of QRS axis with overweight, due at least in part to increased abdominal fat pushing the diaphragm up. This is probably a dominant factor associated with the reported increase of ECG-LVH by the Cornell voltage criteria.

7A.3.1.2 The LIFE Study

In the Losartan Intervention For Endpoint reduction in hypertension (LIFE) study, the presence of ECG-LVH by either the Cornell product or the Sokolow–Lyon voltage in high risk hypertensive patients was a selection criterion. The ECG-LVH prevalence by the Cornell voltage criteria was 52% in normal weight patients and 62% in overweight as well as pronounced overweight patients.[45] The corresponding prevalence figures for Sokolow–Lyon voltage were 13% in normal weight patients and 16% in overweight patients, and the prevalence decreased to 11% in patients with pronounced overweight.

Reduced ECG-LVH prevalence with overweight is most likely associated with increased distance of cardiac excitation fronts from body surface (inverse square effect with distance). Breast tissue in women has been found to have a significant although relatively modest negative association with QRS voltage in chest leads.[46]

7A.3.1.3 The CHS Population

Comparison of the apparent reported prevalence by commonly used ECG criteria in normal weight and overweight subjects emphasizes the important role of obesity.[41] These data were derived from a report from the CHS population. Echocardiographic LVH prevalence ranged from approximately 13 to 18% in various gender and race groups when Echo-LVM was indexed to BSA. In normal weight subjects, the Sokolow–Lyon as well as the Cornell voltage criteria underestimated LVH prevalence in men, overestimated it in African–American women, and they were more closely in reasonable agreement in white women (Figure 7A.13). In overweight men, both ECG criteria grossly underestimate LVH prevalence in men, and the Sokolow–Lyon criteria also in women (Figure 7A.14). The Cornell voltage criteria were in closer agreement with Echo-LVH prevalence in women.

A note of caution is in place in this connection. The apparent close agreement between any given ECG criteria and echocardiographic criteria in the reported LVH prevalence does not necessarily mean a good performance. The reliability of the

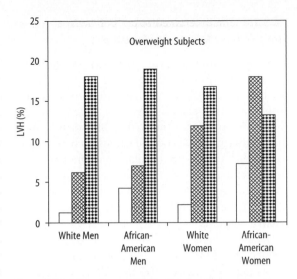

FIGURE 7A.14 Prevalence of LVH by Sokolow–Lyon voltage (*open bars*), Cornell voltage (*bars with diagonal rectangles*) and echocardiographic criteria (*bars with diamonds*) in overweight CHS participants by gender and race.

reported prevalence is often very inaccurate when the correct fraction of "true" LVH (i.e. Echo-LVH) cases is evaluated in the group with reported LVH. This problem will be discussed in detail later on in this chapter.

Body size, body weight in particular, is the primary determinant of Echo-LVM. In the CHS population, the factors associated with Echo-LVM in addition to body weight in stepwise linear regression were, in order of decreasing importance, male sex, systolic blood pressure, prevalent congestive heart failure (CHF), smoking, major and minor ECG abnormalities (including ECG-LVH), treatment for hypertension, and various factors related to valvular heart disease.[47] All these demographic and clinical factors together explained 37% of total LVM variance. Increased LVM and Echo-LVH can be considered a risk and precipitating factor for CHF rather than the other way around. While in multiple regression models systolic blood pressure was associated with Echo-LVM, the association for diastolic blood pressure was equal to that of systolic blood pressure but inverse, and as an obvious consequence, the pulse pressure was a positive correlate of Echo-LVM. High density lipoprotein cholesterol was also an inverse correlate of Echo-LVM.

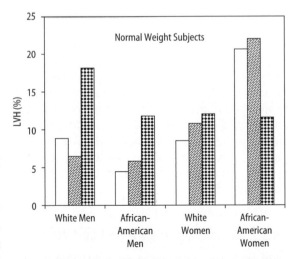

FIGURE 7A.13 Prevalence of LVH by Sokolow–Lyon voltage (*open bars*), Cornell voltage (*bars with diagonal rectangles*) and echocardiographic criteria (*bars with diamonds*) in normal weight CHS participants by gender and race. Compared to echocardiographic LVH, both Sokolow–Lyon and Cornell voltage criteria appear to underestimate LVH prevalence in men and overestimate LVH prevalence in African–American women.

7A.3.1.4 The Veterans Affairs Cooperative Study – the LVM Indexing Problem

The over-riding critical issue in considering the obesity effect in relation to Echo-LVH is the method used for indexing LVM to body size. The results and the conclusions may differ substantially if Echo-LVM is indexed to BSA or to standing height (or some power of height such as $height^2$ or $height^{2.7}$). Left ventricular mass/height is at times referred to as Framingham criteria and LVM/BSA as Cornell criteria. In the Veterans Affairs Cooperative Study Group on Antihypertensive Agents report,[39] adiposity category (normal weight, overweight and obese) was defined by BMI: overweight was significantly associated with Echo-LVH by LVM/BSA criteria ($p < 0.05$ for overweight vs normal weight and for obese vs overweight group) but the intergroup differences were smaller by LVM/height criteria ($p < 0.05$ for overweight vs normal weight and for obese vs normal weight group). Furthermore, the regression slope of LVM/height vs systolic blood pressure was relatively low (approximately $1.25\,g/m$ for a 10-mmHg increment in systolic pressure); the slope was more than threefold in the overweight compared to the normal weight group, suggesting a synergistic effect of overweight and systolic blood pressure on Echo-LVM.

7A.3.1.5 The 1988 Framingham Report

In a 1988 report on 4,976 participants of the Framingham study, Echo-LVH prevalence by LVM/height criteria was 16% in men and 19% in women, showing a strong nonlinear increase with age (from 6% in subjects <30 years old to 43% at age >69 years.[48] Echocardiographic LVM indexed to height was strongly associated with overweight and systolic blood pressure, and the independent effect was additive (not synergistic). Obesity was independently predictive of Echo-LVH, with an approximately 50% increase for each $2\,kg/m^2$ increment in BMI. The apparent association between obesity and Echo-LVM was attenuated for LVM/BSA criteria. The association between LVH (indexed to BSA) was less striking for subscapular skinfold thickness as a measure of obesity.

7A.3.1.6 TOMHS

Multiple logistic regression analysis data in the TOMHS report cited above[40] showed that BMI was significantly associated with LVH by LVM/height criteria, in addition to systolic blood pressure, gender, and urinary sodium excretion. A 10-mmHg blood pressure increment and a $3\,kg/m^2$ increment in BMI were each associated with over 40% increase in odds for LVH. Systolic blood pressure and gender were significantly associated with Echo-LVH by LVM/BSA criteria but BMI was not an independent predictor of Echo-LVH. Interestingly, over one-half of those with LVH by LVM/BSA criteria were classified as having eccentric nondilated hypertrophy, meaning that Echo-LVM is increased with normal relative posterior wall thickness and normal left ventricular diastolic cavity size. This finding is similar to the distribution of LVH patterns in the Framingham study, with one-half of the men and close to two-thirds of the women with Echo-LVH having eccentric nondilated LVH. This raises the question whether LVH at least in the eccentric nondilated category is in part confounded by generation of excessive LVH in short persons when Echo-LVM is divided by height (and particularly by $height^2$ or $height^{2.7}$ as in some studies).

There is a tendency to promote LVMI methods that yield the highest possible prevalence of LVH in overweight persons. By indexing LVM to height to power 2.7, the prevalence may appear to be nearly three times higher in obese normotensive subjects than in normal weight subjects, a difference not detected by indexing LVM to body surface area.[49] The availability of lean body weight data in combination with accurate echocardiographic data is clearly needed to resolve this important issue.

7A.3.2 Gender Differences in ECG-LVH

Okin et al. have performed extensive analyses on gender differences in ECG-LVH criteria, Echo-LVM, and indexing ECG variables to body size and Echo-LVM.[50] The authors concluded that "gender differences in body size and LVM do not completely account for gender differences in QRS duration and voltage measurements, and ECG criteria for LVH have lower accuracy in women even when gender differences in partition value selection are taken into account".

The differing effect of male gender, with a pronounced negative association with ECG-LVH by the Cornell voltage criteria and equally pronounced positive association by the MC criteria, is intriguing.[37] The positive association with the MC criteria is largely explained by the lack of any gender adjustment. The question remains whether the LVH thresholds for the Cornell voltage are optimal. In the CHS population, the correlation between Echo- and ECG-LVM in optimal gender- and race-specific models was actually higher in women than in men.[51] The LVH threshold for the Cornell voltage in men had to be lowered from $2,800\,\mu V$ to $2,650\,\mu V$ to obtain equal specificity (95%). Using these thresholds, there was no appreciable gender difference in sensitivity over a wide range of Echo-LVH severity levels.

7A.3.3 Heredity, ECG-LVH, and Echocardiographic LVH

Among other factors, heritability may possibly play a role in predisposing to LVH. A report from the MONICA Augsburg Center compared the risk of Echo-LVM in 319 siblings and 636 subjects matched for gender and age and found that the relative risk for the septal and posterior wall thickness was significantly increased ($p < 0.05$).[52] The risk of concentric LVH was increased in the siblings with LVH.

Hereditary estimates in 995 members of 229 Caucasian families with a hypertensive proband were evaluated by Mayosi et al.[53] By determining familiar correlations, these investigators concluded that ECG-LVH shows a greater heritability than Echo-LVH.

The Framingham study investigators evaluated intraclass correlations among first-degree relatives, second-degree relatives, and unrelated spouse pairs in adults of the original Framingham cohort and the Framingham Offspring Study using Echo-LVM.[54] The report concluded that heredity explains a small proportion of the LVM variance.

7A.4 Limited Accuracy of ECG-LVH Criteria

Several reports have indicated that the classification accuracy of commonly used ECG-LVH criteria is low, and their reliability particularly in African–American populations may be questionable. A 1990 report from the Framingham study evaluated the accuracy of the Framingham criteria (set 9 in Table 7A.1) in LVH classification in 4,684 subjects with echocardiographic evidence of LVH as the standard.[55] Echocardiographic LVH prevalence was 14.2% in men and 17.6% in women (LVM/height > mean + 2*SD in the healthy reference group). This contrasted with ECG-LVH prevalence of 2.9% in men and 1.5% in women. Comparison of the classification accuracy of ECG-LVH with Echo-LVH as the standard in the quartiles by BMI revealed a striking effect of obesity. The sensitivity declined from 14.2% in the lowest BMI quartile to 5.7% in the highest two quartiles while the specificity increase was less than 1%.

Evaluation of ECG-LVH criteria in the CHS participants using Echo-LVM data as an independent standard yielded higher sensitivity levels for five different LVH criteria evaluated when the classification thresholds were adjusted to obtain 95% specificity.[51] Still, the sensitivity for all five ECG-LVH criteria was 30% or lower, no matter what indexing method was used for adjusting Echo-LVM to body size. The sensitivity was consistently lowest for the Sokolow–Lyon voltage.

Casale et al., using autopsy documentation as the standard for evaluation, reported a higher sensitivity for Sokolow–Lyon voltage, 22% with a specificity of 100%.[17] The sensitivity of the Cornell voltage criteria was higher, 42%, at a specificity of 96%. The Romhilt–Estes 5-point criteria had the sensitivity of 33% and the 4-point criteria 54%, with corresponding specificity 94 and 85%, respectively. The performance was improved with a new multiple logistic regression model derived from the study group using gender, the Cornell voltage, TV1 amplitude and the terminal P wave area in V1: sensitivity 62% and specificity 92%.

In general, clinical study materials with autopsy documentation tend to have a more severe form of LVH than can be expected in populations outside hospital, even in subjects with longstanding hypertension. Casale at al. appropriately commented on the relation of the disease (LVH) prevalence in the population to the overall test accuracy with the observed sensitivity and specificity of the LVH criteria in their study. At 10% LVH prevalence in the population, the overall test accuracy was calculated as 92% for the Sokolow–Lyon and the Cornell voltage. This can be considered quite sufficient from a clinical point of view. The conclusions and the implications of the results are entirely different concerning comparative evaluation of LVH prevalence in many general populations.

The results from the studies cited above will suffice to demonstrate that the sensitivity of ECG-LVH criteria is rather low at an adequate level of specificity when Echo-LVH or autopsy evidence is used as the standard for evaluation. Higher classification accuracy is in general obtained in test and reference groups selected from hospital populations, generally with more severe levels of LVH. As expected, classification accuracy tends to deteriorate when the criteria advocated are subjected to independent testing in different populations.

7A.4.1 Misleading LVH Prevalence Reports from Population Surveys

How realistic are the reported two- and up to threefold differences in LVH prevalence for instance between African–Americans and white

populations, between men and women, and between young and middle-aged men? The following considerations will elucidate some of the reasons for such large differences in reported prevalence between different race, gender and age groups.

The reported prevalence (RP) is related to the true prevalence (P), sensitivity (SE), and specificity by the following expression:

$$RP = SE * P + (1 - SP) * (1 - P). \quad [7A.1]$$

(Note that in the above equation P, SE, SP and RP are expressed as fractions, not as percentages.) A comparison of the reported prevalence for various combinations of the sensitivity and specificity of ECG-LVH criteria reveals some interesting facts (Table 7A.6). The reported prevalence estimates (converted to percentages) in Table 7A.6 are for true LVH prevalence of 10%. If the specificity is 100% (the last row in Table 7A.6), the reported prevalence is equal to the product of the sensitivity and prevalence, and the reported prevalence is equal to sensitivity for combinations with equal levels of sensitivity and specificity (diagonal elements). For low levels of true prevalence (10% and less), the reported prevalence of 20% or more, as commonly observed, can be obtained only if the specificity is 80% or lower at any level of sensitivity.

TABLE 7A.6 Reported left ventricular hypertrophy prevalence (*RP*)* by sensitivity (*SE*) and specificity (*SP*) in a population with true prevalence (*P*) = 10%.

Specificity (%)	Sensitivity (%)										
	0	10	20	30	40	50	60	70	80	90	100
0	90	91	92	93	94	95	96	97	98	99	**100**
10	81	82	83	84	85	86	87	88	89	**90**	91
20	72	73	74	75	76	77	78	79	**80**	81	82
30	63	64	65	66	67	68	69	**70**	71	72	73
40	54	55	56	57	58	59	**60**	61	62	63	64
50	45	46	47	48	49	**50**	51	52	53	54	55
60	36	37	38	39	**40**	41	42	43	44	45	46
70	27	28	29	**30**	31	32	33	34	35	36	37
80	18	19	**20**	21	22	23	24	25	26	27	28
90	9	**10**	11	12	13	14	15	16	17	18	19
100	**0**	1	2	3	4	5	6	7	8	9	10

* Reported prevalence was calculated from Equation 7A.1.
Note that RP = SE * P for SP = 100% (*last row*), RP = SP * P + (1 − SP) for SE = 100% (*last column*), and RP = SE when (SE + SP) = 100 (*bold-faced diagonal elements*). For a low level of true prevalence like 10%, the reported prevalence of 20% or more can be obtained only if the specificity is 70% or less at any level of sensitivity.

Let us assume that the 10% reported prevalence in white men represents the true LVH prevalence and that the sensitivity of the LVH criteria in white men is 36% and specificity 93%. Under what conditions can we get a twofold higher LVH prevalence estimate in African–American compared to white men? Assuming equal sensitivity and specificity in white and in African–American men, it can be determined from Equation 7A.1 above that a twofold higher reported LVH prevalence (20%) in African–American men is obtained if the true LVH prevalence is 50%. Such an LVH prevalence level in African–American men is inconceivable. There is an alternative, more plausible explanation to these rather radical reported LVH prevalence differences. It will be demonstrated next that the sensitivity or the specificity of ECG-LVH criteria has to differ in African–American compared to white men and women.

Using echocardiographic evidence as an independent standard, upper normal limits for Echo-LVM index (LVMI = Echo-LVM/BSA) in a "supernormal" CHS group using strict selection criteria were established as $116 \, g/m^2$ for men and $104 \, g/m^2$ for women. The LVH prevalence by this standard in the CHS population was established as 18.1% in white men, 15.5% in African–American men, 14.7% in white women and 12.8% in African–American women in the subgroups used in a previous study.[41] Thus, ethnic differences in Echo-LVH were relatively small. Taking 15% as the true LVH prevalence, the values for reported

prevalence, and the correct fraction of true LVH in the reported prevalence can be compared for various combinations of the sensitivity and specificity of ECG-LVH criteria (Table 7A.7). Correct fraction (CF) is obtained from the following expression:

$$CF = SE^*P \, / \, (SE^*P + (1 - SP) + (1 - P)), \quad [7A.2]$$

where SE, SP, P, and CF are expressed as fractions and converted to percentages in Table 7A.7.

The options of sensitivity/specificity combinations to obtain a reported LVH within 20% of the true LVH are relatively limited, and even more so if it is desired to have at least 50% true LVH in the reported prevalence. Reported prevalence of 20% is obtained if the sensitivity is 25% or higher combined with specificities from 80 to 86%. Only 45% sensitivity combined with 92% or 94% specificity and 55% sensitivity combined with 92% to 96% specificity will yield true prevalence fraction of 50% or higher.

The true operating points for different ethnic and gender groups according to the echocardiographic standard can be inferred from these models (Table 7A.8). In addition to the false predominance of ECG-LVH in African–American men and women with Sokolow–Lyon criteria, there is also an underestimate in LVH prevalence in all subgroups except the overestimated prevalence in African–American men (Figure 7A.15).

Equally large false ethnic differences in ECG-LVH are present by the unadjusted Cornell voltage

TABLE 7A.7 Reported prevalence (*RP*, %) and correct fraction (*CF*, %) of true left ventricular hypertrophy by sensitivity (%) and specificity (%) of left ventricular hypertrophy criteria for true prevalence of 15%.*

Sensitivity (%)	15		25		35		45		55	
Specificity (%)	RP	CF	RP	CF	RP	CF	RP	CF	RP	CF
80	19.3	12	20.8	18	22.3	24	23.8	28	25.3	33
82	**17.6**	13	19.1	20	20.6	26	22.1	31	23.6	35
84	**15.9**	14	**17.4**	22	18.9	28	20.4	33	21.9	38
86	**14.2**	16	**15.7**	24	**17.2**	31	18.7	36	20.2	41
88	**12.5**	18	**14.0**	27	**15.5**	34	**17.0**	40	18.5	45
90	10.8	21	**12.3**	31	**13.8**	38	**15.3**	44	**16.8**	49
92	9.1	25	10.6	36	**12.1**	44	***13.6***	***50***	***15.1***	***55***
94	7.4	31	8.9	42	10.4	51	***11.9***	***57***	***13.4***	***62***
96	5.7	40	6.3	52	8.7	62	10.2	67	***11.7***	***71***
98	4.0	57	5.5	69	7.0	76	8.5	80	10.0	83
100	2.3	100	3.8	100	5.3	100	6.8	100	8.3	100

* Bold face elements identify prevalences that are within 20% of the true LVH prevalence, and bold face italics those elements that in addition have correct fraction of LVH at least 50%.

TABLE **7A.8** Specificity (*SP*, %), sensitivity (*SE*, %), reported prevalence (*RP*, %) and correct fraction (*CF*, %) in the reported prevalence by three sets of left ventricular hypertrophy criteria with echocardiography as the standard.

		White men	Black men	White women	Black women
Sokolow–Lyon	SP	90.6	86.6	96.3	94.6
	SE	21.3	50.0	13.2	23.1
	RP	11.2	18.9	5.1	8.1
	CF	28.6	39.7	38.6	43.0
Cornell voltage	SP	95.5	95.8	91.6	85.3
	SE	15.8	46.2	27.8	53.8
	RP	6.2	10.5	11.3	20.6
	CF	38.3	66.0	36.9	39.2
Adjusted Cornell voltage*	SP	95.0	95.1	95.1	95.1
	SE	18.8	48.0	20.3	41.0
	RP	7.1	11.4	7.2	10.3
	CF	39.9	63.4	42.2	59.6

* Cornell voltage thresholds adjusted for 95% specificity were 2,700 μV in white men, 2,750 μV in black men, 2,200 μV in white women and 2,400 μV in black women.

criteria (Figure 7A.16), although the operating points for various subgroups are considerably different than for the Sokolow–Lyon criteria. As expected, a greater uniformity in the overall per-

formance for ECG-LVH criteria is achieved if the specificity of the criteria is adjusted to an equal level such as 95% (Figure 7A.17). However, this does not eliminate the false racial differences in

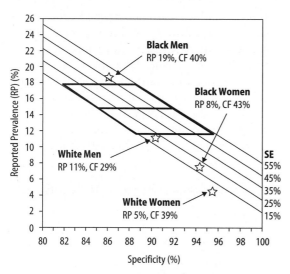

FIGURE **7A.15** Reported prevalence (*RP*) versus specificity at sensitivity (*SE*) ranging from 15 to 55% (*diagonal lines*) for Sokolow–Lyon criteria in subgroups by race and gender for true prevalence equal to 15% according to echocardiographic LVH. The stars at the tips of the arrows indicate the operating points for ECG-LVH. The parallelogram outlines the region where RP agrees with true prevalence within 20%. Echocardiographic LVH prevalence was approximately 15% in all study subgroups. Note the racial difference in the reported prevalence and the underestimate of the prevalence in all subgroups except the overestimate in African–American men.

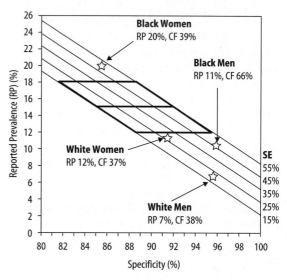

FIGURE **7A.16** Reported prevalence (*RP*) versus specificity at sensitivity (*SE*) ranging from 15 to 55% (*diagonal lines*) for Cornell voltage criteria in subgroups by race and gender for true prevalence equal to 15% according to echocardiographic LVH. The stars at the tips of the arrows indicate the operating points for ECG-LVH. The parallelogram outlines the region where RP agrees with true prevalence within 20%. Echocardiographic LVH prevalence was approximately 15% in all study subgroups. Note the reported twofold higher prevalence in African–American men and women and the underestimate of the prevalence in all subgroups except the overestimate in African–American women. The correct fraction (*CF*) in RP was <50% in all subgroups except 66% in black men.

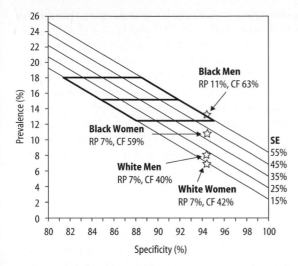

FIGURE 7A.17 Reported prevalence (*RP*) versus specificity at sensitivity (*SE*) ranging from 15 to 55% (*diagonal lines*) for Cornell voltage criteria with specificity adjusted to 95% in subgroups by race and gender for true prevalence equal to 15% according to echocardiographic LVH. The stars at the tips of the arrows indicate the operating points for ECG-LVH. The parallelogram outlines the region where RP agrees with true prevalence within 20%. Echocardiographic LVH prevalence was approximately 15% in all study subgroups. Note the reported twofold higher prevalence in African–Americans than in whites. The prevalence is an underestimate (the stars at the tips of the arrows) by 20% or more in all subgroups except in black men.

ECG-LVH prevalence. Also, LVH prevalence is considerably underestimated in all subgroups, although interestingly, in African–American men, the estimated prevalence is within 20% of the true prevalence and the correct fraction of true LVH in the estimate (63%) is much higher than in other groups.

Wide variations in the sensitivity and specificity by echocardiography as the standard have been reported in other studies, including the Italian Progretto Ipertensione Umbria Monitoraggio Ambulatoriale (PIUMA) study.[25] In that study, for instance, the Cornell voltage had a sensitivity of 16% and a specificity of 97%, and the Perugia score had a sensitivity of 34% and a specificity of 93%. The operating points for various criteria can be expected to be quite different in hypertensive hospital populations compared to community-dwelling populations.

In summary, specificity and sensitivity levels of ECG-LVH criteria vary widely in various race and

gender groups. This creates formidable problems for comparative estimation of ethnic and gender differences in LVH prevalence by ECG criteria, and the adjustment of specificity to equivalent levels does not eliminate the problems. Of course, LVH by echocardiographic criteria would have similar although less serious problems if some independent evaluation method were available to be used as a more accurate "gold standard".

7A.5 ECG-LVH and Mortality Risk

7A.5.1 Prognostic Value of ECG-LVH in General Populations

7A.5.1.1 The Copenhagen City Heart Study

A well-documented 2002 report from the Copenhagen City Heart Study on a large cohort of men and women aged 35–74 years evaluated the risk of MI and mortality for five groups of mutually exclusive ECG abnormalities, including high voltage ECG (MC 3.1–3.3) with and without ST-T abnormalities.[56] There was no significant interaction between gender and ECG abnormalities in individual categories of ECG abnormalities evaluated, and the gender groups were pooled for risk analyses. The study confirmed the common observation that Sokolow–Lyon type high voltage ECG alone is not associated with excess risk, except perhaps in special high risk groups like hypertension clinic patients with LVH by ECG criteria. Isolated T wave and combined ST-T abnormalities had a significantly increased risk for cardiovascular disease (CVD) mortality (Figure 7A.18). The multivariable-adjusted risk of CVD mortality was significantly increased for isolated T wave and combined isolated ST-T abnormalities, and the risk was increased approximately two- to over threefold for high voltage QRS with T wave and for high voltage QRS with combined ST-T abnormalities. A similarly increased risk was also observed for ischemic heart disease mortality for these combinations of high voltage QRS and repolarization abnormalities.

7A.5.1.2 The Framingham Study

Evaluation data for CVD risk are presented here from six other general populations (Table 7A.9).

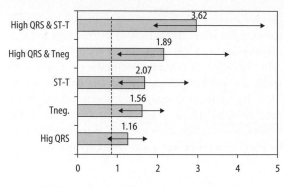

FIGURE 7A.18 Relative risk of 7-year ischemic heart disease mortality in a large combined group of men and women free of ischemic heart disease at the baseline for five mutually exclusive hierarchic (*from bottom to top*) combinations of ECG abnormalities. (Source: Larsen et al.[56] Eur Heart J 2002;23:315–24. © 2002 The European Society of Cardiology. Reproduced with permission.)

Data for the first study come from a 1994 Framingham report.[57] In that report, CVD event risk was evaluated for men and women of the Framingham cohort who were classified as having possible LVH by Framingham voltage criteria (the last set in Table 7A.1) at the initial examination. Data for CVD risk were extracted from subsequent 18 biennial examinations. Risk evaluation was performed for the Cornell voltage stratified into quartiles for subjects who were CVD-free at any given index examination for outcome events occurring through the subsequent scheduled biennial examination ($n + 1$). The subjects in the first Cornell voltage quartile were used as the reference group for other quartiles.

Incident CVD outcome events included CHD (CHD death, angina pectoris, MI), other cardiovascular deaths, CHF, stroke, or transient isch-

TABLE 7A.9 Electrocardiographic left ventricular hypertrophy and cardiovascular disease mortality risk in population samples extracted from general populations.

Study/baseline	Age (years)	Follow-up	Criteria*	Endpoint	Gender/race	RR (95% CI)	Comments
Framingham; CVD-free[57]/ 1948	28–62	18 biennials	Cornell voltage quartiles	CVD events	Men Women	3.08 (1.87–5.07) 3.29 (1.78–6.09)	Age-adjusted 2-year risk for incident LVH (quartile 4 vs 1)
BIRNH, CHD-free at baseline[59]/ 1981–84	25–74	≥10 years	High R + ST-T (2A)	CVD mortality	Men Women	3.14 (1.36–7.26) 2.20 (0.53–9.16)	RR multivariable-adjusted
RIFLE Pooling Project, heart disease-free[60]/ 1978–87	30–69	6 years	High R MC (3A) High QRS + ST-T MC (3B)	CVD mortality CVD mortality	Men Women Men Women	1.86 (1.13–3.07) 3.66 (0.96–14.0) 6.33 (3.02–13.3) 5.91 (0.70–49.9)	Multivariable-adjusted, also for other ECG abnormalities
NHANES 1 CHD-free[16]/ 1971–75	35–74	7–13 years	High QRS + ST-T MC (3B)		White men Black men White women Black women	3.26 (1.91–5.56) 4.29 (2.00–9.18) 2.59 (1.29–5.19) 1.90 (0.64–5.65)	RR age-adjusted
Survivors of the Finnish cohort of the Seven Countries Study[61]/1984	65–84	5 years	High QRS MC (2A) with or without Q, ST-T codes	All-cause mortality	Men	1.27 ($p = 0.034$)	p value from Chi-square test adjusted for age and geographic area
			High QRS alone MC (2A)	All-cause mortality	Men	0.68 (0.22–1.45)	Men without other ECG abnormalities
Bronx Longitudinal Aging Study[62]/1980	75–85	10 years	High QRS, ST-T MC (3B)	CVD mortality All-cause mortality	Men and women Men and women	2.72 (0.53–2.09) 2.18 (1.06–4.45)	Risk for LVH without regression

* Criteria identified in brackets refer to those listed in Table 7A.1. *CHD* coronary heart disease, *CVD* cardiovascular disease, *RR* relative risk.

emic attack, intermittent claudication. The CVD event rate increased progressively in groups stratified by the Cornell voltage. The increase in event rates was particularly pronounced for the highest quartile of the Cornell voltage (RaVL + SV3 >2.4mV) in both gender groups and for LVH-strain pattern in men. In the age-adjusted risk model, the odds ratio for the fourth quartile of the Cornell voltage with the first quartile as the reference was 3.08 (1.87–5.07) for men and 3.29 (1.78–6.09) for women.

Framingham risk data for the Cornell voltage suggest a considerably higher risk than most other studies. The cohort in the report had possible LVH by Framingham QRS amplitude criteria at the onset of the study. Most other studies have evaluated the risk for ECG-LVH at the onset of the study for outcome events during the subsequent whole follow-up period whereby each subject contributes only one observation. In the pooled logistic regression used in the Framingham study, each subject contributes multiple observations until the first outcome event occurs, and it is not clear how the results would differ if risk evaluation were performed just for the study-onset baseline Cornell voltage quartiles when the proportion of subjects with LVH is smaller and the follow-up period longer. However, statistical evaluation suggested that the results from pooled logistic regression are similar to those from time-dependent Cox regression.[58] In any case, the results indicate a graded risk throughout the range of increased Cornell voltage.

7A.5.1.3 The BIRNH Study

The Belgian Inter-University Research on Nutrition and Health (BIRNH) study classified ECG-LVH by the MC high amplitude R waves combined with ST-T changes (set 3 in Table 7A.1).[59] The study population consisted of 5,208 men and 4,746 women 25–74 years of age considered free from CHD at baseline, with a follow-up of at least 10 years. The age-adjusted and multivariable-adjusted relative risk (including adjustment for other major ECG abnormalities) was significantly increased for ECG-LVH in men for CVD mortality but not for CHD mortality or total mortality, and the risk was not significantly increased in women for any of the three major endpoints. For the sig-

nificant CVD mortality risk in men, the multivariable-adjusted risk ratio for ECG-LVH was 3.14 (1.36–7.26).

7A.5.1.4 NHANES 1 Follow-up

Risk data for CVD mortality from a 5- to 12-year follow-up of the NHANES 1 population in Table 7A.9[16] had considerable variations in risk estimates by gender and race and by various LVH criteria. Minnesota Code high amplitude QRS waves combined with repolarization abnormalities were associated with significantly increased risk in all subgroups except in African–American women. The excess risk was over threefold in white men and over fourfold in African–American men. Relative risk was 2.59 (1.29, 5.19) in white women and 1.90 (0.64, 5.65) in African–American women.

7A.5.1.5 The RIFLE Project

The Risk Factors and Life Expectancy (RIFLE) pooling project reported data from four of the nine different population surveys initiated between 1978 and 1987 in various geographical regions in Italy.[60] Men ($n = 12,180$) from 23 cohorts and women ($n = 10,373$) from 22 cohorts included in the report were 30–69 years old. Excluded were subjects with clinically diagnosed heart disease. In multivariate models adjusted for common risk factors including ECG abnormalities related to MI, there was a significant excess CVD mortality risk in men for high amplitude QRS alone (RR 1.86) and high QRS amplitude combined with abnormal ST-T (RR 6.33). The corresponding risk levels were increased also in women but did not reach statistical significance.

7A.5.1.6 An Older Cohort from the Finnish Seven Countries Study

A 5-year follow-up of 697 survivors aged 65–85 years subsequent to the 25-year examination of the initial Finnish cohort of the Seven Countries Study[61] examined the mortality risk for high amplitude QRS waves and other MC items, first separately for each abnormality and then according to a clearly defined hierarchic scheme. The latter scenario included high QRS codes (MC 3.1–3.3) without significant Q, ST and T codes were entered into logistic regression models. Both models were also adjusted for age and survey area. High QRS amplitude codes entered without considering other coexisting codes were associated with a significant excess risk of all-cause mortality, and also with the risk of fatal and nonfatal MI. The risk for isolated high R waves alone in the absence of ST-T abnormalities was not significant for any of the study endpoints. This finding again suggests that investigators formulating new criteria for LVH for risk analysis should consider the inclusion of repolarization abnormalities with high amplitude QRS variables.

7A.5.1.7 The Bronx Aging Study

The Bronx Longitudinal Aging Study had 459 elderly men and women (aged 75–85) with a 10-year follow-up.[62] Those with ECG-LVH (MC 3.1–3.3 with 4.1–4.3 or 5.1–5.3) had a significantly higher CVD mortality than those without ECG-LVH, with risk ratio 2.65 (1.58–4.41). In a multivariate model adjusting for common risk factors, including hypertension and prior MI by history or ECG, CVD mortality risk was similarly increased but it was not statistically significant. The study also evaluated the risk for new ECG-LVH and the regression of the baseline LVH, to be discussed later.

Using ECG predictors of LVM as continuous variables should, in principle, improve the risk prediction power. One of the models in Table 7A.2 (model 2) was used in an early study to evaluate mortality risk using NHANES 1 data.[16] Left ventricular mass index was used as a continuous variable and relative risk was determined for an increment from the 20th to the 80th percentile. Age-adjusted risk for CVD mortality was 1.39 (1.21, 1.60) in white men, 1.67 (1.21, 2.29) in African–American men, 1.62 (1.17, 2.24) in white women, and 2.08 (1.27, 3.42) in African–American women. With an additional adjustment for systolic blood pressure and history of heart attack, a significant CVD mortality risk was retained in white men (RR = 1.21 [1.03, 1.43]), in white women (RR = 1.36 [1.08, 1.70]), and in African–American women (RR = 1.95 [1.44, 2.66]) but not in African–American men (RR = 1.26 [0.81, 1.96]). These data with LVMI estimate as a continuous variable

suggest that the risk is graded across a wide range of the estimated values.

7A.5.2 ECG-LVH and Mortality Risk in Special Populations

7A.5.2.1 A Framingham Cohort

The first of the four data sets compared here (Table 7A.10) comes from an early report from the Framingham cohort.[63] Incident ECG-LVH by high QRS amplitude with LV strain in the heart disease-free subgroup at the onset of each biennial examination was associated with a substantial excess of CVD, CHD, and all-cause mortality. Ten-year age-adjusted mortality in men and in women with ECG-LVH was more than threefold compared with the general Framingham sample as the reference group. Mortality rates for men with ECG-LVH were similar as for MI by ECG, and in women they were always higher for ECG-LVH than for women with MI by ECG, and these differences were retained after the exclusion of subjects with hypertension at baseline.

Subjects with ECG-LVH by the strict Framingham criteria used in the study may be prone to have simultaneous complications due to coronary problems; although very few were stated as having ECG evidence of both conditions at baseline. Two-year age-adjusted incidence of ECG-MI and particularly ECG-LVH increased sharply in both men and women with hypertensive status classified as mild and definite, compared with nonhypertensive groups.

7A.5.2.2 The Glasgow Blood Pressure Clinic Study

Dunn et al. from the Glasgow Blood Pressure Clinic[64] estimated mortality risk for high amplitude R waves with and without ST-T abnormalities in a group of 3,275 hypertensive patients with an average follow-up of 6.5 years. Using patients with normal ECG as the reference group, the age-adjusted ishemic heart disease mortality risk for isolated high amplitude R waves was 2.7 for men ($p < 0.001$) and 2.0 for women ($p < 0.05$). The risk was also significantly increased for all-cause mortality in men and in women ($p < 0.001$ for both). As expected, the risk was higher for high R waves

TABLE 7A.10 Electrocardiographic left ventricular hypertrophy and the risk of adverse cardiovascular events in special populations.

Study population/ baseline year	Age (years)	Follow-up	Criteria/variables	Endpoint	Gender/race or subgroup	RR (95% CI or p value)	Comments
Framingham, CVD-free[63]/1948	>28	18 biennials	High QRS, ST strain (9B)*	CVD mortality	Men Women	3.4 ($p < 0.05$) 3.9 ($p < 0.05$)	RR = age-adjusted mortality rate vs general Framingham sample; risk for incident LVH
Dunn et al.[64]/1990 Patients of a hypertension clinic	–	Mean 6.5 years	S-L, or max R + max S >4,000 µV	IHD mortality	Men Women	2.7 ($p < 0.001$) 2.0 ($p < 0.05$)	RR = age-adjusted mortality rate vs reference group (patients with normal ECG)
				Total mortality	Men Women	1.6 ($p < 0.001$) 2.4 ($p < 0.001$)	
			High R + ST, T	IHD mortality	Men Women	4.0 ($p < 0.001$) 2.3 ($p < 0.05$)	
				Total mortality	Men Women	2.1 ($p < 0.001$) 2.6 ($p < 0.001$)	
Verdecchia et al.[65]/1998 Hypertension clinic referral patients (PIUMA)	Mean 52 years	Mean 3.3 years	Cornell voltage	CVD mortality	Men and women	2.02 (0.87–4.69)	Risk for other ECG-LVH criteria in Table 7A.11
Sullivan et al.[66]/1972–85; coronary arteriography patients		5 years	Age-specific criteria for high R	All-cause mortality	CAD patients CAD-free patients	81.0 vs 87.7 ($p = 0.001$) 84.4 vs. 95.5 ($p < 0.05$)	Survival rates (LVH vs. nonLVH)

* See Table 7A.1. *CAD* coronary artery disease, *CVD* cardiovascular disease, *IHD* ischemic heart disease, *RR* relative risk.

combined with repolarization abnormalities. The excess risk could not be explained by age, blood pressure level upon referral, or cigarette smoking, and the authors concluded that ECG-LVH, with or without repolarization abnormalities, is an independent risk factor for mortality in hypertensive patients.

7A.5.2.3 The PIUMA Study

Prognostic data for Cornell voltage criteria from an Italian study involving hypertension clinic patients (PIUMA)[65] listed in Table 7A.10 indicated a twofold but nonsignificant CVD mortality risk increase.

The PIUMA study also evaluated CVD risk for five sets of ECG-LVH criteria in 1,717 hypertensive patients referred for evaluation and treatment by various antihypertensive regimens and followed up for an average of 3.3 years (up to 10 years). The reported results reproduced in Table 7A.11 show that CVD mortality risk was significant only for the criteria that combine high QRS waves with abnormal ST-T.

The PIUMA investigators also reported population-attributable risk for various ECG criteria for LVH. As a consequence of large variations of LVH prevalence, the estimated population-attributable risk varied from 6 to 37%, with the highest value reported for the Perugia score. The reported population-attributable risk (AR) was determined as $AR = p * (HR - 1) * 100 / (p * (HR - 1) + 1)$, where HR = hazard ratio and p = number of patient-years of observation until event with ECG-LVH present/total patient-years of observation. This kind of attributable risk has the connotation of a causal relationship between CVD mortality and LVH, by some plausible mechanism such as possibly may exist between LVH and CHF. The expectation that attributable fraction might indicate the fraction of CVD deaths that possibly could be averted if the occurrence of ECG-LVH could be prevented appears at first fight a bit unrealistic in view of the weak association between ECG-LVH and increased LVM. Such an expectation will be reconsidered at the end of this chapter in connection with the LIFE study. Statistical aspects of population-attributable risk are considered in Chapter 9B.

TABLE 7A.11 Prevalence of left ventricular hypertrophy by seven electrocardiographic criteria, cardiovascular disease (*CVD*) mortality, hazard ratio, and population-attributable risk in a hypertension clinic population.

		CVD mortality (per 100 patient-years)		Hazard ratio		Attributable risk (%)
	Prevalence (%)	No LVH	LVH	Unadjusted	Adjusted[†] (95% CI)	
Sokolow–Lyon voltage	14.3	0.53	0.74	1.40	1.81 (0.71, 4.58)	10.5
Cornell voltage	9.1	0.48	1.53	3.19	2.02 (0.87, 4.69)	16.9
Framingham	3.9	0.49	2.13	4.34	2.45 (0.92, 6.53)	5.7
Romhilt–Estes score ≥5	4.9	0.44	2.76	6.27	4.46 (1.91, 10.38)[†]	15.2
Romhilt–Estes Score >4	5.9	0.43	2.60	6.04	4.89 (2.16, 11.3)[†]	19.3
Left ventricular strain	6.5	0.40	3.00	7.50	4.58 (2.18, 9.61)[†]	19.3
Perugia score[‡]	17.8	0.30	1.75	5.83	4.21 (2.05, 8.66)[†]	37.0

* Adjusted for age, diabetes and previous CVD events; [†] $p < 0.001$; [‡] Cornell voltage >24 mm in men and >20 mm in women OR Romhilt–Estes score >5 OR left ventricular strain. Source: modified from Verdecchia et al.[65] J Am Coll Cardiol 1998;31:383–90. © 1998 the American College of Cardiology Foundation. Reproduced with permission.

7A.5.2.4 Coronary Arteriography Patients

Sullivan et al. examined 5-year survival for ECG-LVH in 18,969 patients undergoing coronary arteriography.[66] The patients were stratified into two groups: those with and those without coronary artery disease (CAD). The 5-year survival was significantly lower in both stratified groups among patients with ECG-LVH compared to those without: 84.4 vs 94.5% ($p = 0.016$) in patients without CAD and 81.0 vs 87.7% ($p < 0.001$) in patients with CAD. The survival was worse in CAD patients with ECG-LVH who also had ST abnormalities, although the presence of ST abnormalities did not significantly influence the survival in patients free from CAD. Electrocardiographic amplitude criteria from the Marquette 12SL program (essentially age-adjusted Sokolow–Lyon and RV5 criteria) were used in the study.

7A.5.3 Impact of Gender and Race on ECG-LVH Mortality Risk

7A.5.3.1 Framingham 1986 Report

Data in Tables 7A.9 and 7A.10 do not unequivocally suggest that the impact of ECG-LVH on CVD mortality risk is greater in women than in men. The problem in some studies is that no gender-specific ECG criteria have been used, particularly for the Sokolow–Lyon voltage and for the MC criteria. In the 1986 Framingham report,[63] excess risk

for CVD mortality was equally high for men and women. In the 1994 report, progressive increase in CVD event incidence with Cornell voltage quartiles was nearly identical in men and women.[57] This special study group had possible ECG-LVH at the onset of the study by the Framingham QRS amplitude criteria. The Cornell voltage quartiles were formed from the pooled group of men and women, apparently because the mean Cornell voltage in the gender groups was practically equal, possibly because of the selection criteria.

7A.5.3.2 The NHANES 1 Mortality Follow-up Study

In the NHANES 1 mortality follow-up study,[16] relative risk of CVD mortality was reported for the Sokolow–Lyon, the Cornell voltage and the MC criteria, and also for LVMI from set 2 in Table 7A.2 used as a dichotomized variable (Table 7A.12). Like in the PIUMA study, the data show considerable variations between various ECG criteria in ECG-LVH prevalence and relative risk of CVD mortality. The Sokolow–Lyon LVH was not significantly associated with CVD mortality risk in any of the groups stratified by race and gender. The risk for LVH by the Cornell voltage was significant in African–American men and in white women, with over threefold excess in the former group and over twofold excess in the latter group. Excess risk was significant for the last two sets of ECG-LVH criteria (MC and LVMI) in all

TABLE 7A.12 Prevalence of left ventricular hypertrophy by four electrocardiographic criteria and age-adjusted relative risks of cardiovascular disease mortality by race and gender in the NHANES 1 population.

Race/gender	Criteria	Prevalence (%)	Relative risk
White men	Sokolow–Lyon	6.3	1.26 (0.75–2.11)
	Cornell voltage	2.3	1.68 (0.79–3.58)
	MC 1.1, 1.3 + 5.1–5.3	1.9	3.26 (1.91–5.56)
	ECG-LVMI	15.4	2.48 (1.77–3.46)
Black men	Sokolow–Lyon	30.1	1.74 (0.99–3.44)
	Cornell voltage	12.2	3.10 (1.49–6.45)
	MC 1.1, 1.3 + 5.1–5.3	8.3	4.29 (2.00–9.18)
	ECG-LVMI	36.6	3.03 (1.49–6.16)
White women	Sokolow–Lyon	2.6	1.47 (0.60–3.61)
	Cornell voltage	8.5	2.18 (1.36–3.47)
	MC 1.1, 1.3 + 5.1–5.3	1.8	2.59 (1.29–5.19)
	ECG-LVMI	20.1	1.86 (1.21–2.87)
Black women	Sokolow–Lyon	15.5	1.42 (0.57–3.56)
	Cornell voltage	18.8	1.56 (0.67–3.63)
	MC 1.1, 1.3 + 5.1–5.3	6.6	1.90 (0.64–5.65)
	ECG-LVMI	17.4	2.05 (0.83–5.05)

LVMI left ventricular mass index, *MC* Minnesota Code, *NHANES* National Health and Nutrition Examination Survey.

subgroups except in African–American women. By these two sets of criteria that both involve abnormal ST-T patterns, the risk levels were higher in men than in women. Comparing subgroups by race, risk levels were higher in African–American men than in white men. There was no clear trend suggesting that risk levels are higher in African–American than in white women.

7A.5.4 ECG-LVH and Echocardiographic LVH as Independent Mortality Predictors

7A.5.4.1 The Uppsala Health Survey

A report from a health survey in 70-year-old men conducted in the county of Uppsala, Sweden, suggests that ECG-LVH and Echo-LVH both contribute to the prediction of total mortality in risk models adjusted for other CHD risk factors. The median follow-up was 5.2 years (range 0.7 to 6.4 years). Total mortality appeared to increase progressively with quartiles of Echo-LVMI (LVM/BSA). The increase in CVD mortality was rather pronounced for the fourth quartile, and by inspecting the ROC-curve, the cutpoint LVMI $\geq 150 \, g/m^2$ was taken as the definition for Echo-LVH for risk evaluation. By this definition of Echo-LVH, 134 men (28.2%) had Echo-LVH. Con-

ventional cutpoints were taken for the Sokolow–Lyon voltage and the Cornell voltage for ECG-LVH. The cutpoint for the Cornell product was taken as ECG-LVH = Cornell product $>244 \mu V.s$. Of interest is that by the latter definition for ECG-LVH, 15% of men with and 15% without Echo-LVH had ECG-LVH.

Echocardiographic LVH was associated with a four-fold increased risk of CVD mortality and morbidity (crude, unadjusted risk), but the risk was not significant when adjusted for nine other clinical variables. Echocardiographic LVMI evaluated as a continuous variable was a strong predictor of all-cause mortality, CVD mortality, and CVD morbidity, and the multivariable-adjusted (nine clinical risk factors) risk was not diminished. It thus seemed that risk information was lost if Echo-LVMI was used as a dichotomized variable for risk analysis.

Crude risk of all-cause and CVD mortality was significantly increased for ECG-LVH by the Cornell product criteria (HR 3.82 and 3.56, respectively). With the adjustment for Echo-LVMI, it remained over threefold for all-cause mortality but the risk of CVD mortality diminished to nonsignificant. The crude risk of all-cause mortality for ECG-LVH by the Cornell voltage was significant and remained significant in a risk model that included an adjustment for nine clinical risk factors (other than Echo-LVMI). The risk for CVD morbidity was not significant for the Cornell product, nor for CVD mortality, nor for CVD morbidity for the Cornell voltage or the Sokolow–Lyon voltage criteria, even in the unadjusted risk models.

7A.5.5 Spontaneous Progression and Regression of ECG-LVH and Mortality and Morbidity Risk

7A.5.5.1 The 1994 Framingham Report

The 1994 Framingham study report cited before[57] also evaluated the 2-year risk for CVD events (CHD death, other cardiovascular deaths, angina pectoris, MI, CHF, stroke or transient ischemic attack, and intermittent claudication) for ECG-LVH progression and regression. Although subjects with hypertension were probably treated for hypertension, the progression and repression may perhaps be characterized as spontaneous to contrast it with the data from controlled clinical trials.

A transition of the Cornell voltage to a higher quartile between any two successive biennial examinations was classified as progression and a transition to a lower quartile regression of ECG-LVH. The risk was evaluated for CVD events during the subsequent 2-year period. The age-adjusted risk was approximately one-half in the voltage regression group compared with the group with no voltage transition, with odds ratio 0.46 (0.26, 0.84) in men and 0.56 (0.30, 1.04) in women. The risk of CVD events for voltage progression was 1.86 (1.14, 3.03) for men and 1.61 (0.91, 2.84) for women. Thus, there were no appreciable gender differences in the relative risk levels for Cornell voltage transitions, although the associations with CVD events were not significant in women, apparently due to fewer endpoint events in women.

Stratification of ECG-LVH level into quartiles is better than using just one threshold for LVH classification. Changes that are well within normal variability will cause fewer transitions that are counted as (false) regression or progression. The decline in ECG-LVH prevalence and improved hypertension control has apparently weakened

the prognostic value of ECG-LVH in general populations so that ECG-LVH was removed in 1998 from the Framingham risk score categories.[68]

7A.5.6 Echocardiographic LVH and Mortality Risk in Men and Women

7A.5.6.1 The Cornell Study

Echocardiographic data, although limited, indicate increased risk associated with LVH. In an observational study from the Cornell Medical Center, 280 hypertensive patients without preexisting cardiac disease were followed-up for mortality for 10 years.[69] The patients with Echo-LVH (LVM $>125\,g/m^2$) were at a significantly higher risk than those without LVH, both for CVD death (14 vs 0.5%, $p = 0.001$) and all-cause mortality (16 vs 2%, $p = 0.001$). In contrast, ECG-LVH was not significantly associated with mortality risk. In multivariate analysis, gender was not predictive of mortality.

7A.5.6.2 Framingham Studies

In a 4-year follow-up of the Framingham study participants 40 years old and older who were free of clinical CVD and who had echocardiographic data, the relative risk of CVD death for each increment of $50\,g/m$ was 1.73 (1.19, 2.52) in men and 2.12 (1.28, 3.49) in women.[70] The risk model was adjusted for demographic and clinical risk factors, including ECG-LVH. Similarly, the risk of all-cause mortality was higher in women than in men, 2.01 (1.44, 2.81) versus 1.49 (1.14, 1.94), respectively.

In a third Framingham study, mortality risk was evaluated for Echo-LVH in 163 African–American men and 273 African–American women.[71] Left ventricular hypertrophy was defined by the commonly used clinical thresholds (LVM/BSA $\geq 117\,g/m^2$ in men and $104\,g/m^2$ in women). In a Cox regression model comparing LVH versus non-LVH and adjusting for age, hypertension, and ejection fraction, the mortality risk was strikingly higher in women than in men. For total mortality, RR was 2.0 (0.8, 5.0) in men and 14.3 (1.6, 11.7) in women, and for cardiac death, 1.3 (0.4, 3.7) in African–American men and 7.5 (1.6, 33.8) in African–American women. In an earlier report from Framingham, there was no significant gender difference in relative risk for 50 g/m increment in LVM per height.[72]

7A.6 Clinical Trials for Intervention on Hypertension

7A.6.1 The MRFIT Trial

The MRFIT trial was designed as a controlled clinical trial with intervention on smoking, serum cholesterol and with hygienic and pharmacological therapy in study participants who were hypertensive. The MRFIT data agree with the Framingham data with respect to the importance of incident progression of ECG-LVH related voltages for CVD risk.[73] Participants of MRFIT were 35- to 57-year-old men and they were considered at high risk of future heart attack according to the traditional risk factors (diastolic blood pressure, smoking, and serum cholesterol). Men with a history or ECG evidence of MI were excluded. The threshold for a significant increase was defined on the basis of short-range variability data for each continuous variable established by Zhou et al.[74] The increases evaluated were the average individual changes from the baseline during the initial 6 years of the study, and the mortality risk was determined for the subsequent 10 years (Figure 7A.19). Cardiovascular disease mortality included CHD mortality and stroke death, endpoint items of interest with respect to LVH. Progression of ECG-LVH was significantly associated with excess CVD mortality for all incident LVH criteria except for the Sokolow–Lyon voltage.

The incidence rates for significant increase differed substantially for significant increases by different criteria. For CVD death it was 7.9% for a 900-μV increase in Sokolow–Lyon voltage, 13.2% for a 400-μV increase in Cornell voltage, 18.6% for a 41-μV.s increase in the Cornell product, 15.1% for a 356-μV.s increase in 12-lead QRS voltage-duration product, and 28.9% for a 26-g/m² increase in Novacode LVM.

The higher relative risk for the Novacode LVM may reflect the fact that the earlier Novacode model used in the study contained some repolarization variables together with QRS amplitudes.[16] Altered repolarization may reflect altered

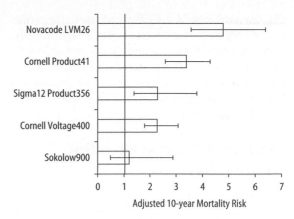

FIGURE 7A.19 Ten-year cardiovascular disease mortality risk with 95% confidence interval for a significant 6-year increase in each of the ECG-LVH criteria. The bars show the lower and upper 2.5% confidence limits. Significant increase was defined as an increase exceeding short-range variability for each criterion. Adjusted for age, diastolic blood pressure, cholesterol, smoking, study group, and average change in body mass index. (Source: modified from Prineas et al.[73] J Electrocardiol 2001;34:91–101. © 2001. Reproduced with permission from Elsevier.)

myocardial structure (fibrosis) or subclinical CAD in LVH.

A different story emerged from MRFIT concerning regression of ECG-LVH (Figure 7A.20).

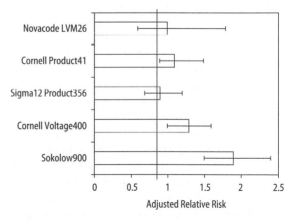

FIGURE 7A.20 Relative risk of 10-year cardiovascular disease mortality in MRFIT men for a 6-year decrease in five LVH-related variables exceeding short-range variability threshold. The bars show the 95% confidence intervals. Adjusted for age, diastolic blood pressure, cholesterol, smoking, study group, and average change in body mass index. Note that risk reduction with reduction of ECG-LVH variables is not significant for any of the criteria, and the risk is actually increased for a reduction in Cornell voltage and Sokolow–Lyon voltage. (Source: Prineas et al.[73] J Electrocardiol 2001;34:91–101. © 2001. Reproduced with permission from Elsevier.)

Electrocardiographic LVH regression by none of the criteria was associated with a significantly reduced risk. In fact, a significant reduction in Sokolow–Lyon LVH was associated with a nearly twofold increase in CVD mortality risk, and by the Cornell voltage criteria with a 30% increase in CVD mortality risk.

7A.6.2 Heart Outcomes Prevention Evaluation Study

The Heart Outcomes Prevention Evaluation (HOPE) study compared ECG-LVH regression in relation to CVD outcomes in 8,281 patients randomly assigned to angiotensin-converting enzyme (ACE) inhibitor ramipril or placebo and followed up for 4.5 years.[75] At baseline, ECG-LVH prevalence by Sokolow–Lyon voltage criteria was 7.8% in the ramipril group and 8.6% in the placebo group. Electrocardiographic LVH persisted or new ECG-LVH developed in 8.1% in the ramipril group and 9.8% in the placebo group. Electrocardiographic LVH regressed or no new ECG-LVH developed in 91.9% in the ramipril group and 90.2% in the placebo group. Although these differences appear relatively small, they were significant ($p = 0.007$). Furthermore, patients with ECG-LVH regression or no progression to new ECG-LVH had a significantly lower risk of primary pre-defined study outcome (CVD death, MI, or stroke) compared to patients with persistent or new ECG-LVH (12.3 vs 15.8%, $p = 0.006$). Similarly, these patients had a lower risk of CHF (9.3 vs 15.4%, $p < 0.0001$).

A single threshold was used for LVH progression/regression classification. Short-range variability of Sokolow–Lyon voltage is approximately $900\,\mu V$, and a significant proportion of the transitions may have been within random variation and secondly, due to regression to the mean. The difference in BMI may have caused a significant number of apparent LVH regressions (BMI was one full unit lower in the LVH "development/persistent" group than in the "LV regression/prevention" group). Random transitions may have significantly weakened the power to detect true progression or regression of LVH. Overall, it is difficult to conceive what really happened to LVH status with ramipril administration. The ultimate question is whether the observed association

between LVH regression with Sokolow–Lyon criteria and reduced risk is real.

Echocardiographic LVH regression was evaluated in the PIUMA study on 430 hypertensive patients cited before.[25] This relatively small study compared LVH patients (26% of the patients) with Echo-LVH regression versus those with no regression. Echocardiographic LVH was defined as LVM >125 g/m² at the baseline and regression by LVM decrease below the LVH threshold in the second echocardiographic examination after 1–10 years of follow-up (average 2.8 years). The rate of all cardiovascular events was lower among patients with LVH regression than among those with persistent LVH (1.58 vs 6.27 events per 100 person-years, $p = 0.002$).

Although LVM is a predictor of CVD, few studies have evaluated factors that determine Echo-LVH progression over time. The CARDIA study reported data from a 5-year follow-up of 1,189 study participants who had two M-mode echocardiographic examinations at 5-year intervals.[76] The participants were young African–American and white men and women aged 23–35 years at the time of their echocardiographic study. Significant independent predictors of the Echo-LVM in the follow-up in all race and gender groups included initial LVM, initial BMI, and the increase in BMI. An increase in LVM (mean increase 5.9 g) was a significant predictor of the follow-up Echo-LVM only in African–American women, with initial systolic blood pressure and systolic blood pressure increase as additional predictors. African–American women also had the largest increase in BMI and systolic blood pressure.

The CARDIA study is one of the very few where the impact of regression to the mean was evaluated and reported. As expected, participants with low initial LVM had a significant (7.3 g) 5-year increase and participants with high initial LVM a significant decrease (8.1 g) in LVM ($p < 0.0001$ for both). In the middle reference group, there was a relatively small (2.55 g) increase in LVM ($p = 0.04$).

7A.6.3 Ramipril Cardioprotective Evaluation Study

Beta-blockers are widely used in hypertension control although diuretics have been shown to be more appropriate first-line therapy of uncomplicated hypertension, at least in elderly patients.[77] Some studies have compared the effectiveness of β-blockers with other antihypertensives in reducing LVM as well as blood pressure. The Ramipril Cardioprotective Evaluation (RACE) group compared ACE inhibitor ramipril with β-blocker atenolol in 193 patients at 16 centers.[78] Echocardiographic LVM was blindly evaluated at a single reading center at 3 and 6 months from the initiation of the therapy. Adequate quality echocardiograms were obtained in 111 out of the 193 patients (58%). Although there was no significant difference in blood pressure reduction by the two drugs, LVM was significantly reduced only by ramipril.

A meta-analysis of randomized double-blind studies by Schmieder et al. in 1996 concluded that the database in published papers is limited and incomplete and that most of the published papers are of poor scientific quality.[79] Based on analysis of data from 33 trials that qualified for the meta-analysis (out of 471 studies searched), ACE inhibitors reduced LVM by 13%, calcium channel blockers by 9%, diuretics by 7%, and β-blockers by 6%.

7A.6.4 Losartan Intervention For Endpoint Reduction in Hypertension Study

Regression of LVH has been the ultimate goal of hypertension control and the ultimate evidence of successful intervention. Results from the LIFE study in diabetic, hypertensive patients at an early phase of the study suggested that LVM reduction may not produce any benefits as far as reduction of the risk of CVD is concerned.[80] The LIFE study was a double-blinded, randomized trial comparing β-blocker atenolol with ACE inhibitor losartan therapy in over 9,000 hypertensive patients with ECG-LVH and with a 4-year follow-up. Electrocardiographic LVH, one of the selection criteria, was defined by Sokolow–Lyon voltage (>3,800 μV) or by Cornell product criteria (>24.4 μV.ms) – a rather strange combination of choices! For a similar reduction in systolic and diastolic blood pressure, regression of ECG-LVH was significantly higher in the losartan than in the atenolol group ($p < 0.0001$). There was no signifi-

cant difference in CVD mortality, fatal, or nonfatal MI.

In the ECHO substudy on 960 patients (754 with serial echocardiographic measurements), losartan significantly reduced LVM and anatomic LVH despite relatively small decreases in blood pressure, and LVH reduction continued at least for 2 years.[81] In spite of the LVM reduction, the risk reduction was nonsignificant (odds ratio 0.87 [0.67, 1.17]). Fatal and nonfatal strokes were reduced by >20% both in the whole study population and in the ECHO substudy.

More recent reports from the LIFE trial have ended up with more positive conclusions. Compared to patients with progression of ECG-LVH, those with no significant change or a decrease in ECG-LVM had a greater absolute and relative reduction in Echo-LVM.[82] Furthermore, less severe in-treatment ECG-LVH by Cornell product or Sokolow–Lyon criteria was associated with 14 and 17% lower rates, respectively, of study composite endpoint (cardiovascular death, nonfatal MI, or stroke).[83] The hazard ratios were 0.86 (0.82, 0.90) for incremental decrease of 105 μV.s of Cornell product and 0.83 (0.78, 0.88) for a decrease by 1.05 mV of Sokolow–Lyon voltage. The Cox regression model was adjusted for treatment modality, baseline Framingham risk score, baseline and in-treatment blood pressure, and severity of baseline ECG-LVH.

Blood pressure control remains, of course, an important goal for CVD risk reduction. If the LIFE study results are confirmed in other independent studies, it may indicate that antihypertensive therapy with ECG-LVH reduction as an endpoint may be more effective than hypertension control, at least with some drug intervention modalities. Echocardiographic and ECG-LVH are different entities, with different associations with CVD risk factors and mortality risk. Electrocardiographic LVH reflects increased excitable, living muscle mass, with less cancellation and a stronger excitation wave front producing increased QRS amplitudes. Anatomic/Echo-LVM increase may be associated with fibrosis as a consequence of LVH, often concomitant ischemic myocardial injury with CHD, and diminished net strength of cardiac potentials may induce a discrepancy between anatomic/Echo-LVH and ECG-LVH.

References

1. Wilson PW, D'Agostino RB, Levy D et al. Prediction of coronary heart disease using risk factor categories. Circulation 1998;97:1837–47.

2. Ashley EA, Raxwal VK, Froelicher VF. The prevalence and prognostic significance of electrocardiographic abnormalities. Current Problems in Cardiology 2000;25:5–70.

3. Milliken JA, MacFarlane PW, Lawrie TDV. Enlargement and hypertrophy. In: MacFarlane PW, Lawrie TDV (eds). Comprehensive Electrocardiology. New York: Pergamon Books Ltd, 1988, pp 631–70.

4. Rautaharju PM. Electrocardiogram in epidemiology and clinical trials. In: MacFarlane PW, Lawrie TDV (eds). Comprehensive Electrocardiology. New York: Pergamon Books Ltd, 1988, pp1219–66.

5. Vakili BA, Okin PM, Devereux RB. Prognostic implications of left ventricular hypertrophy. Am Heart J 2001;141:334–41.

6. Lewis T. Observations upon ventricular hypertrophy, with especial reference to preponderance of one or the other chamber. Heart 1914;5:367–403.

7. Hermann GR, Wilson FN. Ventricular hypertrophy. Comparison of electrocardiographic and postmortem observations. Heart 1922;9:91–147.

8. Sokolow M, Lyon TP. The ventricular complex in left ventricular hypertrophy as obtained by unipolar precordial and limb leads. Am Heart J 1949;37:161–86.

9. Blackburn H, Keys A, Simonson E et al. The electrocardiogram in population studies. A classification system. Circulation 1960;21:1160–75.

10. Casale PN, Devereux RB, Kligfield P et al. Electrocardiographic detection of left ventricular hypertrophy: development and prospective validation of improved criteria. J Am Coll Cardiol 1985;6:572–80.

11. Molloy TJ, Okin PM, Devereux RB, Kligfield P. Electrocardiographic detection of left ventricular hypertrophy by the simple QRS voltage-duration product. J Am Coll Cardiol 1992;20:1180–6.

12. Romhilt DW, Estes EH Jr. A point-score system for the ECG diagnosis of left ventricular hypertrophy. Am Heart J 1968;75:252–8.

13. Schillaci G, Verdecchia P, Borgioni C et al. Improved electrocardiographic diagnosis of left ventricular hypertrophy. Am J Cardiol 1994;74:714–9.

14. Norman JE, Levy D, Cambell G, Bailey JJ. Improved detection of echocardiographic left ventricular hypertrophy using a new electrocardiographic algorithm. J Am Coll Cardiol 1993;21:1680–6.

15. Wolf HK, Burggraf GW, Cuddy E, Milliken JA et al. Prediction of left ventricular mass from the electrocardiogram. J Electrocardiol 1991;24:121–7.

16. Rautaharju PM, LaCroix AZ, Savage DD et al. Electrocardiographic estimate of left ventricular mass vs. radiographic cardiac size and the risk of cardiovascular disease mortality in the epidemiologic follow-up study of the First National Health and Nutrition Examination Survey. Am J Cardiol 1988; 62:59–66.

17. Casale PN, Devereux RB, Alonso DR et al. Improved sex-specific criteria of left ventricular hypertrophy for clinical and computer interpretation of electrocardiograms: validation with autopsy findings. Circulation 1987;75:565–72.

18. Rautaharju PM, Manolio TA, Siscovick D et al. Utility of new electrocardiographic models for left ventricular mass in older adults. Hypertension 1996;28:8–15.

19. Kannel WB, Gordon T, Offutt D. Left ventricular hypertrophy by electrocardiogram. Prevalence, incidence, and mortality in the Framingham study. Ann Int Med 1969;71:89–105.

20. Multiple Risk Factor Intervention Trial Research Group. Baseline rest electrocardiographic abnormalities, antihypertensive treatment and mortality in the Multiple Risk Factor Intervention Trial. Am J Cardiol 1985;55:1–15.

21. Keys A, Aravanis C, Blackburn H et al. Epidemiological studies related to coronary heart disease: characteristics of men aged 40–59 in seven countries. Acta Med Scand 1966;460(Suppl):1–392.

22. Karvonen MJ, Blomqvist G, Kallio V et al. Epidemiological studies related to coronary heart disease: characteristics of men aged 40–59 in seven countries. C4. Men in rural east and west Finland. Acta Med Scand 1966;460(Suppl):169–90.

23. Karvonen MJ, Rautaharju PM, Orma E et al. Cardiovascular studies on lumberjacks. J Occupational Med 1961;3:46–53.

24. Rautaharju PM, Karvonen MJ, Keys A. The frequency of arteriosclerotic and hypertensive heart disease among ostensibly healthy working populations in Finland. An electrocardiographic and clinical study. J Chronic Dis 1961;13:426–38.

25. Verdecchia P, Schillaci G, Borgioni C et al. Prognostic significance of serial changes in left ventricular mass in essential hypertension. Circulation 1998; 97:48–54.

26. Rautaharju PM, Neaton JD for the MRFIT Research Group. Electrocardiographic abnormalities and coronary heart disease mortality among hypertensive men in the Multiple Risk Factor Intervention Trial. Clin Invest Med 1987;10:606–15.

27. Wolf HK, MacInnis PJ, Stock S. The Dalhousie Program. A comprehensive analysis program for rest and exercise electrocardiograms. In: Zywiets C,

Schneider B (eds). Computer Application on ECG and VCG analysis. Amsterdam, London: North Holland Publishing Co., 1973, pp 231–40.

28. Rautaharju PM, MacInnis PJ, Warren JW et al. Methodology of ECG interpretation in the Dalhousie program; NOVACODE ECG classification procedures for clinical trials and population health surveys. Methods Inf med 1990;29:362–74.

29. Östör E, Schnohr, Jensen G, Nyboe J, Tybjærg Hansen A. Electrocardiographic findings and their association with mortality in the Copenhagen City Heart Study. Eur Heart J 1981;2:317–28.

30. Beaglehole R, Tyroler HA, Cassel JC, Deubner DC. An epidemiological study of left ventricular hypertrophy in the biracial population of Evans County, Georgia. J Chron Dis 1975;28:549–59.

31. Strogatz DS, Tyroler HA, Watkins LO, Hames CG. Electrocardiographic abnormalities and mortality among middle-aged black men and white men of Evans County, Georgia. J Chron Dis 1987;40: 149–55.

32. Arnett DK, Strogatz DS, Ephross SA et al. Greater incidence of electrocardiographic left ventricular hypertrophy in black men than in white men in Evans County, Georgia. Ethn Dis 1992;2:10–17.

33. Sorlie PD, Garcia-Palmitieri MR, Costas R. Left ventricular hypertrophy among dark and light skinned Puerto Rican men: the Puerto Rico Heart Health Program. Am Heart J 1988;116:777–83.

34. Xie X, Liu K, Stamler J, Stamler R. Ethnic differences in electrocardiographic left ventricular hypertrophy in young and middle-aged employed American men. Am J Cardiol 1994;73:564–7.

35. Arnett DK, Rautaharju P, Sutherland S et al. Validity of electrocardiographic estimates of left ventricular hypertrophy and mass in African Americans (The Charlston Heart Study). Am J Cardiol 1997;79:1289–92.

36. Huston SL, Bunker CH, Ukoli FAM. Electrocardiographic left ventricular hypertrophy by five criteria among civil servants in Benin City, Nigeria: prevalence and correlates. Int J Cardiol 1999;70:1–14.

37. Rautaharju PM, Zhou SH, Calhoun HP. Ethnic differences in electrocardiographic amplitudes in North American white, black and Hispanic men and women: effect of obesity and age. J Electrocardiol 1994;27(Suppl):20–30.

38. Lee DK, Marantz PR, Devereux RB et al. Left ventricular hypertrophy in black and white hypertensives. Standard electrocardiographic criteria overestimate racial differences in prevalence. JAMA 1992;267:3294–9.

39. Gottdiener JS, Reda DJ, Materson BJ et al. Importance of obesity, race and age to the cardiac structural and functional effects of hypertension. The Department of Veterans Affairs Cooperative Study Group on Antihypertensive Agents. J Am Coll Cardiol 1994;24:1492–8.

40. Liebson PR, Grandits G, Prineas R et al. Echocardiographic correlates of left ventricular structure among 844 mildly hypertensive men and women in the Treatment of Mild Hypertension Study (TOMHS). Circulation 1993;87:476–86.

41. Rautaharju PM, Park LP, Gottdiener JS et al. Race- and sex-specific ECG models for left ventricular mass in older populations. Factors influencing overestimation of left ventricular hypertrophy prevalence by ECG criteria in African–Americans. J Electrocardiol 2000;33:205–18.

42. Gardin JM, Wagenknecht LE, Anton-Culver H et al. Relationship of cardiovascular risk factors to echocardiographic left ventricular mass in healthy young black and white men and women. The CARDIA Study. Circulation 1995;92:380–7.

43. Hypertension Detection and Follow-up Program Cooperative Group. Five-year findings of the Hypertension Detection and Follow-up Program. Prevention and reversal of left ventricular hypertrophy with antihypertensive drug therapy. Hypertension 1985;7:105–12.

44. Mosterd A, D'Agostino RB, Silbershatz H et al. Trends in the prevalence of hypertension, antihypertensive therapy, and left ventricular hypertrophy from 1950 to 1989. N Engl J Med 1999;340: 1221–7.

45. Okin PM, Jern S, Devereux RB et al. Effect of obesity on electrocardiographic left ventricular hypertrophy in hypertensive patients: the Losartan Intervention for Endpoint (LIFE) reduction in hypertension study. Hypertens 2000;35:13–18.

46. Rautaharju PM, Park L, Rautaharju FS, Crow R. A standardized procedure for locating and documenting ECG chest electrode positions. Consideration of the effect of breast tissue on ECG amplitudes in women. J Electrocardiol 1998;31:17–29.

47. Gardin JM, Arnold A, Gottdiener JS et al. Left ventricular mass in the elderly. The Cardiovascular Health Study. Hypertension 1997;29: 1095–103.

48. Levy D, Anderson KM, Savage DD, Kannel WB et al. Echocardiographically detected left ventricular hypertrophy: prevalence and risk factors. The Framingham Study. Ann Intern Med 1988; 108:7–13.

49. De Simone GM, Devereux RB, Roman MJ et al. Relation of obesity and gender to left ventricular hypertrophy in normotensive and hypertensive adults. Hypertension 1994;23:600–6.

50. Okin P, Roman MJ, Devereux RB, Kligfield P. Gender differences and the electrocardiogram in left ventricular hypertrophy. Hypertension 1995; 25:242–9.

51. Rautaharju PM, Manolio TA, Siscovick D et al. The CHS Collaborative Research Group. Classification accuracy of electrocardiographic criteria for left ventricular hypertrophy in older adults. Ann Noninvasive Electrocardiol 1996;1:121–32

52. Schunkert H, Brockel U, Hengstenberg C et al. Familial predisposition of left ventricular hypertrophy. J Am Coll Cardiol 1999;33:1685–91.

53. Mayosi BM, Keavney B, Kardos S et al. Electrocardiographic measures of left ventricular hypertrophy show greater heritability than echocardiographic left ventricular mass. Eur Heart J 2002;23:1963–71.

54. Post WS, Larson MD, Mayers RH et al. Heritability of left ventricular mass: the Framingham Heart Study. Hypertension 1997;30:1025–8.

55. Levy D, Labib SB, Anderson KM et al. Determinants of sensitivity and specificity of electrocardiographic criteria for left ventricular hypertrophy. Circulation 1990;81:815–20.

56. Larsen CT, Dahlin J, Blackburn H et al. Prevalence and prognosis of electrocardiographic left ventricular hypertrophy, ST segment depression and negative T-wave. Eur Heart J 2002;23:315–24.

57. Levy D, Salomon M, D'Agostino RB et al. Prognostic implications of baseline electrocardiographic features and their serial changes in subjects with left ventricular hypertrophy. Circulation 1994; 90:1786–93.

58. D'Agostino RB, Lee ML, Belanger AJ et al. Relation of pooled logistic regression to time-dependent Cox regression analysis: the Framingham Heart Study. Stat Med 1990;9:1501–15.

59. De Bacquer D, De Backer G, Kornitzer M, Blackburn H. Prognostic value of ECG findings for total, cardiovascular disease, and coronary heart disease death in men and women. Heart 1998;80:570–7.

60. Menotti A, Seccaraccia F, and the RIFLE Research Group. Electrocardiographic Minnesota Code findings predicting short-term mortality in asymptomatic subjects. The Italian RIFLE Pooling Project (Risk Factors and Life Expectancy). G Ital Cardiol 1997;27:40–9.

61. Tervahauta M, Pekkanen J, Punsar S, Nissinen A. Resting electrocardiographic abnormalities as predictors of coronary events and total mortality among elderly men. Am J Med 1996;100:641–5.

62. Kahn S, Frishman WH, Weissman S et al. Left ventricular hypertrophy on electrocardiogram: prognostic implications from a 10-year cohort study of older subjects: a report from the Bronx Longitudinal Aging Study. J Am Geriatr Soc 1996;44: 524–9.

63. Kannel WB, Abbott RD. A prognostic comparison of asymptomatic left ventricular hypertrophy and unrecognized myocardial infarction: the Framingham study. Am Heart J 1986;111:391–7.

64. Dunn FG, McLenachan J, Isles CG et al. Left ventricular hypertrophy and mortality in hypertension: an analysis of data from the Glasgow Blood Pressure Clinic. J Hypertens 1990;8:775–82.

65. Verdecchia P, Schillaci G, Borgioni C et al. Prognostic value of new electrocardiographic method for diagnosis of left ventricular hypertrophy in essential hypertension. J Am Coll Cardiol 1998;31: 383–90.

66. Sullivan JM, vander Zwaag R, El-Zeky F et al. Left ventricular hypertrophy: effect on survival. J Am Coll Cardiol 1993;22:508–13.

67. Sundström J, Lind L, Ärnlö J et al. Echocardiographic and electrocardiographic diagnoses of left ventricular hypertrophy predict mortality independently of each other in a population of elderly men. Circulation 2001;103:2346–51.

68. Wilson PW, D'Agostino RB, Levy D et al. Prediction of coronary heart disease using risk factor categories. Circulation 1998;97:1837–47.

69. Koren MJ, Devereux RB, Casale PN et al. Relation of left ventricular mass and geometry to morbidity and mortality in uncomplicated essential hypertension. Ann Intern Med 1991;114:345–52.

70. Levy D, Garrison RJ, Savage DD et al. Prognostic implications of echocardiographically determined left ventricular mass in the Framingham Heart Study. N Engl J Med 1990;322:1561–6.

71. Liao Y, Cooper RS, Mensah GA, McGee DL. Left ventricular hypertrophy has a greater impact on survival in women than in men. Circulation 1995; 92:805–10.

72. Levy D, Garrison RJ, Savage DD et al. Left ventricular mass and incidence of coronary heart disease in an elderly cohort: the Framingham Heart Study. Ann Intern Med 1989;110:101–7.

73. Prineas RJ, Rautaharju PM, Grandits G, Crow R, for the MRFIT Research Group. Independent risk for cardiovascular disease predicted by modified continuous score electrocardiographic criteria for 6-year incidence and regression of left ventricular hypertrophy among clinically disease free men: 16 year follow-up for the Multiple Risk Factor Intervention Trial. J Electrocardiol 2001;34:91–101.

74. Zhou SH, Rautaharju PM, Prineas RJ et al. Improved ECG models for estimation of left ventricular hypertrophy progression and regression incidence by redefinition of the criteria for a significant

change in left ventricular hypertrophy. J Electrocardiol 1994;26(Suppl):108–13.

75. Mathew J, Sleight P, Lonn E et al. Reduction of cardiovascular risk by regression of electrocardiographic markers of left ventricular hypertrophy by angiotensin-converting enzyme inhibitor ramipril. Circulation 2001;104:1615–21.

76. Gardin JM, Brunner D, Schreiner PJ et al. Demographics and correlates of five-year change in echocardiographic left ventricular mass in young black and white adult men and women: the Coronary Artery Risk Development in Young Adults (CARDIA) Study. J Am Coll Cardiol 2002;40: 529–35.

77. Messerly FH, Grossman E, Goldbourt U. Are β-blockers efficacious as first-line therapy for hypertension in the elderly? A systematic review. JAMA 1998;279:1903–7.

78. Agabiti-Rosei E, Ambrosioni E, Dal Palu C et al. ACE inhibitor ramipril is more effective than beta-blocker atenolol in reducing left ventricular mass in hypertension. Results of the RACE (ramipril cardioprotective evaluation) study on behalf of the RACE group. J Hypertens 1995;13:1325–34.

79. Schmieder RE, Martus P, Klingbell A. Reversal of left ventricular hypertrophy in essential hypertension. A meta-analysis of randomized double-blind studies. JAMA 1996;275:1507–13.

80. Lindholm LH, Ibsen H, Dahlöf B et al. Cardiovascular morbidity and mortality in patients with diabetes in the Losartan Intervention For Endpoint reduction in hypertension study (LIFE): a randomised trial against atenolol. Lancet 2002;359: 1004–10.

81. Devereux RB, Gerdts E et al. Regression of hypertensive left ventricular hypertrophy by angiotensin receptor blockade versus beta-blockade: the LIFE trial (abstract). Am J Hypertens 2002;15:15A.

82. Okin PM, Devereux RB, Jern S et al. Regression of electrocardiographic left ventricular hypertrophy during antihypertensive treatment and the prediction of major cardiovascular events. JAMA 2004;292:2343–9.

83. Okin PM, Devereux RB, Liu JE et al. Regression of electrocardiographic left ventricular hypertrophy predicts regression of echocardiographic left ventricular mass: the LIFE study. J Hum Hypertens 2004;18:403–9.

7B
Normal Standards for Cornell Voltage, Cornell Product and Sokolow–Lyon Voltage

In this chapter, normal standards are reproduced for ECG variables in commonly used left ventricular hypertrophy (LVH) criteria, Cornell voltage, Cornell product and Sokolow–Lyon voltage (Tables 7B.1, 7B.2 and 7B.3). Considering the differences between African–American and white subgroups, the differences are significant in both gender groups except that the difference in Sokolow–Lyon voltage is not significant in women.

A comparison of the Cornell voltage, Cornell product and the Sokolow–Lyon voltage between normal weight (body mass index [BMI] $\leq 25.4\,kg/m^2$) and obese (BMI $30.5\,kg/m^2$) subjects in Table 7B.4 shows again similar differences as documented previously. The Cornell voltage and

Cornell product are higher and the Sokolow–Lyon voltage is lower in obese than in normal weight subjects. The differences between obese and normal weight subjects are significant in all subgroups ($p < 0.001$ except $p < 0.01$ for the Sokolow–Lyon voltage in African–American women).

An argument could be made that normal standards should perhaps be established from subgroups with normal body weight, particularly for evaluating the effect of obesity on ECG variables used in LVH criteria. Normal standards for the Cornell voltage, Cornell product and Sokolow–Lyon voltage are listed in Tables 7B.5, 7B.6 and 7B.7 for normal weight subjects by gender and ethnicity. Table 7B.5 indicates that for Cornell voltage the racial differences in normal weight

TABLE 7B.1 Normal standards for Cornell voltage* by ethnicity, age and gender.

Ethnic group		40–59 years		60+ years	
		Males ($N = 1,478$)	Females ($N = 2,252$)	Males ($N = 2,337$)	Females ($N = 3,312$)
White	Mean; SD	1,323; 495.7	983; 412.8	1,431; 541.8	1,229; 473.0
	2%→98%	436→2,432	273→1,899	438→2,689	419→2,337
	5%→95%	571→2,193	383→1,710	614→2,391	544→2,074
African–American		Males ($N = 452$)	Females ($N = 778$)	Males ($N = 459$)	Females ($N = 639$)
	Mean; SD	1,461; 592.8	1,152; 479.9	1,526; 630.4	1,373; 569.0
	2%→98%	370→2,708	342→2,391	464→3,060	409→2,706
	5%→95%	567→2,433	433→2,012	585→2,714	575→2,300
	$p^\dagger$	<0.001	<0.001	<0.001	<0.001

* Cornell voltage (μV) = (RaVL + SV3).
† Two-tailed t-test for the significance of the difference between the mean values of African–Americans and whites.

TABLE 7B.2 Normal standards for Cornell product* by ethnicity, age and gender.

Ethnic group		40–59 years		60–79 years	
		Males ($N = 1,478$)	Females ($N = 2,252$)	Males ($N = 2,337$)	Females ($N = 3,312$)
White	Mean; SD	128; 52.9	87; 39.9	135; 57.8	106; 45.8
	2%→98%	39→252	22→182	38→273	34→222
	5%→95%	53→227	32→159	52→242	44→192
African–American		Males ($N = 452$)	Females ($N = 778$)	Males ($N = 459$)	Females ($N = 639$)
	Mean; SD	137; 61.0	100; 45.6	142; 67.3	120; 57.0
	2%→98%	29→268	28→232	35→320	34→269
	5%→95%	51→239	37→187	51→273	47→221
	$p^{\dagger}$	<0.01	<0.001	<0.05	<0.001

* Cornell product (μV.s) = (RaVL + SV3)*QRSdur.
† Two-tailed t-test for the significance of the difference between the mean values of African–Americans and whites.

TABLE 7B.3 Normal standards for Sokolow–Lyon voltage* by ethnicity, age and gender.

Ethnic group		40–59 years		60+ years	
		Males ($N = 1,478$)	Females ($N = 2,252$)	Males ($N = 2,337$)	Females ($N = 3,312$)
White	Mean; SD	2,235; 633.6	2,036; 521.4	2,217; 706.6	2,154; 674.3
	2%→98%	1,124→3,799	1,118→3,281	1,055→3,940	1,044→3,879
	5%→95%	1,316→3,343	1,298→2,941	1,228→3,472	1,229→3,314
African–American		Males ($N = 452$)	Females ($N = 778$)	Males ($N = 459$)	Females ($N = 639$)
	Mean; SD	2,832; 785.9	2,470; 649.4	2,716; 893.8	2,558; 802.3
	2%→98%	1,395→4,623	1,330→4,075	1,260→5,169	1,273→4,632
	5%→95%	1,592→4,266	1,522→3,716	1,440→4,296	1,472→4,058
	$p^{\dagger}$	<0.001	<0.001	<0.001	<0.001

* Sokolow–Lyon voltage (μV) = RV5 + max (SV1 or SV2 or QSV1 or QSV2).
† Two-tailed t-test for the significance of the difference between the mean values of African–Americans and whites.

TABLE 7B.4 The effect of obesity on Cornell voltage, Cornell product and Sokolow–Lyon voltage* by ethnicity and gender.

Ethnicity/gender	Obesity status	Cornell voltage Mean; SD	Cornell product Mean; SD	Sokolow–Lyon voltage Mean; SD
White men	Normal	1,267; 538.3	120; 55.9	2,350; 736.3
	Obese	1,525; 507.0	147; 56.0	2,008; 563.0
	Difference	258‡	28‡	−342‡
African–American men	Normal	1,360; 599.4	125; 59.2	2,949; 890.7
	Obese	1,580; 638.0	159; 69.3	2,522; 773.6
	Difference	220‡	26‡	−427‡
White women	Normal	1,014; 450.0	88; 41.8	2,150; 646.2
	Obese	1,266; 443.3	112; 44.7	2,037; 530.0
	Difference	252‡	24‡	−113‡
African–American women	Normal	1,150; 573.6	99; 56.8	2,625; 840.5
	Obese	1,357; 506.9	119; 49.7	2,425; 630.8
	Difference	207†	21‡	−200‡

* Cornell voltage (μV) = RaVL + SV3; Cornell product ($\mu V.s$) = CV*QRSdur(s); Sokolow–Lyon voltage (μV) = RV5 + max (SV1 or SV2 or QSV1 or QSV2).

† $p < 0.01$, ‡ $p < 0.001$; t-test (two-tailed) for the significance of the difference between obese and normal weight subjects.

TABLE 7B.5 Normal standards for Cornell voltage* in normal weight subjects by ethnicity, age and gender.

Ethnic group		40–59 years		60+ years	
		Males	Females	Males	Females
White	N	460	1,022	792	1,346
	Mean; SD	1,220; 500.2	865; 381.9	1,295; 558.1	1,128; 464.4
	2%→98%	347→2,371	209→1,740	322→2,605	326→2,176
	5%→95%	521→2,095	327→1,552	476→2,355	493→1,972
African–American	N	153	179	162	153
	Mean; SD	1,371; 607.4	998; 453.1	1,350; 593.5	1,327; 645.8
	2%→98%	126→2,647	276→1,825	338→2,738	430→3,299
	5%→95%	439→2,385	399→1,688	537→2,420	553→2,504
	$p^\dagger$	<0.01	<0.001	ns	<0.001

* Cornell voltage (μV) = (RaVL + SV3).

† Two-tailed t-test for the significance of the difference between the mean values of African–Americans and whites; ns nonsignificant.

TABLE 7B.6 Normal standards for Cornell product* in normal weight subjects by ethnicity, age and gender.

Ethnic group		40–59 years		60+ years	
		Males	Females	Males	Females
White	N	460	1,022	792	1,346
	Mean; SD	118; 53.4	76; 36.0	121; 57.4	97; 43.6
	2%→98%	30→249	17→160	29→254	27→206
	5%→95%	45→215	27→144	42→236	40→173
African–American	N	153	179	162	153
	Mean; SD	127; 59.8	85; 41.5	123; 58.9	115; 67.4
	2%→98%	11→252	21→173	29→271	33→342
	5%→95%	41→234	31→154	45→248	46→219
	$p^†$	ns	<0.01	ns	<0.001

* Cornell product (μV.s) = (RaVL + SV3)*QRSdur.
† Two-tailed t-test for the significance of the difference between the mean values of African–Americans and whites.

TABLE 7B.7 Normal standards for Sokolow–Lyon voltage* in normal weight subjects by ethnicity, age and gender.

Ethnic group		40–59 years		60+ years	
		Males	Females	Males	Females
White	N	460	1,022	792	1,346
	Mean; SD	2,383; 680.3	2,041; 538.0	1,295; 558.1	1,128; 464.4
	2%→98%	1,252→3,893	1,068→3,271	322→2,605	326→2,176
	5%→95%	1,404→3,557	1,283→2,997	476→2,355	493→1,972
African–American	N	153	179	162	153
	Mean; SD	3,077; 861.7	2,515; 727.2	1,350; 593.5	1,327; 645.8
	2%→98%	1,579→4,921	1,384→4,103	338→2,738	430→3,299
	5%→95%	1,870→4,931	1,511→3,961	537→2,420	553→2,504
	$p^†$	<0.001	<0.001	<0.001	<0.001

* Sokolow–Lyon voltage (μV) = RV5 + max (SV1 or SV2 or QSV1 or QSV2).
† Two-tailed t-test for the significance of the difference between the mean values of African–Americans and whites.

subjects are significant except in males 60 years old and older. Racial differences in Cornell product are not significant in men in either age group. Considering racial differences in normal weight subjects in Tables 7B.5–7B.7, these differences are significant except for Cornell voltage and Cornell product in men 60 years old and older and for Cornell voltage also in men 40–59 years old. In women, all of these differences are significant.

As discussed in Chapter 7A, ECG and echocardiographic estimates of LVH differ substantially. The key issue concerning echocardiographic LVH estimation is the left ventricular mass indexing to body size. The effect of overweight on LVH will remain largely unresolved until lean body mass data become available. This question is also unresolved concerning models for ECG estimates of left ventricular mass as a continuous variable. In spite of all these problems, it is possible that the changes in these LVH variables as a response to intervention on hypertension will be more important than their use for LVH estimation per se. It is also hoped that some new imaging modality better than echocardiography (magnetic resonance imaging?) will become a standard for LVH evaluation.

8
Prolonged Ventricular Excitation

Synopsis

Significance

Complete bundle branch blocks, particularly left bundle branch block (LBBB) and indeterminate type ventricular conduction delay (IVCD), commonly signify the presence of a generalized gradual degenerative process involving the main ventricular conduction pathways and the myocardium.

Mechanism

Ventricular excitation is prolonged when excitation pathways are altered because of a block in the conduction system. Excitation time can also be prolonged when excitation pathways are altered because of structural alterations in myocardial infarction (MI), chronic ischemic injury, or left ventricular hypertrophy. Altered excitation pathways cause secondary repolarization abnormalities (ST deviation, T wave inversion, QT prolongation).

Classification Problems

Criteria for fascicular blocks are not as clearly delineated as those for a complete LBBB or right bundle branch block (RBBB). Small R-prime wave in V1 and J point elevation in early repolarization may cause problems in defining the endpoint of QRS.

Prevalence and Incidence

The reported prevalence of LBBB is low in community-based populations, ranging from approximately 0.5 to 1.5%. The prevalence of RBBB is higher in younger age groups, with the reported RBBB/LBBB prevalence ratio up to four at age <30 years, decreasing to approximately unity in age groups ≥70 years. The male/female prevalence ratio for LBBB ranges from less than one to 1.4 and that for RBBB from 1.4 to 2.8. The reported incidence rates are low in younger age groups. Incidence rates of LBBB and RBBB are over 1.5 times and three times higher, respectively, in men than in women. There is a progressive up to over tenfold increase in LBBB incidence from age <50 years to age 70 years and older, and a similar progressive increase has been reported for RBBB incidence. The overall RBBB/LBBB incidence ratio is approximately two. However, the RBBB incidence reaches its peak 10 years earlier than that for LBBB and then decreases substantially. The reported incidence rates in older age groups vary, between approximately 40 and 100 or higher/10,000 per year at age 70 years and older.

Precursors

Hypertension, diabetes mellitus and cardiomyopathies have been reported as significant precursors of bundle branch blocks. In community-based populations, acute MI preceding incident bundle branch block is uncommon; conduction defects of various degrees are more common in hospital patients with acute MI.

Associated Risk

Many studies have not found a significant association between prevalent bundle branch block and mortality, mostly due to a limited statistical power to detect morbidity and mortality risk because of small sample size and relatively low prevalence. Some larger studies have identified LBBB as a very strong predictor of coronary heart disease mortality in men. In women, LBBB in one large study was reported as a strong predictor of cardiovascular disease (CVD) mortality, and LBBB and RBBB both as strong predictors of incident congestive heart failure. Data on mortality risk for incident bundle branch block are scarce. In the Framingham study, the 10-year CVD mortality risk ratio was 3.4 for incident LBBB in men and in women, 3.4 for incident RBBB in men and 2.9 for incident RBBB in women, compared to age- and gender-matched reference groups with no bundle branch block. Bundle branch blocks in admission ECGs of patients with acute MI are associated with increased in-hospital and 30-day mortality. There is no clear evidence in asymptomatic subjects for increased risk associated with isolated fascicular blocks or even with bifascicular blocks (RBBB with left anterior fascicular block).

Abbreviations and Acronyms

CDP – Coronary Drug Project
CHD – coronary heart disease
CHF – congestive heart failure
CHS – the Cardiovascular Health Study
CVD – cardiovascular disease
GUSTO – the Global Utilization of Streptokinase and t-PA (tissue-type plasminogen activator) for Occluded Coronary Arteries
IVCD – indeterminate type ventricular conduction delay
LAFB – left anterior fascicular block
LBBB – left bundle branch block
LMFB – left midfascicular block
LPFB – left posterior fascicular block
MI – myocardial infarction
RBBB – right bundle branch block
TAMI – Thrombolysis and Angioplasty in Myocardial Infarction

8.1 Categories of Ventricular Conduction Defects

Prolonged ventricular excitation includes (complete) bundle branch blocks and borderline delay of right and left ventricular excitation. Bundle branch blocks include the left bundle branch block (LBBB), the right bundle branch block (RBBB), and the indeterminate type ventricular conduction delay (IVCD). A bundle branch block is classified whenever QRS duration is $\geq 120\,ms$ in the absence of ventricular pre-excitation (Wolf-Parkinson-White) pattern. Borderline ventricular conduction delays are categorized when QRS duration is from $115\,ms$ to $<120\,ms$ with LBBB or RBBB pattern. R-prime patterns in V1 are clinically labeled as incomplete RBBB. Left anterior fascicular block (LAFB) and left posterior fascicular block (LPFB) are also included in the category of prolonged ventricular excitation.

Aberrations of ventricular conduction can occur in various combinations of blocks, including RBBB and LBBB, RBBB and LAFB or RBBB and LPFB (bifascicular block), and occasionally also as RBBB, LAFB and LPFB combination (trifascicular block). Differentiation between trifascicular block and RBBB combined with LBBB is not possible from body surface ECG.

8.1.1 Criteria for Ventricular Conduction Delay

The criteria for ventricular conduction defects adapted from the Novacode classification system[1] are summarized in Table 8.1. The criteria for some of the combinations of blocks are more complex and not covered in detail. A RBBB pattern in one ECG and LBBB in another is a sign of a bilateral block. A complete bilateral or trifascicular block is associated with a complete AV block. Right bundle branch block combined with LAFB in one ECG and combined with LPFB in another is also a sign of a trifascicular block. Right bundle branch block combined with LAFB is the most common form of bifascicular block and is defined as follows: RBBB + LAFB = RBBB and QaVL $25–100\,\mu V$ and QRS II mainly negative and QRS I mainly positive. The last two conditions imply that QRS mean frontal plane axis is from $-30°$ to $-90°$.

TABLE 8.1 Criteria for ventricular conduction defects.

Category	Definition
Left bundle branch block (LBBB)	QRS duration $\geq$125 ms and R peak time in lateral leads I or aVL or V5 or V6 $\geq$60 ms
Right bundle branch block (RBBB)	QRS duration $\geq$120 ms and (R peak time $\geq$60 ms in V1 or V2 or S duration $\geq$R duration in I or V6)
Indeterminate type ventricular conduction delay (IVCD)	QRS $\geq$120 ms and no LBBB or RBBB. Note that LBBB pattern with QRS duration less than 120 ms is classified in this category
Borderline delay of right ventricular excitation*	QRS duration 115–119 ms and the presence of R2 (R-prime wave) in V1
Borderline delay of left ventricular excitation†	QRS duration 115–119 ms and none of the other criteria above are met
Left anterior fascicular block (LAFB)	The presence of the following five criteria: 1. QRS <120 ms 2. QRS deflection in II mainly negative and I mainly positive (i.e. QRS mean angle −31° to −90°) 3. Initial R present in II with an amplitude <100 µV 4. Q wave in aVL with an amplitude 25–100 µV 5. RaVL $\geq$100 µV and R peak time $\geq$40 ms
Left posterior fascicular block (LPFB)	The presence of the following five criteria: 1. QRS <120 ms 2. QRS I mainly negative and QRS aVF mainly positive (i.e. QRS axis 91–179°) 3. In leads III and aVF, a Q wave with amplitude 25–100 µV and an R $\geq$100 µV 4. Q <40 ms in III and aVF 5. No right ventricular hypertrophy

* Often labeled as incomplete right bundle branch block.

† In the absence of LAFB and normal septal Q waves in I, aVL and V6, this category is often called incomplete left bundle branch block.

Characteristic patterns of the LBBB and RBBB always involve secondary repolarization abnormalities due to alterations of ventricular conduction pathways, the timing of the onset of excitation, and the consequent alteration of the sequence of ventricular repolarization.

8.2 Clinical Factors Associated with Ventricular Conduction Defects

Clinical conditions commonly reported as attributing factors for ventricular conduction defects include male gender, older age, hypertension, and the presence of an AV block. Hypertension, diabetes, and cardiomyopathies have been identified as precursors for ventricular conduction defects.

8.3 The Mechanism of Bundle Branch Blocks

Left bundle branch block and RBBB appear when myocardial damage, an ischemic or other injury, ventricular hypertrophy or fibrosis or other histological change or functional condition produces a conduction blockage in the left or the right main branch of the ventricular conduction system. The IVCD is generally due to a more diffuse conduction delay in the myocardium rather than a more localized problem in the ventricular conduction system. In general, bundle branch blocks occur in the presence of a gradually developing degenerative disease involving both the conduction system as well as myocardial structures. Right bundle branch block may be more localized and is often associated with prolongation of the AV conduction time (PR interval).[2] Acute myocardial infarction (MI) is at times reported to induce LBBB. The presence of a pre-existing conduction defect is often not possible to exclude in these patients.

Bundle branch blocks are generally permanent, less commonly transient or intermittent. Intermittent bundle branch blocks can be independent of the ventricular rate but are often rate dependent, occurring when a critical rate is reached and the conduction in the bundle is blocked because it is still in the functional refractory period. Occasionally, the reverse takes place and a bradycardic episode produces the block. The disappearance of the block is possibly due to the induction by a higher sinus rate, with the so-called supernormal phase (Wedensky facilitation) in the bundle branch cells.

Repolarization patterns are always drastically changed in complete bundle branch blocks. This occurs even if there are no other abnormalities that cause changes in the distribution of regional action potential durations. These are so-called secondary repolarization abnormalities due to altered sequence of excitation. In complete bundle branch blocks, there is a loss of the normal relatively close synchronization of the onset of excitation in various endocardial regions and as a consequence, there is an increased dispersion in the onset of excitation. This increased dispersion exceeds the normal and even abnormal variations in regional action potential duration and thus the sequence of repolarization tends to follow more closely the direction of excitation than normally, i.e. repolarization becomes more concordant than normally. This is the case especially in LBBB where the normal fast, synchronized onset of left ventricular endocardial excitation does not occur and the start of excitation proceeds slowly from the right side across the septum and the anterior and posterior walls all the way to the basal portions of the left ventricle. Repolarization follows nearly the same path, and thus the T waves are deep and of opposite polarity compared to the main QRS deflection.

Hereditary bundle branch blocks have been reported,[3] with various manifestations of ECG patterns in affected family members: RBBB, right or left axis deviations and AV blocks. A worsening of the defect may take place in 5–15% of the affected family members. In a subgroup demonstrating various aberrations in V1 with small R and R-prime waves, over one-half were mutation carriers.

8.4 The Mechanism of Generation of ECG Patterns in Fascicular Blocks

Fascicular blocks are generally associated with fibrosis of the fascicles of the left main bundle. Precipitating clinical conditions include ischemic injury/MI, myocarditis, Chaga's disease, cardiomyopathy, and hyperkalemia. In LAFB, the ischemic injury is generally associated with left anterior descending coronary artery problems and anterior MI. Demoulin et al. performed a quantitative assessment of the relative density of the fibrosis in anterior fascicular blocks and observed that fibrosis was diffuse with lesions distributed throughout the ramifications of the left bundle branch in four of the eight hearts studied.[4] In the remaining four hearts, fibrosis was dominant in the anterior and midseptal fibers. The authors concluded that LAFB is a reliable marker of the left main bundle disease but that the underlying lesions are generally not limited to the anterior fascicle. Left posterior fascicular block as a complication of acute MI suggests a larger MI size involving the septum or both the anterior and inferior walls and acute changes predominantly in the posterior and midseptal fascicles.[5] Prevalence of LPFB is considerably lower than that of LAFB, attributed to less vulnerability to damage in case of coronary atherosclerotic processes due to a more substantial anatomical structure and better perfusion.[6]

8.4.1 Left Anterior Fascicular Block

The dominant feature in LAFB is the delayed excitation (by up to 20 ms) of the left anterior paraseptal area normally activated by the Purkinje fibers arising from the left anterior fascicle. Thus, the wave front components parallel to the left septal surface originating from the left posterior fascicle and propagating in the inferior–right direction dominate. In addition, the normal septal excitation from the midseptal fibers propagates anteriorly and to the right. The net initial cardiac vector is thus oriented inferiorly, to the right and anteriorly. The apex and the inferior–posterior endocardial surface of the left ventricle are activated and the posterior left ventricle is excited in an apex-to-base direction. Combined source events from the excitation of the posterior wall and from the delayed excitation of the anterior and lateral left ventricle generate mid-portion QRS vectors in the left–posterior direction, producing left axis deviation. There is also a pronounced superior shift during the mid and terminal periods of QRS.

8.4.2 Left Posterior Fascicular Block

In LPFB, excitation of the left posterior inferior paraseptal regions is delayed. The initial wave fronts generate net cardiac vectors oriented to the left and anteriorly, for a short moment with an upward component. After that, excitation initiated in the superior anterior paraseptal area propagates in the inferior direction and the corresponding cardiac vectors are directed inferiorly throughout the rest of QRS, first anteriorly and to the left and then shifting prominently to the right and posteriorly, producing a right axis deviation.

There are a number of diagnostic difficulties in identification of LPFB, including right axis deviation due to right ventricular hypertrophy and anterolateral MI. From an epidemiological point of view it is noteworthy that LPFB is rare in comparison with LAFB.

8.4.3 Left Midseptal Block

Intermittent aberration of ventricular conduction producing prominent R waves in V1 and V2 with no other ECG abnormalities and a normal frontal plane QRS axis has been suggested possibly to represent left midfascicular block.[5] This does not quite fit with the assumed role of the midseptal fibers in producing septal excitation in the right anterior direction. This dilemma can perhaps be reconciled by considering that there are always anastomosing fibers to the midcentral septum from the left anterior and posterior fascicles that are not interrupted by a block in the midseptal fascicle. This being the case, septal excitation from left to right may take slightly longer than normally. Septal excitation from the right side of the septum originating from the more limited distribution of the branches of the right main bundle on the right lower septal area is dominated by the excitation fronts from the left, even in case of possible block in the midseptal fascicle.

8.5 Prevalence of Bundle Branch Blocks in Men and Women in Community-dwelling Populations

Earlier population studies tended to select men only in their surveys, and they often pooled all bundle branch blocks in their prevalence esti-

mates because of the low prevalence of each individual category. Some studies did not have a category for classification of IVCD, and IVCD was in most instances forced into LBBB count. Prevalence data from several population studies are listed in Table 8.2, with mortality risk data shown for those studies that reported results from risk analysis.

In Finland's Social Insurance Institution's coronary heart disease survey of 12 communities, the prevalence of all bundle branch blocks combined (LBBB, RBBB and IVCD) in men aged 50–59 years was 2.5% and in women 1.3%.[7] In age groups <50 years, the prevalence was 0.9% in men and 0.4% in women. In age groups 30–59 combined, the prevalence of LBBB in men was 0.4%, of RBBB 0.5%, and of IVCD 0.4%. The corresponding prevalence values in women were 0.3, 0.2, and 0.1%, respectively. The male-to-female ratios were 1.3, 2.5 and 4.0 for LBBB, RBBB and IVCD, respectively. The RBBB/LBBB ratio was 1.25 in men and 0.67 in women.

Pooled prevalence data from the 12th biennial examination of the original Framingham cohort and from the first examination of the Framingham offspring study between 1970 and 1973 show a strong dependence of the prevalence (QRS $\geq$120 ms) on age.[8] The prevalence of all bundle branch blocks combined was less than 0.6% in men and 0.3% in women in age groups less than 40 years, progressively increased with age and reached nearly 11% in men and nearly 5% in women 70 years and older. The proportion of RBBBs decreased from over 80% in age group less than 30 years to 50% in age group 70 years and older. It is evident that the prevalence of bundle branch blocks is relatively high in older age groups. The low prevalence of bundle branch blocks in the younger age groups indicates that congenital bundle branch blocks are relatively uncommon. The report does not give gender ratios separately for LBBB and RBBB prevalence. However, the incident LBBB was 1.6 times higher and the incident RBBB three times higher in men than in women.

In the Reykjavik area population aged 41–72 years screened in various stages of the study, the prevalence of RBBB was 1.4% in men and 0.7% in women.[9] The prevalence was 0% both in men and in women under 40 years of age, and it increased

TABLE 8.2 Prevalence of complete bundle branch blocks in community-based populations and mortality risk if reported.

Study/cohort assembly	Gender/age group considered (years)	Prevalence (%)	Comments
Studies in men and women			
Finnish Social Insurance Institution's survey from four geographical areas in Finland/ 1966–1972[7]	5,738 men and 5,224 women, ages 30–59	Age-adjusted prevalence LBBB: Men 0.4 Women 0.3 RBBB: Men 0.5 Women 0.2 IVCD: Men 0.4 Women 0.1	Mortality risk data not reported
Survivors of a CHD-free subgroup of the Framingham original cohort at 12th biennial, and the offspring study combined/ 1970–1973[8]	3,867 men, 4,529 women, 5 to 83 years old	QRS ≥120 ms: Men 2.6 Women 1.2 Prevalence nearly 11% in men and nearly 5% in women ≥70 years old. Proportion RBBB: >80% at age <30 years, 50% at age ≥70 years	Mortality risk reported for incident blocks only (Table 7.3)
Reykjavik study/1967–1979[9,10]	8,450 men, 9,039 women in LBBB report; 9,039 men, 9,627 women in RBBB report	LBBB: Men 0.4 Women 0.3 RBBB: Men 4.1 Women 1.6 (at age 75–79 years)	Risk of all-cause mortality not significant for LBBB or RBBB Unadjusted risk for CVD mortality significantly increased for RBBB; not significant with adjustment for age and other risk factors
Tecumseh, Michigan/ 1959–1960[11]	1,113 men and 1,159 women aged ≥40	LBBB: Men 0.4 Women 0.3 RBBB: Men 0.9 Women 0.5	Mortality risk not reported
Irish Heart Foundation's Screening Program/ 1968–1993[12]	Case-control design for 310 cases with isolated LBBB or RBBB Mean follow-up 9.5 years	LBBB: Men 0.11 Women 0.08 RBBB: Men 0.23 Women 0.075 Progressive increase in prevalence with age for LBBB and RBBB both in men and in women	Cardiac mortality significantly increased (p = 0.01). All-cause mortality not significantly increased for LBBB or for RBBB, compared with age- and gender-matched control group
Cardiovascular Health Study (CHS), sampled from Medicare eligibility lists in four US communities/1989–1990[13]	2,210 men and 2,940 women, aged ≥65	LBBB: Men 1.6 Women 1.8 RBBB: Men 6.8 Women 2.4 IVCD: Men 4.7 Women 1.2	Mortality risk not reported
Studies in men			
Seven Countries Study 17 male cohorts/1957–1962[14]	11,860 CHD-free men aged 40–59 at baseline	LBBB 0.20 RBBB 0.73 IVCD 0.16	CHD mortality (5-year risk), hazard ratio: LBBB 9.23 (2.91, 29.60) RBBB 7.4 (2.99, 18.30) IVCD 4.2 (0.58, 30.43) Long-term risk (5–25 years) significant for LBBB only, with hazard ratio 2.60 (1.34, 5.02). Adjusted for age, cigarette smoking, serum cholesterol, and cohort indicator variable

TABLE 8.2 *Continued*

Study/cohort assembly	Gender/age group considered (years)	Prevalence (%)	Comments
Gothenburg Study/1963[15]	855 men 50 years old at baseline	Age 50: LBBB 0.4 RBBB 0.8 Age 67: LBBB 1.4 RBBB 4.9 Age 75: LBBB 2.3 RBBB 9.9 Age 80: LBBB 5.7 RBBB 11.3	Nonsignificant trend toward a higher mortality for prevalent BBB evaluated at 50, 67, and 75 years Limited statistical power for risk detection
Baltimore Longitudinal Study on Aging/follow-up since 1958[2]	1,142 men, 24 clinically healthy men with RBBB in a subgroup aged 64 ± 13.5 years	Prevalence of RBBB 2.1%	Prevalent RBBB was not significantly associated with subsequent cardiac mortality or morbidity during an average 8.4 years follow-up compared with age-matched controls without BBB. Limited statistical power for risk detection

CHD coronary heart disease, *IVCD* indeterminate type ventricular conduction delay, *RBBB* right bundle branch block, *LBBB* left bundle branch block.

with age, reaching the level of 4.1% in men and 1.6% in women aged 75–79 years. In an earlier report from the Reykjavik study, the LBBB prevalence was 0.4% in men and 0.3% in women.[10] No breakdown by age for LBBB prevalence was given. Equally low population prevalence was reported in the Tecumseh Study in Michigan[11] and in the Irish Heart Foundation's Screening Program.[12]

In the Cardiovascular Health Study (CHS) population of men and women 65 years and older, the prevalence of bundle branch blocks was relatively high, and significantly higher in men (13.0%) than in women (5.4%).[13] In men, the prevalence of LBBB was 1.6%, 6.8% for RBBB, and 4.7% for IVCD. In CHS women, the prevalence of LBBB was 1.8%, 2.4% for RBBB and 1.2% for IVCD.

8.6 Prevalence of Bundle Branch Blocks in Male Populations

In the Seven Countries study of middle-aged men 40–59 years of age at the baseline, the prevalence ranged from 0.7% in Crete, Greece to 2.4% in Zutphen, Netherlands.[14] It was slightly higher in a smaller subgroup of US executives (2.8%) and nonsedentary clerks (4.5%). In a coronary heart disease (CHD)-free subgroup of the study including 11,721 men, the LBBB prevalence at the baseline by the Minnesota Code criteria was 0.20%, RBBB prevalence 0.73%, and IVCD prevalence 0.16%.

A longitudinal (30-year) prospective study of 955 men born in 1913 in Gothenburg, Sweden, demonstrated a strong dependence of the cross-sectional bundle branch block prevalence on age among the survivors of the cohort available for re-examination at each follow-up.[15] The prevalence was 1.2% at the baseline when the men were 50 years old. It was 6.3% when the cohort was 67 years old, 12.2% at the age of 75 years, and 17.0% at the age of 80 years in the remaining cohort of 212 men after attrition by death and other reasons.

8.7 Incidence of Bundle Branch Blocks

The incidence rates of bundle branch blocks are low in adult general populations, particularly in the younger age groups, and the rates are strongly age-dependent. The low incidence rates require very large populations or a long follow-up time for the assessment of the incidence and the prognostic value. During the 18 years follow-up of the original Framingham Heart Study cohort members who did not have a bundle branch block at the initial examination ($n = 5,171$), a new LBBB was found in the biennial examinations in 55 subjects and a new RBBB in 70.[16] In their risk analyses, the Framingham report clearly identified incident bundle branch block cases separately from those with bundle branch block at the initial examination, and the Framingham results are presented here in some detail.

The Framingham study report mentioned no specific criteria for IVCD, and these cases were possibly classified among LBBB. The approximate incidence rates are listed in Table 8.3, estimated from Figure 8.3 of the Framingham report. Expressed as annual rates per 10,000, the incidence of LBBB in men was approximately 2 per 10,000 per year in age groups <50 years, between

TABLE 8.3 Incidence of complete bundle branch blocks and the associated risk, if reported.

Study	Incidence			Mortality risk and comments
Studies in men and women				
Framingham cohort at 18 years of biennial follow-ups, free from BBB at baseline; 5,176 men and women[16]	Annual incidence/10,000			Cumulative 10-year CVD mortality risk ratio for incident blocks:
	LBBB	Men	Women	
	Age 20–29	2	Rare	LBBB, men: 3.6
	Age 30–39	2	<1	LBBB, women: 3.3
	Age 50–59	11	5	RBBB, men: 2.3
	Age 60–69	14	9	RBBB, women 2.8
	Age 70–79	31	26	
	RBBB	Men	Women	Approximate estimates from Figures 1
	Age 28–39	2	Rare	and 7 of reference 16. Reference
	Age 40–49	10	<1	group: age- and sex-matched members
	Age 50–59	13	6	of the Framingham population at large
	Age 60–69	28	6	free from bundle branch block
	Age 70–79	8	16	
Reykjavik Study/1967–1979[8,9,10]	Annual incidence/10,000:			No age breakdown reported for LBBB
	LBBB	Men	Women	incidence. Mortality risk reported for
	(overall)	3.2	3.7	prevalent BBB only (Table 8.2)
	RBBB	Men	Women	
	Age 50	6.8	3.1	
	Age 60	13.3	5.8	
	Age 70	26.2	11.9	
	Age 80	51.4	22.6	
Studies in men only				
Gothenburg Study/1963[15] 855 men, 50 years old 30-year follow up	Cumulative incidence during preceding interval:			Mortality risk reported for prevalent BBB only (Table 8.2)
	Age 67: LBBB 1.5			
	RBBB 5.3			
	Age 75: LBBB 3.1			
	RBBB 10.7			
	Age 80: LBBB 6.5			
	RBBB 12.8			
Manitoba Heart Study, 3,983 male air force personnel, mean age at entry in 1948 31 years; mortality data from 29-year follow-up[17–19]	Incidence/1,000 person-years at age when first detected:			Mortality rate of the cohort (excluding aircraft accidents) 32% lower than in the general Canadian male population, indicating a highly select, physically fit group
	Age 30–39: LBBB 0.1			
	RBBB 0.3			
	Age 40–49: LBBB 0.2			
	RBBB 0.4			5-year risk of sudden death in men ≥45
	Age 50–59: LBBB 0.4			years old over 10-fold for LBBB; not
	RBBB 0.9			significant for RBBB
	Age 60–69: LBBB 1.4			
	RBBB 2.1			
	Age ≥70: LBBB 3.7			
	RBBB 5.9			

BBB bundle branch block, *LBBB* left bundle branch block, *RBBB* right bundle branch block.

10 and 14 in age groups 50–69 years, and it increased to approximately 30 per 10,000 per year in age group 70–79 years. Similarly, the annual incidence rate per 10,000 for RBBB in men increased with age from <2 per 10,000 per year in the youngest age group to a peak level of approximately 28 per 10,000 per year in age group 60–69 years. Overall, the LBBB incidence rates were 1.6 times higher in men than in women and the incidence rates of RBBB three times greater in men than in women. The peak level in the incidence of RBBB in men was reached 10 years earlier than that for LBBB, and the RBBB incidence dropped in men to 8 per 10,000 per year in men aged 70–79 years. For LBBB, the male/female sex ratio decreased progressively from 2 and less, and at age 70–79 the LBBB incidence rates were nearly equally high in men and women. In that age group, the incidence rate of RBBB was nearly twice as high in men as in women.

Antecedent clinical conditions and cardiovascular abnormalities as possible precipitating factors for the onset of bundle branch blocks were also evaluated in the Framingham report. Approximately 20% of the subjects with incident bundle branch block had cardiovascular disease (CVD) and approximately 10% diabetes before the onset of the block, and a small percentage had congestive heart failure (CHF) or a valvular heart disease. Approximately 60% were hypertensive. However, the development of new CHD including clinically suspected MI within 2 years immediately before the onset as a possible precipitating factor was uncommon.

In the Reykjavik screening program, the incidence of LBBB was 3.2 per 10,000 per year in men and 3.7 per 10,000 per year in women.[9,10] The overall incidence rate for RBBB was not given. Like the RBBB prevalence, the RBBB incidence increased progressively with age. In men aged 60–69 years, the incidence was approximately 20 per 10,000 per year and it continued to increase in older age groups, reaching a level over 50 per 10,000 per year in the age group 80–84 years.

The cumulative incidence at age of 80 years in the Gothenburg study during the 30-year follow-up was 18.1% for LBBB and RBBB combined, with RBBB incidence twice as high as that of LBBB.[15]

8.8 Prognostic Value of Prevalent Bundle Branch Blocks in Community-based Populations

The data on the prognostic values of the prevalent bundle branch block from a few studies are listed in Table 8.2. In the 1993 Reykjavik study report for RBBB, the univariate CVD mortality risk in men for prevalent RBBB was significantly increased.[10] After inclusion of age and other risk factors in a multivariate model, the risk was no longer significant. All-cause mortality risk for RBBB was not significant in univariate or multivariate models. The relative risk of all-cause mortality evaluated in 1984 for LBBB was 1.56 (0.6, 4.0), and thus not significant.[9] The authors concluded that with the exception of its association with dilated cardiomyopathy, LBBB is a relatively benign disorder. In the 1979 Reykjavik study report for LBBB, both prevalent and incident bundle branch blocks were apparently combined in risk analysis.

In the Irish Heart Foundation study, a control group without bundle branch blocks matched for age and sex was selected from the ostensibly healthy men and women of the screened population.[12] Both groups were followed-up for an average of 9.5 years. There was no significant difference in actuarial survival at 5, 10, and 15 years between controls and LBBB or RBBB or between RBBB and LBBB. Cardiac death survival at 15 years was worse for LBBB than for controls ($p < 0.001$). Cardiovascular disease mortality risk was significantly higher for LBBB than for RBBB but the difference was not significant when age was entered into a Cox multiple regression model. The difference was also not significant if the subjects aged 60 years and older were excluded from analysis. Cardiovascular disease incidence was marginally higher among subjects with LBBB than in controls ($p = 0.04$). No significant difference was found between RBBB and controls.

The Seven Countries Study evaluated the short-term (0–5 years) and long-term (5–25 years) CHD mortality risk for bundle branch blocks in their pooled sample of 11,721 men who were CHD-free at the baseline.[14] The short-term CHD mortality risk was very high in these men, 40–60 years old at the baseline. The hazard ratios, adjusted for age, cigarette smoking, serum cholesterol, and the cohort were 9.23 for LBBB and 7.4 for RBBB. It was also fourfold but not significant for IVCD because of low prevalence and correspondingly wide confidence limits. The long-term CHD mortality risk was significant only for LBBB, with a hazard ratio 2.60 (1.34, 5.02).

Two other studies in Table 8.2, the Gothenburg Study 5[15] and the Baltimore Aging Study[2] did not find an increased risk for bundle branch block, probably due to the limited statistical power for risk detection.

8.9 Prognostic Value of Incident Bundle Branch Blocks

Information about the risk associated with incident bundle branch blocks is scarce because of the sample size problem. In the Framingham report, the cumulative 10-year CVD mortality rates for men and women indicated an increased risk for incident LBBB as well as for incident RBBB in both sex groups (Table 8.3).[16] The CVD mortality risk ratio in comparison with age- and sex-matched members of the Framingham population at large and free from bundle branch blocks in men was approximately 3.6 and 2.3 for incident LBBB and RBBB, respectively, and in women approximately 3.3 and 2.8 for incident LBBB and RBBB, respectively. The cumulative CVD mortality rates in men and women combined for those with incident LBBB and RBBB were approximately four and three times higher, respectively, than in the matched control group without bundle branch block.

The risk of future CHD and CHF was significantly increased in men and in women for incident LBBB and RBBB compared with the matched Framingham reference group. Multivariate logistic regression analysis with adjustment for age, diabetes status and systolic blood pressure indicated that in women, both incident LBBB and incident RBBB were independent predictors of an increased risk of subsequent CHD and CHF. In men, the association of incident LBBB or RBBB with increased risk for these conditions did not reach statistical significance after adjustment for age, systolic blood pressure and diabetes.

8.10 Long-term Prognosis of Incident Bundle Branch Blocks

In the Manitoba Heart Study, incident LBBB was associated with a significantly increased risk of CVD mortality: 5-year incidence of sudden death as the first manifestation of ischemic heart disease was over tenfold in men 45 years or older compared to men without LBBB. Men with ischemic or valvular heart disease at the time LBBB first appeared were excluded from these analyses. Incident RBBB was not associated with an increased risk of ischemic heart disease or sudden death in analyses of the data from the 29-year follow-up period. When the follow-up period was extended to 35 years, a significant association was found also for RBBB in men 55 years of age.

It is debatable to what extent the results from observations in highly select groups can be generalized. However, the data from the Manitoba Heart Study supports the findings from several more representative community-dwelling populations that LBBB is associated with a higher CVD mortality risk than RBBB. It also showed, like many other studies, that neither the incident LBBB nor RBBB is significantly associated with manifestations of CHD preceding the occurrence of bundle branch block.

8.11 Bundle Branch Blocks and Acute Myocardial Infarction

Ten to 12% of the patients hospitalized for acute MI were reported to have a bundle branch block in their admission ECG or developed a bundle branch block during hospitalization before thrombolytic therapy became common.[20-23] One of the early clinical intervention trials, the Coronary Drug Project (CDP), examined the prognostic significance of various ECG abnormalities in 2,035 survivors of the first heart attack.[23] After adjustment for major CHD risk factors and clinical risk indicators, complete bundle branch blocks, with the exception of RBBB, had a significant independent association with mortality during the 3-year or longer follow-up period of the study.

In a 1984 study of 1,013 consecutive patients with acute MI, 104 (10.0%) with a bundle branch block at admission or appearing during the first 24 hours after admission, the RBBB and LBBB occurred with approximately equal frequency.[22] The in-hospital mortality rate of the patients with a bundle branch block was high, 32%.

A more recent clinical trial, the Global Utilization of Streptokinase and t-PA (tissue-type plasminogen activator) for Occluded Coronary Arteries (GUSTO-1), reported a considerably lower prevalence of bundle branch blocks in the admission ECGs of acute MI patients: 1.6%.[24] The selection criteria and the trial design in GUSTO-1 may have differed from other studies, and there may also have been a selection bias. Of all bundle branch blocks, 31.2% were LBBB and 69.8% RBBB. Of all RBBB, 50.2% were combined with LAFB and 3.8% with LPFB. Infarct location was the anterior wall in 65% of the patients with RBBB and in 35% of the patients with LBBB.

Bundle branch block in the admission ECG was associated with a 53% increased risk of 30-day mortality (odds ratio 1.53 (1.0, 2.33), $p = 0.050$) compared to the control group of acute MI patients without bundle branch block after adjusting for all relevant risk factors (age, systolic blood pressure, anterior MI location, Killip class, heart rate and diabetes).

The incidence of bundle branch blocks (LBBB and RBBB) developing after hospital admission in acute MI patients receiving thrombolytic therapy was 23.6% in the combined GUSTO-1 and Thrombolysis and Angioplasty in Myocardial Infarction (TAMI) trials.[25] The high bundle branch block incidence, including transient bundle branch blocks, was in part due to the 36- to 72-hour monitoring period of these patients. The majority of the bundle branch blocks were transient (77.6%). Of all bundle branch blocks, 55.2% were RBBB, 29.8% LBBB, and the remaining 14.9% were alternating between RBBB and LBBB.

Incident bundle branch blocks had a strong association with increased 30-day mortality risk. The mortality rate was 3.5% for acute MI patients without bundle branch block and 8.7% for patients with bundle branch block. The increased risk was particularly high for persistent bundle branch block, with an odds ratio 6.0 (2.6, 13.5). The relatively high incidence of transient bundle branch

blocks in the study population may in part be due to an effective monitoring of the patients. It can also mean that thrombolytic therapy reduced the incidence of persistent bundle branch blocks by converting them into transient bundle branch blocks with a more favorable prognosis. Persistent bundle branch block in acute MI patients still appears to carry a high risk of short-term mortality.

8.1 Prognostic Significance of Fascicular Blocks

In selected clinical populations such as those referred to coronary angiography, LAFB may be a marker of significant obstruction of the left anterior descending coronary artery. De Padua et al, in their comprehensive review of ventricular conduction defects,[6] concluded that prognosis depends on the severity of the underlying clinical or subclinical heart disease, and that isolated LAFB does not seem to affect prognosis, even in old age. Prognostic information about LPFB is scanty due to the low prevalence and incidence of this condition.

References

1. Rautaharju PM, Calhoun HP, Chaitman BR. Novacode serial ECG classification system for clinical trials and epidemiological studies. J Electrocardiol 1992;24:179–87.
2. Fleg JL, Das DN, Lakatta E. Right bundle branch block: long-term prognosis in apparently healthy men. J Am Coll Cardiol 1983;1:887–92.
3. Stephan E, deMeeus A, Bouvagnet P. Hereditary bundle branch block: right bundle branch blocks of different causes have different morphologic characteristics. Am Heart J 1997;133:249–56.
4. Demoulin JC, Simar LJ, Kulbertus HE. Quantitative study of left bundle branch fibrosis in left anterior hemiblock: a stereologic approach. Am J Cardiol 1975;36:751–6.
5. Rizzon P, Rossi L, Baissus C et al. Left posterior hemiblock in acute myocardial infarction. Br Heart J 1975;37:711–20.
6. De Padua F, Pereirinha A, Lopes M. Conduction defects. In: MacFarlane PW, Veitch Lawrie TD (eds). Comprehensive Electrocardiography. Theory and Practice in Health and Disease. New York,

Oxford, Beijing, Frankfurt, Sao Paolo, Sydney, Tokyo, Toronto: Pergamon Press, 1989, pp 459–510.

7. Reunanen A, Aromaa A, Pyorala K et al. The Social Insurance Institution's Coronary Heart Disease Study. Baseline data and 5 year mortality experience. Acta Med Scand 1983;21(Suppl 673):1–120.

8. Kreger BE, Anderson KM, Kannel WB. Prevalence of intraventricular block in the general population: The Framingham Study. Am Heart J 1989;117:903–10.

9. Trainsdottir IS, Hadarson T, Thorgeirsson G et al. The epidemiology of right bundle branch block and its association with cardiovascular morbidity – the Reykjavik Study. Eur Heart J 1993;14:1590–6.

10. Hadarson T, Arnason A, Eliasson GJ et al. Left bundle branch block: prevalence, incidence, follow-up and outcome. Eur Heart J 1987;8:1075–9.

11. Ostrander LD Jr, Brandt RL, Kjelsberg MO, Einstein FH. Electrocardiographic findings among the adult population of a total natural community, Tecumseh, Michigan. Circulation 1965;31:888 98.

12. Fahy GJ, Pinski SL, Miller DP et al. Natural history of isolated bundle branch block. Am J Cardiol 1996; 77:1185–90.

13. Furberg CD, Manolio TA, Psaty BM et al. Major electrocardiographic abnormalities in persons aged 65 years and older (the Cardiovascular Health Study). Am J Cardiol 1992;69:1329–35.

14. Menotti A, Blackburn H, Jacobs DR et al. The predictive value of resting electrocardiographic findings in cardiovascular disease-free men. Twenty-five-year follow-up in the Seven Countries Study. Internal document, Division of Epidemiology, School of Public Health, University of Minnesota, 2001.

15. Eriksson P, Hansson PO, Eriksson H, Dellborg M. Bundle-branch block in a general male population: the study of men born 1913. Circulation 1998;98:2494–500.

16. Schneider JF, Thomas HE Jr, Sorlie P et al. Comparative features of newly acquired left and right bundle branch block in the general population: the Framingham study. Am J Cardiol 1981;47:931–40.

17. Rabkin SW, Mathewson FA, Tate RB. Natural history of left bundle-branch block. Br Heart J 1980;43:164–9.

18. Rabkin SW, Mathewson FAL, Tate RB. The natural history of right bundle branch block and frontal plane QRS axis in apparently healthy men. Chest 1981;2:191–6.

19. Mathewson FAC, Manfreda J, Tate RB, Cuddy TE. The University of Manitoba Follow-up Study – an investigation of cardiovascular disease with 35 years of follow-up (1948–1983). Can J Cardiol 1987; 40:149–55.

20. Dubois C, Pierard LA, Smeets JP et al. Short- and long-term prognostic importance of complete bundle-branch block complicating acute myocardial infarction. Clin Cardiol 1988;11:292–6.

21. Roos JC, Dunning AJ. Bundle branch block in acute myocardial infarction. [Review] Eur J Cardiol 1978; 6:403 24.

22. Klein RC, Vera Z, Mason DT. Intraventricular conduction defects in acute myocardial infarction: incidence, prognosis, and therapy. Am Heart J 1984;108:1007–13.

23. The Coronary Drug Project Research Group. The prognostic importance of the electrocardiogram after myocardial infarction: experience in the Coronary Drug Project. Ann Intern Med 1972;77: 677–89.

24. Sgarbossa EB, Pinski SL, Topol EJ et al. Acute myocardial infarction and complete bundle branch block at hospital admission: clinical characteristics and outcome in the thrombolytic era. J Am Coll Cardiol 1998;31:105–10.

25. Newby KH, Pisano E, Krucoff M et al. Incidence and clinical relevance of the occurrence of bundle-branch block in patients treated with thrombolytic therapy. Circulation 1996;94:2424–8.

9A
Old Myocardial Infarction

Synopsis

Significance

Old myocardial infarction (MI) by ECG criteria has been used as evidence for coronary heart disease (CHD) in epidemiological studies for comparing cross-sectional MI prevalence and for risk evaluation in contrasting populations. Myocardial infarction by ECG is the only manifestation of past silent MI.

Mechanism

Coronary arteries are endarteries. Obstruction of an artery in the coronary bed results in acute ischemic injury, and if not resolved, a subsequent loss of electrical activity and death of damaged myocardial cells. Abnormal QS or Q waves usually appear following or concomitant with ST deviations in acute phase and evolving ST-T changes. Dead or fibrosed myocardial tissue alters excitation pathways around the damaged region causing other QRS changes, and occasionally blocking conduction in major conduction pathways of the His–Purkinje system.

Risk Factors

These include CHD risk factors in general: cigarette smoking, age, male gender, serum cholesterol and improper lipoprotein balance, hypertension, impaired glucose tolerance, and heredity. Elevated homocysteine, C-reactive protein, fibrinogen, and other factors promoting plaque forma-

tion in coronary arteries have been identified as newer risk factors for MI.

Classification Problems

Abnormal Q waves in survivors of acute MI may not develop and when present, they tend to diminish or even disappear with time. In older studies using ventriculography as a standard, the sensitivity of Minnesota Code 1.1–1.3 Q waves in detecting wall motion abnormalities was reported as 51% at a specificity of 84%. Equally low sensitivity has been reported in autopsy studies or using ECG-independent evidence in the acute phase as a standard. Low specificity reduces the utility of some more sensitive ECG criteria such as poor R wave progression in anterior MI. Up to a quarter to a third of MIs by ECG criteria have been found to be unrecognized, one-half of them without any reported symptoms. The limited classification accuracy of ECG criteria based solely on ECG evidence reduces the utility of comparative evaluation of MI prevalence in contrasting populations.

Prevalence

The reported prevalence of Minnesota Code 1.1–1.3 Q waves in community-based populations at age 40–59 years ranges from less than 1% to 6.6% in men and from 1% to 4.5% in women. In CHD-free cohorts of 40- to 59-year-old men, the prevalence ranges from 1.6 to 2.1%. Definite old MI prevalence by strict Q-wave criteria is low at age 40–59 years, even in countries with high CHD mortality like Finland (1.3% in men and 0.5% in women).

Mortality Risk

Independent short-term risk for CHD mortality for MI by the Minnesota Code 1.1–1.3 combination varies in contrasting populations from nonsignificant to over fourfold risk increase. Long-term risk is not significant. Short-term excess mortality risk for large Q waves in CHD-free and in total male cohorts has been 13- to nearly 20-fold in some studies. For strict MI criteria combining major Q waves and major ST-T codes, the reported multivariable-adjusted short-term risk for CHD mortality ranges from sevenfold up to 19-fold, and also the reported long-term risk is over threefold. Prevalence of MI by such stricter criteria is low, reducing the corresponding utility in identifying high-risk subgroups. In most studies, mortality risk has been similar for non-recognized and recognized MI in men. Mortality risk in women has been reported to be marginally lower for unrecognized than for recognized MI.

Abbreviations and Acronyms

BARI – Bypass Angioplasty Revascularization Investigation
CABG – coronary artery bypass grafting
CAD – coronary artery disease
CHD – coronary heart disease
CVD – cardiovascular disease
LAD – left anterior descending (coronary artery)
LCX – left circumferential (coronary artery)
LBBB – left bundle branch block
LVH – left ventricular hypertrophy
LPD – left posterior descending (coronary artery)
MI – myocardial infarction
RCA – right coronary artery

9A.1 Introduction

Objective coding of ECG abnormalities associated with coronary heart disease (CHD), particularly old myocardial infarction (MI), has been one of

the primary requirements in cardiovascular epidemiological studies. Acute MI, of primary concern in clinical applications, is rarely encountered in community health surveys. The sequels of myocardial damage following the acute MI phase, the residual abnormal Q waves and repolarization abnormalities, provide primary evidence for an old MI. Abnormal Q waves do not develop in a certain fraction of patients, and when they do, they tend to become smaller or even disappear with time because of cardiac remodeling in the healing and adaptation phase following acute MI. While ST elevation is the primary marker of acute ischemic injury, negative or "flat" T waves, often with borderline-abnormal Q waves, remain as chronic manifestations of old ischemic injury. Some degree of residual ST elevation is often retained particularly in old anterior MI. Sustained ST depression may indicate the presence of a chronic ischemic state.

There are several other clinical conditions that may induce secondary repolarization abnormalities, including in particular left ventricular conduction defects and left ventricular hypertrophy (LVH). In CHD, repolarization abnormalities may be secondary, due to altered sequence of ventricular excitation with scar formation and fibrosis (often combined with compensatory LVH in post-MI states), or they can be primary signs of derailed ionic channel function in ischemic regions. Clinically so-called non-Q-wave MI in the acute phase may occur particularly in smaller MIs when clearly abnormal Q waves do not develop. Repolarization abnormalities evolve characteristically in the acute phase in Q-wave and in non-Q-wave MI.

This chapter covers ECG abnormalities that are most directly associated with an old MI. Various studies have used quite diverse definitions for MI and ischemic abnormalities. In the Minnesota Code, abnormal Q waves are covered under Code 1. Abnormalities in ST and T waves are coded under Codes 4 and 5. In the Minnesota Code in general, various categories are coded as independent entities without a clear hierarchy in relation to other coding categories. Many newer studies have used various combinations of Q wave and ST-T codes to identify an old MI. At times left bundle branch block (Code 7.1) is included with Q wave and ST-T codes in a pooled category characterized as "ischemic abnormalities".

Studies that have used reasonably similar definitions for abnormalities for risk evaluation are grouped together here when considering the risk associated with these abnormalities.

9A.2 The Mechanism of Generation of Abnormal Q Waves

Coronary arteries are endarteries, and an ischemic injury following a total occlusion results in death of a smaller or larger myocardial segment normally perfused by the arterial bed distal to the site of the occluded artery. Consequent loss of electrical activity of the injured myocardial tissue alters cardiac potential gradients generated during the early phase of ventricular excitation. This loss is manifested as the loss of initial R waves or the appearance of QS waves or Q waves that are wider in duration and larger in amplitude than Q waves that are seen in normal ventricular excitation. In vectorcardiographic terms, the direction and the magnitude of the initial QRS vectors are altered. Alterations at some later parts of QRS can also take place, depending on the location of the MI.

The combinations of possible occlusion sites and the locations and extent of myocardial damage are numerous and complex (Table 9A.1).[1] Fascicular blocks often occurring with acute MI further complicate the problem (Table 9A.2). Most commonly occurring MIs can be categorized into three groups: (1) anterior MI following occlusion of the left anterior descending artery (LAD) or its branches; (2) posterior MI from occlusion of the left posterior circumflex artery or its branches, with MI located mainly in the posterolateral wall; and (3), inferior MI from occlusion of the posterior inferior descending coronary artery arising usually from a dominant right coronary artery (RCA) as its proximate coronary. (A dominant left posterior circumflex coronary artery can also have the posterior inferior descending coronary artery as one of its branches.) Circumferential extension around the apex seen in larger MIs is most common in anterior MI, at times also in posterior and inferior MI.

The traditional simple vectorcardiographic "rule" is that in old Q-wave MI, the initial QRS vector points away from the infarcted area. Thus, in anterior MI, initial R waves disappear and QS waves are present in anterior chest leads V1 and V2. It should be noted that there is a QS wave (no initial R wave) in V1 in a small percentage of normal adult men and women, and the initial R wave in V2 is missing or is $\leq 100\,\mu V$ in 2% of men

TABLE 9A.1 QRS abnormalities in old myocardial infarction (MI) in various myocardial segments, and possible occlusion site in acute phase.

Segments involved in MI	Q waves or equivalents	Possible occlusion site in acute phase
Anterior	QS V1–V3	Distal LAD, small MI often in anterior-apical segment
Apical	Q or diminished R in I, V5, V6, or no QRS involvement	
Larger anterior MI, may extend to anterior-lateral, anterior-basal segments	QS V1–V4; Q I, aVL, V5, V6	Diagonal or proximal LAD
Posterior	Enhanced initial R V1, V2; increased R/S ratio	LCX
Middle posterior, extending to postero-lateral segments	Q I, aVL, V5, V6	MI size varies even in total proximal LCX occlusion
Inferior (diaphragmatic)	Q II, aVF	Anywhere proximal, middle third or PDA branching point of RCA, or PDA arising from dominant LCX
Right ventricular; lateral-posterior aspects, usually with inferior MI.	Initial R aVR. Q waves in anterior leads absent. Normal small initial R waves in right precordial leads V3R and V4R may be replaced by QS or Q with small initial R waves	RCA, commonly proximal third
Thin anterior wall less involved (patchy scar formation), protected by collaterals, Thebesian vessels (?)		Note: ECG signs of right ventricular failure (P V1 $\geq 75\,\mu V$) with inferior MI suggests right ventricular MI

LAD left anterior descending coronary artery, *LCX* left circumflex coronary artery, *RCA* right coronary artery, *PDA* posterior descending artery.
Residual ST elevation may be present in leads with ST elevation in acute phase; T-wave changes can be in any lead group; fascicular block will alter QRS patterns.

TABLE 9A.2 Examples of fascicular blocks modifying QRS abnormalities in myocardial infarction.

Fascicular block occurrence in combination with infarcted segment and occlusion site	QRS prolongation	ECG pattern
Anterior MI in LAD occlusion and LAFB occlusion (in about 8%)	QRS slightly prolonged, 105–110 ms (wider if LVH)	Prominent QR pattern in aVL, Pronounced LAD (−45° to −90°), wide frontal plane angle between initial and terminal QRS vectors
Anterior MI in LAD occlusion and RBBB with LAFB; anterior MI is often large	QRS prolongation ≥120 ms	The additional RBBB does not considerably alter ECG criteria
Inferior MI in RCA (PID) occlusion and LPFB (develops in 85% of patients; recent onset LBBB may also occur)	20 ms QRS prolongation, 100–120 ms, may be intermittent	High-frequency notches in mid- and terminal QRS
	Initial QRS vectors superior, left; form a smooth arc	If LPFB disappears, QRS shortens to 80–90 ms, axis shifts superiorly (due to inferior MI)

LAD left anterior descending coronary artery, LAFB left anterior fascicular block, LPFB left posterior fascicular block, PID posterior inferior descending coronary artery, RBBB right bundle branch block, LBBB left bundle branch block, RCA right coronary artery.

and women aged 40–59 years and in 5% at age 60 years and older. With a more extensive anterior MI, QS waves are seen also in V3 and to the left.

Left septal involvement disrupts the normal septal excitation spread from left to right. The septal excitation starting from the right side of the septum proceeds undiminished because of the missing left side excitation. This eliminates or reduces the normal septal Q waves in the left lateral leads I, aVL and V6. Anterior MI with apical extension generates more pronounced Q waves than normally in inferior leads II, III, and aVF in addition to the Q waves in anterior chest leads.

Inferior MI generates Q waves of longer duration than normally in inferiorly oriented leads II, III, and aVF. The largest Q wave is generally in lead III. The lead vector of lead aVR is oriented along the long axis of the left ventricular cavity, directed from apex to base. A wider than normal initial R wave in aVR is equivalent to Q waves in inferior leads III and aVF.

Posterior MI can occasionally have apical extension. The lead vectors of the lateral chest leads also have a small inferior component so that they can reflect apical extension of anterior or inferior MI (or posterior MI).

Strictly posterior MI can be expected to produce more prominent initial R waves in anterior chest leads V1 and V2 (equivalent to Q waves in inverted leads –V1 and –V2).

Dead or fibrosed myocardial tissue also alters the propagation of excitation fronts that have to go around the damaged region. Peripheral Purkinje subendocardial network is partially perfused by ventricular cavity blood (Thebesian vessels) and it remains generally intact even in large MI over the Purkinje network.[2] If the damage includes a fascicle, QRS patterns will change. When MI damages a major branch of the conduction system most profound overall changes in QRS and ST-T patterns will occur, resembling bundle branch blocks.

9A.2.1 Left Anterior Descending Artery Occlusion and Anterior Myocardial Infarction

When small, an MI caused by LAD artery occlusion is commonly localized in the anterior apex, and when moderately sized, in the middle anteroseptal and anterior segments of the left ventricle. A large MI in the anteroseptal and anterosuperior segments also involves circumferential extension around the apex. Occlusion of the diagonal branch of the LAD artery with high lateral, lateral or superior MI produces Q waves in lateral leads I, aII, or V5,V6, or in a combination of these leads. Loss of amplitudes in the middle and later QRS may occur together with these Q waves.[1]

9A.2.2 Left Circumflex Artery Occlusion and Posterior Myocardial Infarction

Occlusion of the left circumferential (LCX) artery or its branches produces an MI mainly in the posterolateral wall. Myocardial infarction in LCX occlusion, usually near its proximal third, is mostly small or moderately sized and located in the middle posterolateral segment. With increasing size, MI extends into the adjacent myocardial segments. Small basal posterior MI is seen in more distal LCX occlusion. The size of MI varies even in total proximal occlusion of LCX from barely noticeable to moderate size and occasionally large, including an extension into the inferior wall.

The left LCX artery is dominant in a smaller fraction of patients (10–15%), supplying perfusion of the inferior (posterior) descending artery.[1]

9A.2.3 Right Coronary Artery Occlusion

Right coronary artery occlusions are commonly in the proximal third of the artery, less frequently in the middle third or at the branching point of the posterior descending branch. Right ventricular MI is frequently seen in the proximal but not in distal occlusions of RCA. Electrocardiographic manifestations of the inferior MI of the left ventricle are similar with RCA occlusion at all three sites. The occlusion of the posterior (inferior) descending branch of RCA produces Q waves in the inferiorly oriented leads. In the majority of patients, a block in the posterior fascicular branch of the left bundle branch develops. The proximal branch of the left bundle has a blood supply from the septal perforator branch of the LAD and the inferior branch of the RCA, but LBBB is more commonly associated with an inferior than with an anterior MI. The inferior branches of the left main bundle get their blood supply from the atrioventricular nodal branch and the septal branches of RCA. The initial portion of the Q waves in inferior MI is generated by the normal left-to-right and upwards directed septal excitation, followed by abnormal, superiorly oriented QRS vectors of the inferior MI.

9A.3 Risk Factors for Myocardial Infarction

The risk factors for old MI are the same as for acute MI, including cigarette smoking, age, male gender, serum cholesterol and improper lipoprotein balance, hypertension, impaired glucose tolerance, and heredity. Newer factors include

elevated homocysteine, C-reactive protein, fibrinogen, and other factors promoting plaque formation in coronary arteries.

9A.4 Sensitivity and Specificity of Old Myocardial Infarction Classification Criteria

As already mentioned, Q waves in MI tend to diminish or disappear with time in survivors of acute MI with the healing process and a gradual improvement of perfusion with collateral development.[3,4] The relative volume of dead tissue may also diminish with left ventricular remodeling in compensatory hypertrophy.

Evaluation data on classification accuracy of the Minnesota Code MI-related categories is limited. Older pathological studies with autopsy evidence in hospitalized patients documented relatively low sensitivity of MI classification criteria.[5,6] The sensitivity in detecting wall motion abnormalities in ventriculography in patients with coronary angiography for suspected MI was reported as 21% for Minnesota Code 1.1 Q waves, with a specificity of 93%.[7] For Minnesota Code 1.1–1.3 Q waves, the sensitivity was 51% at a specificity of 84%.

Pipberger et al. used ECG-independent clinical data in acute phase to evaluate the sensitivity of MI criteria.[8] The sensitivity of the quite strict Minnesota Code 1.1 criterion was only 49% although the specificity was rather high, 94%. Low specificity reduces the utility of some more sensitive ECG criteria such as poor R wave progression in anterior MI, with false positive findings in other conditions such as in ventricular hypertrophy, emphysema, and also in women.[9,10]

Startt/Selvester et al. summarized the reasons why in 40–50% of the patients an MI 2 cm or larger does not produce Q waves that could be classified as an old MI.[1] These reasons include small MI size (30% of MIs less than 2–3 cm in diameter), cancellation effects due to multiple MIs, and major ventricular conduction defects masking ECG signs of Q-wave MI. Small MIs tend to produce QRS alterations other than Q waves, such as R wave attenuation, notching, or slurring. The Selvester score developed using computer simulation and making extensive use of empirical observations of various QRS features[1] has been reported to produce superior accuracy in classification, sizing, and locating old MIs. The utility of a simplified version of the score for risk prediction has also been suggested.[11]

Computer algorithms developed using scalar and vectorcardiographic variables with nuclear cardiac imaging as the standard have been reported to enhance prior MI detection accuracy up to the level of 79% sensitivity and 97% specificity.[12] Although such a high level of classification accuracy probably reflects selection and exclusion criteria and other characteristics of the MI and non-MI groups of the study population (100 patients with MI and 98 without MI), it suggests potential power of model-based MI classifiers. Simple statistical models derived from body surface potential maps have also shown that diagnostic information in MIs missed by the standard 12-lead ECG criteria are located in ECG leads outside the standard chest and the limb leads.[13] Diagnostic performance of the standard 12 leads can also be considerably enhanced by multivariate discriminant models by choosing optimal temporal locations in QRS and ST-T patterns of best discriminating leads. None of the more advanced MI classification schemes mentioned above have found a way for use in epidemiological studies or clinical trials.

The present state-of-the art in MI classification is perhaps best represented by the results from a large European evaluation study including MI classification in a data base documented by wall motion abnormalities in left ventriculogram as ECG-independent evidence (akinesia or dyskinesia).[14] Sensitivity was determined for independent classification of 547 MIs by eight cardiologists and 16 computer programs, and the specificity in classification of 382 control patients. The control group consisted of 286 ambulatory patents. The inclusion criteria were based on medical history and chest x-ray. The control group also included 96 patients referred for cardiological examination, most with coronary angiography for evaluation of atypical chest pain or repolarization abnormalities in their rest or exercise ECG.

The specificity determined from the classification of the control group was high. The median value was 97.1% for the cardiologists and 96.7%

for the programs. The best program for epidemiological applications with a specificity of 97% had a sensitivity of 67%. One of the programs with a sensitivity of 82% and a specificity of 92% appeared particularly attractive for clinical applications. The best programs reached performance levels similar to those of the best cardiologists, a rather remarkable result considering that the cardiologists tested were experienced electrocardiographers with a strong research background.

9A.5 Prevalence and Mortality Risk for Old Q-Wave Myocardial Infarction

Several studies have documented increased mortality risk for Q/QS waves in diverse study populations. Health survey data in some studies have provided data on ECG-MI in more or less unselected population samples with no or minimal exclusions on the basis of ECG or clinical findings. Some other studies have dealt primarily with healthy or CHD-free subgroups.

Table 9A.3 summarizes data from some of the well-documented studies related to the mortality risk for Q-wave MI.

9A.5.1 Mortality Risk in Three Populations

9A.5.1.1 Old Q-Wave Myocardial Infarction in CHD-free Men of the Seven Countries Study

Two recent reports from the Seven Countries Study evaluated baseline prevalence and short-term and long-term mortality risk for old Q-wave MI in CHD-free men.[15,16] Excluded from the study group were men with a history of any heart disease, peripheral arterial or cerebrovascular disease. Electrocardiographic findings were not used as exclusion criteria. Risk data were reported for two MI-related categories: (1) Minnesota Code 1.1–1.3 Q waves; and (2), Q-wave MI defined by the presence of diagnostic Q waves (Minnesota Code 1.1; with or without ST-T codes), or category 1.2 Q waves combined with major ST-T codes 4.1, 4.2 or 5.1, 5.2. The prevalence of any Q-wave codes in the CHD-free subgroup of the male cohort aged 40–59 years at baseline was 2.1% (2.4% in Northern Europe and USA, 2.1% in Southern Europe and 1.2% in Japan), compared to 2.4% in the

TABLE 9A.3 Three population studies with evaluation of the mortality risk for ECG manifestations of an old myocardial infarction.

	Seven Countries Study[15,16]	Finland's Social Insurance Institution's CHD study[17]	Italian RIFLE Pooling Project[18]
Geographic location	Finland, Greece, Italy, the Netherlands, former Yugoslavia, Japan, USA	South-western, western, central and eastern districts of the country	Eight regions in Italy
Source population	12,763 men (11 cohorts from rural areas of Finland, Greece, Japan and Yugoslavia; three other more diverse cohorts from Yugoslavia; the town of Zutphen, the Netherlands; and cohorts of railroad employees from the USA and Italy)	Men and women of the districts. Participation rate 90% (5,738 men and 5,224 women)	Reported four out of nine studies, 23 cohorts total. Participation rate 65–70%
Baseline	1958–1964	1966–1972	1978–1987
Exclusions	Sampling goal: total male population from selected geographic areas Participation rate ≥60%. For CHD-free sample, excluded 854 with prevalent CHD at baseline; no ECG exclusions	All participants included	History of angina pectoris by Rose questionnaire, hospitalization with discharge diagnosis of MI, history of other heart disease
CHD-free sample	11,860		12,180 men, 10,373 women
Age range	40–59 years	30–59 years	30–69 years
Follow-up	Initial 5 years and subsequent 6–25 years	5 years	6 years
Q-wave MI-related ECG findings evaluated for risk	1. Any Q wave codes, with or without other ECG abnormalities (MC 1.1– 1.3) 2. Diagnostic Q-wave MI (MC 1.1 OR (MC 1.2 and MC 5.1– 5.2)	1. Diagnostic Q-wave MI (MC 1.1 OR (MC 1.2 and MC 5.1–5.2) 2. Other "ischemic" categories (MC 1.2–1.3, 4.1–4.3, 5.1–5.3, 6.1–6.2, 7.1, 7.2, 7.4, 8.3)	1. Any Q-wave codes (MC 1.1–1.3) 2. Any Q-wave codes with any T-wave codes (5.1–5.3) 3. Q-wave codes 1.1–1.2 with T-wave codes 5.1, 5.2
Baseline prevalence	MC 1.1–1.3 (all men combined): 2.7% CHD-free men: 2.1%	1. Diagnostic Q-wave MI Men 40–59 years: 1.3% Women 40–59 years: 0.5% 2. Other "ischemic" ECG Men 40–59 years: 10.4% Women 40–59 years: 12.8%	Men: any Q codes 30–49 years: 0.6% 50–69 years: 1.1% Women: any Q codes 30–49 years: 0.5% 50–59 years: 1.2%
Follow-up (years)	5 and 25	5	6
Associated risk (hazard ratio HR)	Short-term (years 0–5) risk for CHD Death (CVD-free men) 1. Any Q: HR 4.1 (2.20, 7.61) 2. Large Q or major Q with ST-T: HR 15.6 (7.2, 34.1) (not significant if large Q category excluded) Long-term (years 6–25) risk for CHD death 3. Any Q: HR 1.2 (0.84, 1.58) 4. Large Q or major Q with ST-T: HR 3.4 (1.9, 6.2)	1. Diagnostic Q-wave MI (5-year, age-standardized risk for age group 40–49) Men: CHD mortality RR = 19.5 CVD mortality RR = 13.3 All-cause mortality RR = 5.6 Women: too few events for risk evaluation 2. "Other ischemic" ECG: Men: CHD mortality RR = 7.2 CVD mortality RR = 6.4 All-cause mortality RR = 3.1 Women: CVD mortality RR = 3.0 All-cause mortality 2.2 Symptom-free men with "other ischemic" ECG CHD mortality RR = 4.4 CVD mortality RR = 3.9	CHD mortality 1. Any Q waves: not significant in men or in women 2. Any Q waves with any T waves: not significant for men or for women 3. Major Q waves with major T waves: Men: RR 17.2 (1.54, 1.92) Women: too few events for RR calculations CVD mortality 1. Any Q waves: RR 2.77 (1.08, 7.07) in men, not significant in women 2. Any Q waves with any T waves: RR 7.24 (1.98, 26.4) in men, too few events in women

CHD coronary heart disease, *CVD* cardiovascular disease, *HR* hazard ratio, *MC* Minnesota Code, *RR* relative risk.

whole cohort before selection of the CHD-free subgroup. The low prevalence and relatively low event rates indicate that very large pooled samples of subjects are required for risk analysis to yield adequate statistical power.

Risk evaluation for the short-term follow-up (5 years after baseline) and subsequently for the long-term follow-up from 6 to 25 years was done for men who remained CHD-free at the examination after the initial 5-year follow-up. The endpoint evaluated was CHD death. For 5-year CHD death for any Q-wave code 1.1–1.3, the relative risk was 4.1 (2.20, 7.61). The long-term risk was not significant. For the strict Q-wave MI criteria, the multivariable-adjusted short-term relative risk for CHD mortality was very high, 15.6 (7.2, 34.1), and also the long-term risk was 3.4 (1.9, 6.2).

In spite of the high risk for men with strict ECG evidence of old MI, the prevalence, and the associated population-attributable risk is too low for the use of these criteria for selection of high-risk subgroups of otherwise healthy men for intervention as a public health measure.

9A.5.1.2 Finland's Social Insurance Institution's Coronary Heart Disease Study

The second cohort in Table 9A.3 is the total population sample of the CHD survey of Finland's Social Insurance Institution, comprising 5,738 men and 5,224 women aged 30–59 years.[17] The report used the same combination of Q-wave and T-wave criteria for Q-wave MI for risk evaluation as the Seven Countries Study (Code 1.1 Q waves or Code 1.2 Q waves with major T-wave codes, 5.1 or 5.2). As in other similar populations, there was a progressive increase in the prevalence with age both in men and in women. The prevalence of Q-wave MI in the age group used for risk evaluation (40–59 years) was 1.3% in men and 0.5% in women. The total age-adjusted prevalence of any Q waves was 6.6% in men and 4.5% in women, and the prevalence of major Q waves (Minnesota Code 1.1, 1.2) was 2.6% in men and 1.5% in women.

There was a significantly increased risk in men for Q-wave MI for all mortality endpoints: relative risk was 19.5 for CHD mortality, 13.3 for cardiovascular disease (CVD) mortality, and 5.6 for all-cause mortality. There were too few events in

women for risk evaluation in this ECG category. The risk for Minnesota Code 1.1 large Q waves in men was 13.4, and for smaller Q waves in codes 1.2, 1.3 approximately threefold compared to men without significant Q waves. The relative risk of CVD mortality for the combined category of "other ischemic" ECG was 6.4 for men and 3.0 for women.

9A.5.1.3 CHD-free Men and Women from the Italian RIFLE Pooling Project

The third study in Table 9A.3 comes from the Italian Risk Factors and Life Expectancy (RIFLE) pooling project, which included a group of 12,180 CHD-free men and 10,373 women aged 30–69 years.[18] The CHD-free group was selected by excluding subjects with angina pectoris by Rose questionnaire, hospitalization with discharge diagnosis of MI or history of any other heart disease. Like in the Seven Countries Study, the prevalence of any Q waves by the Minnesota Code was low. In the age group 50–69 years, it was 1.1% in men and 1.2% in women, and approximately 50% lower in the younger age groups.

Risk of CHD mortality for any of the Minnesota Code Q-wave codes with or without ST-T codes was not significant in men or in women. It was significant for CVD mortality in men, with relative risk 2.77 (1.08, 7.07).

Although prevalence data were not reported for combinations of Q- and T-wave codes, they can be assumed to be even lower than those for any Q-wave codes. Risk of CHD mortality was not significant in men or in women for Q waves in Codes 1.1–1.3 combined with T waves in Codes 5.1–5.3 (possible MI). For major Q waves combined with major T waves (definite MI), the CHD mortality risk was significantly increased, with relative risk 17.2 (1.54, 1.92). There were too few events in the women for relative risk determination.

9A.5.2 Some Other Studies on Mortality Risk for Old Myocardial Infarction

There are several other reports from epidemiological studies in diverse populations with evaluation of the mortality risk for ECG-MI. The Whitehall study on 18,403 male civil servants 40–60 years old in the early 1970s evaluated the 5-year

CHD mortality risk for Q waves coded from limb lead ECGs.[19] The study population contained a subgroup of 15,974 nonsymptomatic men with no history of angina pectoris or MI and who were not under medical care for heart disease or hypertension. The prevalence of Codes 1.1–1.3 was 2.0% in the whole group and 1.6% in the nonsymptomatic group. Approximately two-thirds of the Q waves were minor, Minnesota Code 1.3. The age-adjusted CHD mortality ratio for men with any Q waves was 6.1, with all men in the study as the reference. In the nonsymptomatic group, the mortality ratio was 4.0.

The Busselton study on 2,119 unselected subjects reported that the 13-year standardized CVD mortality rate was significantly higher in the pooled group of men and women with Minnesota Code 1.1–1.3 Q waves than among those with a normal ECG.[20]

The cross-sectional data from the Copenhagen City Heart Study involved a random sample of 9,384 men and 10,314 women aged 20 years and older.[21] In the age group 60–69 years, 92 men (5.9%) and 38 women (2.4%) had Minnesota Code 1.1–1.3 Q waves. Among 25 men who died, 21 had major Q waves (Minnesota Code 1.1, 1.2), a highly significant difference between the observed and expected number of deaths compared to men without Q waves. There was only one death among women with Q waves.

9A.5.3 Unrecognized Compared to Recognized MI

Comparative data on the mortality risk data for recognized versus unrecognized MI from three studies are listed in Table 9A.4. Unrecognized MI in these studies consisted of subjects who were either totally asymptomatic (silent MI) or reported symptoms atypical for acute MI.

9A.5.3.1 The Reykjavik Study

The first of the studies in Table 9A.4 summarizes data of the Reykjavik study male cohort aged 33–80 years.[22] The study was performed in five stages, 3–5 years apart, with the last one conducted during 1983–1987. The overall prevalence of unrecognized MI at the first stage of the study was 0.5%, increasing sharply with age. It was 0.5% at

age 50 years and increased to over 5% at age 75 years. The prevalence of unrecognized MI increased at the later phases of the study, with the last phase prevalence being 2.8% in 1987.

About 30% of all MIs in the pooled data from all phases of the study were unrecognized. As expected, angina pectoris was strongly associated with recognized and unrecognized MI. Other factors from logistic regression associated with both types of MI were age, smoking, serum cholesterol level, cardiomegaly, and diuretic therapy. Impaired glucose tolerance and digoxin therapy were significantly associated only with prevalent recognized MI. Factors with predictive power for incident unrecognized and recognized MI from Poisson regression included age, diastolic blood pressure, and hypertension medication. Digoxin therapy was significantly predictive for future unrecognized MI. Current smoking had a more consistent association with future recognized than with unrecognized MI.

Relative risk of CHD mortality for MI without angina pectoris was 4.6 (2.4, 8.6) for unrecognized MI and 6.3 (3.7, 10.6) for recognized MI. For all-cause mortality, the corresponding risks were 2.7 (1.5, 4.8) and 2.9 (1.8, 4.6), respectively. Life table analysis for participants with MI in the first four stages of the study confirmed relatively similar survival probabilities for both types of MI. Ten-year survival probabilities for unrecognized and recognized MI were 49 and 45%, respectively, and 15-year survival probabilities 62 and 48%, respectively.

9A.5.3.2 The Framingham Study

A 1986 report from Framingham in Table 9A.4 indicated that patients with unrecognized MI were as likely as those with recognized MI to be at increased risk of death, heart failure, and stroke.[23] The baselines for the evaluation were the onsets of the three successive 10-year periods since the start of the Framingham study in 1948. Of all MIs detected in 5,127 subjects at the initial examination, 130 out of 469 MIs among men (27.7%) and 83 out of 239 MIs among women (34.7%) were unrecognized, almost half without any symptoms. Almost these same proportions of incident MI during the three 10-year follow-up periods were unrecognized. As seen from Table 9A.4,

TABLE 9A.4 Mortality risk for recognized versus unrecognized myocardial infarction.

	The Reykjavik study[22]	The Framingham study[23]	The Honolulu Heart Program[25]
Geographic location	Reykjavik area, Iceland	Framingham, Massachusetts, USA	Oahu Island, Hawaii
Source population	Male residents born between 1907 and 1934. Response rate 64–75%	Town's adult population, 2,336 men, 2,873 women	Men of Japanese ancestry born between 1900 and 1919. Participation rate 73%
Baseline	1967–1968	Onset of each of the three successive 10-year periods starting 1948	1965–1968
Selection criteria	Whole cohort included	Free from overt CHD at baseline, excluding from next follow-up subjects with MI during the preceding period	CHD-free at baseline, with at least one follow-up examination
Sample size	9,141	5,127 men and women	7,331
Age range	33–80 years	30–62 years	45–68 years
Follow-up period	4–24 years (in four stages, at 3- to 5-year intervals)	30 years	10 years from the examination where incident MI was detected
Definition of MI	1. Recognized MI: MONICA criteria (patients with MC 1.1, 1.2 Q waves, or with MI by enzymes, chest pain, borderline Q waves) 2. Unrecognized MI: MC 1.1, 1.2 with no history of MI	Appearance of pathologic ($\geq$40 ms) Q waves or loss of initial R waves Unrecognized MI: incident MI when neither the patient nor the attending physician had considered heart attack	1. Serial ECG changes at follow-up considered diagnostic for old or age-undetermined MI 2. Hospitalization with acute chest pain with evolving ECG changes and/or elevated enzymes 3. Serial ECG changes at hospital surveillance considered as old or age-undetermined MI
Prevalence/ incidence of MI	Prevalence of unrecognized MI 0.5% at first stage, increased at later stages to 2.8% in 1980. Prevalence increased sharply with age, from 0.5% at age 50 years to over 5% at age 75 years. About 30% of all MI unrecognized (in pooled data from all phases)	Incidence of all MIs (during three 10-year periods): Age 45 to 54 years: Men 7.1%, women 1.3% Age 75 to 84 years: Men 11.3%, women 12.8%	Average annual rate/1,000 for recognized MI (in category 1 above) 1.46, for unrecognized MI 0.71, with significant age trend in both Unrecognized MIs 32.6%
Associated risk	CHD death, MI without angina: RR = 4.6 (2.4, 8.6) for unrecognized MI RR = 6.3 (3.7, 10.6) for recognized MI CHD death, MI with angina: RR = 16.9 (9.4, 30.3) for unrecognized MI RR = 8.5 (5.8, 12.6) for recognized MI	Ten-year age-adjusted mortality risk ratio (unrecognized MI vs recognized MI) from proportional hazards model Men: CHD death 1.0 CVD death 1.2 Sudden coronary death 0.6 All deaths 1.2 Women: CHD death 0.6 CVD death 0.5[†] Sudden coronary death 0.8 All deaths 0.7	Ten-year CHD mortality 33 vs 25% ($p = 0.107$), CVD mortality 39 vs 28% ($p = 0.045$), total mortality 45 vs 35% ($p = 0.055$), for unrecognized vs recognized MI, respectively
Multivariate adjustment	Age, cholesterol level, antihypertensive medication, diastolic pressure and smoking associated with risk of unrecognized MI; not clear if adjustment was made for these factors in risk analysis	Age-adjusted, controlling also for the effect of the loss of subjects to follow-up because of death from unrelated causes	Unadjusted for age (age distribution similar in both groups)
Comments	Survival probabilities for CHD death 10 years: 49% for unrecognized MI, 62% for recognized MI 15 years: 45% for unrecognized MI, 48% for symptomatic MI		

CHD coronary heart disease, *CVD* cardiovascular disease, *MI* myocardial infarction, *MC* Minnesota Code, *RR* relative risk.
[†] $p < 0.05$; not significant difference for other recognized vs nonrecognized MI

cause-specific mortality, and all-cause mortality in men was similar for unrecognized and recognized MI. In women, the mortality was lower for unrecognized compared to recognized MI, and the difference was significant ($p < 0.05$) for CVD mortality.

A later report in 1984 from Framingham evaluated the risk for cumulative 2-year incident unrecognized MI in comparison with asymptomatic LVH.[24] In the subgroup free from ECG-MI, ECG-LVH, and who were CHD-free at the beginning of each biennial follow-up period, incident MI was identified from biennial serial ECG comparisons by the appearance of pathological Q waves or "unequivocal loss of R wave potential". The overall 2-year MI incidence rate was 3.8/1,000 in men and 1.9/1,000 in women, showing male dominance and a progressive highly significant increase with age and hypertensive status. The striking observation was that within 10 years of the appearance of either ECG-MI or ECG-LVH, more than 45% of men and 30% of women had died, which was double the mortality rate in the general Framingham population sample.

9A.5.3.3 The Honolulu Heart Program

The Honolulu Heart Program data summarized in Table 9A.4 focused attention to the comparison of the prognosis of recognized and unrecognized MI during a 10-year follow-up among 7,331 men.[25] Risk evaluation included only men who were CHD-free at baseline examination and who had serial ECG changes classified as incident Q-wave MI at the second or third examinations (2 and 6 years following the baseline). There were a total of 89 Q-wave MIs classified from serial ECG changes, 33% of them asymptomatic. This proportion was 22% when men who were classified as MI from hospital surveillance were included in the group of all non-fatal MIs. The average annual incidence rate (per 1,000) for all nonfatal MIs was 3.29. The unrecognized MI group had a consistently higher (60–70%) total mortality, CVD mortality, and CHD mortality than the group with recognized MI. The number of events in the comparison group was rather small and the difference in risk was not significant. In any case, the results suggested that the mortality risk for silent MI was at least as high as for recognized, symptomatic MI.

9A.5.3.4 An Older Finnish Cohort from the Seven Countries Study

The Finnish cohorts of the Seven Countries Study had 697 men who had survived at the time of the 23-year follow-up examination.[26] These men were followed up for the next 5-year period. At the time of the beginning of the follow-up, 98 of the men (14.1%) had Minnesota Code 1.1–1.3 Q waves. Q waves combined with ST depression (Codes 4.1–4.3) or negative T waves (Codes 5.1 or 5.2) were significantly associated with excess risk of fatal MI, nonfatal MI, and total mortality. Isolated Q waves were not associated with independent risk of any of the endpoints.

9A.5.3.5 The Bronx Aging Study

The Bronx Aging Study assessed the prognosis of recognized and unrecognized MI in 390 old (75–85 years) community-based men and women in an 8-year prospective evaluation.[27] In this older group, baseline prevalence of MI was 18.5%, over one-third (34.7%) of them unrecognized (completely silent and with atypical symptoms). During the follow-up, the proportion of unrecognized MIs of all incident MIs was 44%. The total mortality rate in subjects with recognized and unrecognized MI combined was 5.9/100 person-years compared with 3.9/100 person-years in the group without MI ($p = 0.059$). The sample size is small and the events in study subgroups are low but the mortality rates were similar among those with recognized and unrecognized MI. The report reviewed other studies on unrecognized MI and noted that in more recent reports more often from prospective studies, the proportion of unrecognized MI has averaged 30%.

9A.6 Time Trends – are Risk Evaluation Results from Older Studies still Valid?

Controlled clinical trials have demonstrated a reduced mortality in acute MI with more common use of primary angioplasty and improved treatment of acute MI with coronary reperfusion procedures and antiplatelet therapy. A survey of patients hospitalized for acute Q-wave MI in Worcester, Massachusetts, metropolitan area hospitals comparing two periods a decade apart (1995–1995 versus 1986–1988) showed that in-hospital case fatality rate had declined from 19 to 14%.[28]

It is appropriate to ask to what extent risk evaluation results reported from the older studies are still valid. It is apparent that the short-term risk in acute MI patients has improved, at least in industrialized countries that have benefited from improved acute care. The question remains to what extent the long-term prognosis has improved. Already before the introduction of the major improvements in the care of CHD patients, factors other than ECG evidence of old MI seemed to determine the long-term outcome. Unrecognized and silent MI may be less likely to benefit from improved care until a later phase of the evolution of the disease. The proportion of unrecognized MI has been approximately one-third of all MIs in the studies cited above. This proportion was also 30% in one of the early major epidemiological investigations, the Western Collaborative Group Study.[29]

Epidemiologists face a twofold problem in producing evidence for possibly improved long-term prognosis for ECG-MI. It will again take a prolonged period of time to produce results from long-term studies. Secondly, it will take a much larger sample size to gain enough power for the study if the prevalence of ECG-MI has decreased. Finally, the traditional population studies are perhaps no longer as popular among investigators as they used to be, in part because obtaining funding for them is nowadays more difficult. Investigators are having problems in getting their manuscripts from long-term studies published in first-class medical journals because of the questions raised about the validity of the conclusions, with steadily changing acute care and population health profiles. Clinical drug trials have taken a higher priority than descriptive population-based epidemiological studies.

9A.7 Coronary Artery Disease: Intervention Strategies

Coronary artery bypass grafting (CABG) and coronary angioplasty (clinically denoted as percutaneous transluminal coronary angioplasty) are the current intervention strategies in established coronary artery disease (CAD).

The Bypass Angioplasty Revascularization Investigation (BARI) used 5-year cardiac mortality and MI rates to compare the efficacy of CABG and coronary angioplasty in a randomized trial involving 1,829 patients (353 diabetics on drug therapy) with multivessel CAD.[30] The trial used strictly standardized criteria for incident MI based on an adaptation of the Novacode.[31] The intervention groups had similar event rates for the combined endpoint of cardiac death or MI. The 5-year cardiac mortality rate was 8.0 and 4.9% in patients assigned to the coronary angioplasty and the CABG groups, respectively (relative risk = 1.55 [1.07–2.23]; $p = 0.022$). Subgroup analysis indicated that the difference was due to the diabetic subgroup. There were no significant differences between the intervention groups in overall cardiac mortality or in subgroups based on symptoms, left ventricular function, number of stenotic vessels, or stenotic left anterior descending coronary artery.

References

1. Startt/Selvester RH, Wagner G, Ideker R. Myocardial infarction. In: MacFarlane PW, Lawrie TDV (eds). Comprehensive Electrocardiology. New York: Pergamon Books Ltd, 1988, pp 565–629.
2. Cox JL, Daniel TM, Boineau JP. The electrophysiological time course of acute myocardial ischemia and the effects of early coronary artery reperfusion. Circulation 1973;48:971–83.
3. Willems J, Draulans J, Geest H. An appraisal of the Minnesota Code in "inferior" myocardial infarction. J Electrocardiol 1970;3:147–53.
4. Pyörälä K, Kentala E. Disappearance of Minnesota Code Q/QS patterns in the first year after myocardial infarctions. Ann Clin Res 1974;6:137–41.
5. Sullivan W, Vlodaver Z, Tuna N et al. Correlation of electrocardiographic and pathological findings in healed myocardial infarctions. Am J Cardiol 1978;42:724–32.
6. Uusitupa M, Pyörälä K, Raunio H et al. Sensitivity and specificity of the Minnesota Code Q/QS abnormalities in the diagnosis of myocardial infarction verified at autopsy. Am Heart J 1983;106: 753–7.
7. Heinbuch S, Koenig W, Gehring J. Assessment of global and regional myocardial function using the Minnesota Q/QS codes. J Electrocardiol 1993;26: 137–45.

8. Pipberger HV, Simonson E, Lopez EA Jr et al. The electrocardiogram in epidemiologic investigations. A new classification system. Circulation 1982;65: 1456–64.

9. Zema MJ, Collins M, Alonso DR, Kligfield P. Electrocardiographic poor R-wave progression. Correlation with postmortem findings. Chest 1981;79: 195–200.

10. Colaco R, Reay P, Beckett C et al. False positive ECG reports of anterior myocardial infarction in women. J Electrocardiol 2000;33(Suppl):239–44.

11. Bounous EP Jr, Califf RM, Harrell FE Jr et al. Prognostic value of the simplified Selvester QRS score in patients with coronary artery disease. J Am Coll Cardiol 1988;11:35–41.

12. Andersen A, Dobkin J, Maynard C et al. Heart rate variability parameters correlate with functional independence measures in ischemic stroke patients. J Electrocardiol 2001;34(Suppl):243–8.

13. Kornreich F, Montague TJ, Rautaharju PM et al. Identification of best electrocardiographic leads for diagnosing anterior and inferior myocardial infarction by statistical analysis of body surface potential maps. Am J Cardiol 1986;58:863–71.

14. Willems JL, Abreu-Lima C, Arnaud P et al. The diagnostic performance of computer programs for the interpretation of electrocardiograms. N Engl J Med 1991;325:1767–73.

15. Menotti A, Blackburn H. Electrocardiographic predictors of coronary heart disease in the Seven Countries Study. In: Kromhout D, Menotti A, Blackburn H (eds). Prevention of Coronary Heart Disease. Diet, lifestyle and risk factors in the Seven Countries Study. Norwell, Massachusetts: Kluver Academic Publishers, 2002, pp 199–211.

16. Menotti A, Blackburn H, Jacobs DR et al. The predictive value of resting electrocardiographic findings in cardiovascular disease-free men. Twenty-five-year follow-up in the Seven Countries Study. Internal document, Division of Epidemiology, School of Public Health, University of Minnesota, 2001.

17. Reunanen A, Aromaa A, Pyörälä K et al. The Social Insurance Institution's Coronary Heart Disease Study. Acta Med Scand 1983;Suppl 673: 1–120.

18. Menotti A, Seccaraccia F, and the RIFLE Research Group. Electrocardiographic Minnesota Code findings predicting short-term mortality in asymptomatic subjects. The Italian RIFLE Pooling Project (Risk Factors and Life Expectancy). G Ital Cardiol 1997;27:40–9.

19. Rose G, Baxter PJ, Reid DD, McCartney P. Prevalence and prognosis of electrocardiographic findings in middle-aged men. Br Heart J 1978;40: 636–43.

20. Cullen K, Stenhouse NS, Wearne KL, Cumpston GN. Electrocardiograms and 13 year cardiovascular mortality in Busselton study. Br Heart J 1982;47: 209–12.

21. Larsen CT, Dahlin J, Blackburn H et al. Prevalence and prognosis of electrocardiographic left ventricular hypertrophy, ST segment depression and negative T-wave. Eur Heart J 2002;23:315–24.

22. Sigurdsson E, Sigfusson N, Sigvaldason H, Thorgeirsson G. Silent ST-T changes in an epidemiologic cohort study – a marker of hypertension or coronary artery disease, or both: the Reykjavik study. J Am Coll Cardiol 1996;27:1140–7.

23. Kannel WB, Abbott R. A prognostic comparison of asymptomatic left ventricular hypertrophy and unrecognized myocardial infarction: the Framingham Study. Am Heart J 1986;111:391–7.

24. Kannel BW, Abbott R. Incidence and prognosis of unrecognized myocardial infarction. An update on the Framingham Study. N Engl J Med 1984;311: 1144–7.

25. Yano K, MacLean CJ. The incidence and prognosis of unrecognized myocardial infarction in the Honolulu, Hawaii, Heart Program. Arch Intern Med 1989;149:1526–32.

26. Tervahauta M, Pekkanen J, Punsar S, Nissinen A. Resting electrocardiographic abnormalities as predictors of coronary events and total mortality among elderly men. Am J Med 1996;100:641–5.

27. Nadelmann J, Frishman WH, Ooi WL et al. Prevalence, incidence and prognosis of recognized and unrecognized myocardial infarction in persons aged 75 years or older: the Bronx Aging Study. Am J Cardiol 1990;66:533–7.

28. Dauerman HL, Lessard D, Yarzebski J et al. Ten-year trends in the incidence, treatment, and outcome of Q-wave myocardial infarction. Am J Cardiol 2000;86:730–5.

29. Rosenman RH, Friedman M, Jenkins CD et al. Clinically unrecognized myocardial infarction in the Western Collaborative Group Study. Am J Cardiol 1967;19:776–82.

30. Chaitman BR, Rosen AD, Williams DO et al. Myocardial infarction and cardiac mortality in the Bypass Angioplasty Revascularization (BARI) Randomized Trial. Circulation 1997;96:2162–70.

31. Chaitman BR, Zhou SH, Tamesis B et al. Methodology of serial ECG classification using an adaptation of the NOVACODE for Q-wave myocardial infarction in the Bypass Angioplasty Revascularization Investigation (BARI). J Electrocardiol 1996;29: 265–77.

9B
Attributable Risk

In comparison with relative risk, the concept of attributable risk (AR) has only recently received some attention among electrocardiographic investigators, although it was introduced by Levin as early as 1953.[1] The publications of Miettinen in the 1970s have elaborated on the meaning of the concepts of relative risk and attributable risk (etiological fraction) in cohort and case control studies.[2-4]

Levin's attributable risk is best expressed using the notation of conditional probabilities. Key definitions are summarized in Table 9B.1. Incident disease is taken as the outcome measure of the study in the source population from which the "cases" arise, S the survival or disease-free condition at the conclusion of the observation period, P the positive test or the presence of the risk indicator for which we wish to evaluate the AR, and N the negative test or the absence of the risk indicator. Various fractions (f) defining the notation used in expressions for relative risk and AR are as follows:

$f(A)$ = fraction of source population with an abnormal or positive test or risk indicator prevalence fraction (fraction of source population exposed to the risk indicator)

$f(N) = 1 - f(A)$ = fraction of source population with a negative test (nonexposed)

$f(D)$ = case fraction in the source population

$f(S) = 1 - f(D)$ = survival fraction or incidence-free fraction of the source population

$f(D|A)$ = case fraction among those with risk indicator $= f(P|D) * f(D)/f(A)$

$f(D|N)$ = case fraction among those without risk indicator

$f(P|D)$ = indicator prevalence fraction among cases

Table 9B.2 gives the distribution as fractions of the source population into various elements of the contingency table. The fractions (f) can be multiples of those defined for various elements (percentages, etc.), or when expressed for the incidence, as the risk indicator of the outcome, the fraction of defined number of person-years of follow-up.

The "crude" relative risk (RR) is defined as:

$$RR = f(D|P)/f(D|N). \qquad [9B.1]$$

The denominator in the expression for the relative risk is the case fraction among those without the risk indicator as the reference category (called "the referent" by Miettinen).

The AR is excess relative risk that under certain assumptions can conceivably be associated with the risk indicator, with the risk among those without the risk indicator as the "referent". The meaning of the AR differs considerably, depending on exactly how it is defined. First, consider the following expression:

$$AR_1 = [f(D|P)/f(D|N) - 1]/[f(D|P)/f(D|N)]$$
$$= (RR - 1)/RR, \qquad [9B.2]$$

with $f(D|P)/f(D|N) = RR \geq 1$.

AR_1 is the excess relative risk among the higher risk category, those who have the risk indicator (i.e. the subgroup in which the prevalence of the indicator $f(P_1) = 1$). (Note: in clinical terminology $AR_1 = [(PTA/FP) - 1]/(PTA/FP)$, where PTA is positive test accuracy and FP is false positive).

179

TABLE 9B.1 Contingency table defining the notation in terms of conditional probabilities for outcome and risk indicator.

		Risk indicator or exposure	
		Present (P)	Absent Negaative Negative (N)
Outcome	Death or diseased (D)	No. = a	No. = c
		$f(D \mid P) = a / n_1$	Fraction $f(D \mid N) = c / n_2$
	Survival or nondiseased (S)	No. = b	No. = d
		$f(S \mid P) = b / n_1$	$f(S \mid N) = d / n_2$
	Column totals and fractions	No. = $n_1 = a + b$	No. = $n_2 = c + d$
		$f(P) = (a + b) / n_1 = 1$	$f(D \mid P) = 1$

Next, consider the following expression:

$$AR_2 = f(P|D) * (RR - 1)/RR. \qquad [9B.3]$$

It is noted that $f(P|D)$ is the proportion of cases with the risk indicator. Thus, AR_2 is the excess relative risk associated with the risk indicator among those who die or become diseased and who have the risk indicator. It is at times called attributable proportion or etiologic fraction,[5] and indicates, under certain assumptions, the fraction of mortality or morbidity that could be prevented if the risk indicator prevalence in the subgroup of future cases could be reduced to the level of the indicator prevalence in the noncases. AR_2 is of interest in evaluating disease etiology if it is plausible to expect a causal relationship between the risk indicator and the confounding factors are properly under control. Otherwise AR_2 is of little interest from the point of view of the importance of the risk indicator in the source population, from the point of view of prevention. We do not know in advance who is going to die, unless all of those with the risk indicator are going to become fatalities or diseased (i.e. $f(D|P) = 1$).

Next, we have the following expression:

$$AR_3 = f(P_3) * [f(D|P)/f(D|N) - 1]/\{1 + f(P_3) \\ * [(f(D|P)/f(D|N) - 1]\} \\ = f(P_3) * (RR - 1)/[1 + f(P_3) * (RR - 1)], \\ [9B.4]$$

where $f(P_3)$ is the prevalence of the risk indicator in the whole source population from which the cases arise. AR_3 is the excess risk in this source population, at times called population AR or community AR[6] (i.e. excess risk of event among those with risk indicator over overall risk of event in the source population. f(P3) should also be adjusted to the variable observation times with the risk indicator to the event where f(P3) = patient-years of observation with the risk indicator to the event over total patient-years of observation.

Most reports comparing relative merits of various ECG criteria, for instance for left ventricular hypertrophy or myocardial infarction, have used only the relative risk associated with each criterion. The problem is that a high relative risk can be obtained for the indicator in a small fraction of the population by sacrificing the sensitiv-

TABLE 9B.2 Fractions of the total source population in various elements of the contingency table in terms of conditional probabilities.

		Risk indicator or test		
		Present or positive (P)	Absent or negative (N)	Totals and fractions
Outcome	Death or diseased (D)	No. = n_1 $f(D \mid P) * f(P) = [(n_1 / (n_1 + n_2)] * p$	No. = n_3 $f(D \mid N) * f(N) = [(n_3 / (n_3 + n_4)] * n$	No. = $n_1 + n_3$ $f(D) = d = (n_1 + n_3 / (n_1 + n_2 + n_3 + n_4)$
	Survival or nondiseased (S)	No. = n_2 $f(S \mid P) * f(P) = [(n_2 / (n_1 + n_2)] * p$	No. = n_4 $f(S \mid N) * f(N) = [(n_4 / (n_3 + n_4)] * n$	No. = $n_2 + n_4$ $f(S) = s = (n_2 + n_4 / (n_1 + n_2 + n_3 + n_4)$
	Totals and fractions	No. = $n_1 + n_2$ $f(P) = p = (n_1 + n_2 / (n_1 + n_2 + n_3 + n_4)$	No. = $n_3 + n_4$ $f(N) = n = (c + d) / (a + b + c + d)$	No. = $n_1 + n_2 + n_3 + n_4$ $f = p + n + d + s = 1$

ity. In this sense the attributable risk AR_3 has merits by considering the prevalence of the indicator in the source population. However, it needs to be emphasized that AR should be used with caution. It should be reserved for special situations when there is reasonable evidence that the ECG variable is the causative factor, like certain arrhythmias may be for adverse events or when there is reasonable evidence that ECG abnormality is a strong marker of the disease or a marker of subclinical disease. Primary and secondary prevention ordinarily addresses the underlying disease (rather than "treating" an ECG abnormality), to prevent the disease or at least to slow down its evolution.

9B.1 Consideration of Confounding Factors

Cases and noncases in terms of the outcome may differ in characteristics other than the risk indicator, and these characteristics associated with the risk indicator may be significant confounding factors (age, gender, clinically overt or subclinical disease, etc.). In general, it is pretentious to attribute the excess risk to a risk indicator as an *etiologic* fraction of the risk as if confounding was well controlled, as emphasized by Miettinen,[2] who suggests that it would be more prudent to think in terms of etiologic fraction related to the indicator. It is generally prudent to use the term attributable factor rather than etiologic fraction unless there is genetic evidence or strong pathophysiological reason to expect a causal relationship and confounding is well under control.

Consider Equation 9B.1 for the crude relative risk:

$$RR = f(D|P)/f(D|N).$$

RR can be considered as the ratio of the morbidity or mortality fractions, which in this context we can label as M fractions. The numerator $f(D|P)$ is the fraction of all deaths or incident disease in the group with the risk indicator. The denominator is the fraction of all deaths or incident disease in the group free from the indicator. Now, assume that we wish to consider two confounding factors, each stratified at two levels into a total of four strata (i = 4). (Note that $\Sigma P_i = 1$ and $\Sigma_i N_i = 1$ as

shown in Table 9B.2.) The distribution of the "M fractions" across various strata may not be similar in the two groups that we compare, which could cause confounding to be controlled. In the group free from the risk indicator, each stratum i contributes fraction f_i to the total mortality fraction $f(D|N)$. An adjustment for unequal distribution of the mortality fractions in various strata is made by multiplying each f_i $(D|N)$ by the ratio $f(P_i)/f(N_i)$. Then the sum across all four strata i, $\Sigma f_i(D|N) * f(P_i/f(N_i))$, is the "M fraction", which could be expected in the group with the risk indicator due to uncontrolled confounding. The ratio of the observed mortality fraction in the group with risk indicator $f(D|P)$ to the expected mortality fraction obtained with the adjustment for the nonuniform distribution of the mortality fractions across all strata is the standardized mortality (morbidity) ratio (SMR). Thus,

$$SMR = f(D|P)/\Sigma\, f_i(D|N) * f(P_i/f(N_i)).$$

Standardized mortality ratio rather than the "crude" relative risk has to be used in expressions for the AR. Thus, Equation 9B.2 is modified to read:

$$AR_1 = (SMR - 1)/SMR, \qquad [9B.5]$$

(with SMR $\geq$ 1).

Equation 9B.3 becomes:

$$AR_2 = f(P|D) * (SMR - 1)/SMR. \qquad [9B.6]$$

Finally, for Equation 9B.4, Miettinen proposes the following modification:[2]

$$AR_3 = [f(P_3) * (RR - RR/SMR)/ \\ [1 + f(P_3) * (RR - 1)], \qquad [9B.7]$$

where $f(P_3)$ is, as before, the prevalence of the risk indicator in the whole source population from which the cases arise. In this expression, the second term in the numerator is the expected crude relative risk (RR/SMR). This modification is based on the argument that the crude relative risk in the reference group should not generally be taken as unity but instead as RR/SMR.

The risk indicator can be a polytomous multicategory parameter. For instance, when relative risk is evaluated for the quartiles of the risk using the quartile with the lowest risk as the reference category (with $RR_0 = 1$), the AR is calculated for each quartile. The overall AR for the risk indicator is then obtained by summation over all quartiles other than the reference quartile. The corresponding equation is:

$$AR = \sum_i f(P_i) * (PR_I - 1)/PR_I \qquad [9B.8]$$

where $RR_I > 1$ is the relative risk in quartiles other than the reference quartile.

References

1. Levin ML. The occurrence of lung cancer in man. Acta Un Intern Cancer 1953;9:531–41.

2. Miettinen OS. Proportion of disease caused or prevented by a given exposure, trait or intervention. Am J Epidemiol 1974;99:325–32.

3. Miettinen OS. Components of the crude risk ratio. Am J Epidemiol 1972;96:168–72.

4. Miettinen OS. Standardization of risk ratios. Am J Epidemiol 1972;96:383–8.

5. Ahlbom A, Norell S. Modern Epidemiology. Chestnut Hill, MA: Epidemiology Resources Inc., 1984, p 31.

6. Cole PT, MacMahon B. Attributable risk percent in case-control studies. Br Prev Soc Med 1971;25: 242–4.

10A
Primary Repolarization Abnormalities

Synopsis

Significance

Primary repolarization abnormalities may be associated with a variety of clinically overt conditions, or they may be subclinical markers of gradually evolving coronary heart disease (CHD) or left ventricular hypertrophy (LVH) in hypertensive heart disease, or they may be manifestations of a variety of other conditions and nonspecific factors.

Mechanisms

Primary repolarization abnormalities occur as a result of derailed ionic channel mechanisms or dynamic alterations in ionic channel functions, resulting in altered myocardial action potential waveforms and associated changes in the time course of spatial/temporal potential gradients. The characteristics of primary repolarization abnormalities depend to a large degree on the magnitude of the action potential waveform change in amplitude as well as in interval domains.

Classification Problems

Limited information is available on the prevalence of primary isolated repolarization abnormalities in the absence of clinical conditions and other ECG abnormalities that induce secondary ST-T changes. Comparative assessment of the risk data is complicated by differing criteria used, often combining ST and T wave abnormalities as a single category, variable follow-up time, and differences in risk analysis, in stratification of study populations, and in adjustment for clinical and demographic covariates and for other ECG abnormalities.

Prevalence of ST Depression

Minnesota Code 4.1–4.3 prevalence is approximately 4% in community-based adult male population cohorts aged 40–59 years. Some studies have reported no notable gender difference in the prevalence of ST-T abnormalities in their healthy subgroups. Health survey data from populations considered at high risk of CHD have reported an age-adjusted prevalence at age 30–60 years for ST depression codes (MC 4.1–4.3) of 2.2% in men and 4.3% in women, increasing to 6.3% in men and 9.7% in women at age 55–59 years.

Confounding Factors

These include altered ventricular conduction causing secondary ST-T wave abnormalities, intracranial lesions causing autonomic imbalance, meals and glucose ingestion, hyperventilation, tachycardia, hyperkalemia, many drugs (digitalis, etc.), and "juvenile" T wave patterns in young adults.

Mortality Risk

An up to eightfold short-term risk of CHD death has been reported in men for ST-T codes without Q waves. Reported long-term risk for CHD death in men for ST-T codes varies from nonsignificant to a twofold excess risk. Abnormal T wave codes (MC 5.1–5.3) combined with abnormal ST (Minnesota Codes 4.1–4.3) have been found to be associated with an over fivefold excess risk for cardiovascular disease mortality and no significant risk for isolated T wave abnormalities. Mortality risk for ST-T items in the few studies that are available for gender comparisons has been found in general nonsignificant in women, or sample size and adverse events have been too few for evaluation. Abnormal T axis and QRS/T angle has been associated with adverse cardiovascular events, otherwise the question of independent risk for isolated T wave abnormalities still remains largely unanswered. There is no question, however, that primary ST abnormalities as a category carry independent information about the risk of future adverse cardiac events both in men and in women.

Abbreviations and Acronyms

AV – atrioventricular
BIRNH – Belgian Interuniversity Research on Nutrition and Health
CHD – coronary heart disease
CHF – congestive heart failure
CHS – Cardiovascular Health Study
CVD – cardiovascular disease
ECG-LVM – ECG estimate of left ventricular mass
LBBB – left bundle branch block
LVH – left ventricular hypertrophy
MI – myocardial infarction
MRFIT – Multiple Risk Factor Intervention Trial
RBBB – right bundle branch block
WHI – Women's Health Initiative

10A.1 Introduction

Repolarization abnormalities with normal ventricular conduction sequence are denoted primary repolarization abnormalities.

Repolarization abnormalities are commonly described using a limited number of univariate descriptors separately for each ECG lead, sum-marized as ST depression, ST elevation, and negative T wave amplitude. Classic vectorcardiac parameters (orientation and magnitude of the ST-T vectors) have received little attention from the present generation of ECG investigators.

This chapter covers primary repolarization abnormalities. Although of critical clinical importance, ischemic repolarization abnormalities associated with acute myocardial infarction were intentionally excluded from this book, occlusion sites relating to ST deviations in acute MI were considered in Chapter 9 (Table 9A.1). The main focus in this chapter is on ST abnormalities. ST abnormalities occur frequently in combination with T wave abnormalities, although the latter can occur as an isolated primary repolarization abnormality, with manifestations such as an abnormal T axis and an abnormal spatial angle between QRS and T. Interval domain repolarization abnormalities including QT prolongation will be covered in Chapter 11.

10A.1.1 The Mechanism of Primary Repolarization Abnormalities

Primary ST-T abnormalities are ultimately related to changes in myocardial action potential waveforms and durations and the associated alterations in spatial/temporal potential gradients. The characteristics of the associated repolarization abnormalities depend on the degree of the action potential waveform change in amplitude as well as in interval domain with respect to the onset of excitation and the end of repolarization in the region with derailed ionic mechanisms.

Action potential duration changes in acute ischemia incorporated in the ischemic region in a computer model by Miller and Geselowitz in 1978 generated ST-T evolutionary patterns in body surface ECGs.[1] Among more realistic computer models is that of van Oosterom.[2] It incorporates as the cardiac electric generator an equivalent double layer at the boundary of the region with derailed ionic mechanisms and an elegant solution to the forward problem. The model generates epicardial potentials and repolarization patterns in body surface ECGs. This makes it possible to study epicardial potential distributions and body surface ECGs in simulated ischemia in various myocardial regions. The timing of the local depolarization and repolarization in the boundary region of ischemia and the size of the boundary determine the characteristics of the repolarization abnormalities in the body surface ECG.

ST depression as a primary repolarization abnormality is generally taken to indicate residual myocardial ischemia. One possible model for such chronic ischemic ST depression requires the presence of a residual ischemic zone residing in between an infarcted subendocardial layer and healthy cells in the overlaying subepicardial layers (Figure 10A.1). During phase 2 of the action potentials, the membrane potential of the healthy cells transit to zero or slightly positive potential (inside vs outside), and the ischemic cells remain slightly depolarized at a negative level. This generates injury current flow across the ischemic boundary shown by the open block arrow in Figure 10A.1, resulting in ST segment depression in an ECG lead with a lead vector (L) or ECG lead axis in the opposite direction.

In addition to the old nontransmural myocardial infarction (MI) in subendocardial segments with a residual ischemic zone, there are other clinical conditions that can induce ST depression. These include tachycardia, hypokalemia and digitalis. Tachycardia induces J-point depression, in subjects without coronary heart disease (CHD)

generally with an upsloping ST. Early ECG abnormalities in hyperkalemia include ST depression sloping upwards to a peaked T wave with shortened QT. Patients on digitalis often have ST depression in multiple leads, commonly less than $100\,\mu V$, at times more severe in digitalis intoxication, and T amplitude is reduced or negative. Left ventricular hypertrophy produces ST depression with reduced-amplitude T waves in left lateral leads. In more pronounced hypertrophy, there may be an ST strain pattern (downsloping ST and negative T).

In addition to ST depression, primary repolarization abnormalities include ST elevation in the absence of acute myocardial ischemia, the socalled idiopathic early repolarization. It has at times been labeled as a syndrome, although it is really an asymptomatic condition and a normal variant. ST J point is usually elevated in V1 or V2 when there is an RR' pattern with late excitation in the pulmonary cone region. A more serious condition is hypothermia, which may induce atrial fibrillation, QT prolongation, and widening of the QRS, and early ST segment J-point elevation with a hump-like Osborn wave. The mechanism of this J wave has been associated with transient outward potassium current, which is more prominent in epicardial than in endocardial layers.[3] This is one example of the importance of investigating aberrant ionic channel functions as an explanation of primary repolarization abnormalities. The Osborn wave is present also in Brugada syndrome, which has recently received wide attention. This abnormality will not be included here because, overall, it is a rare condition.

10A.2 Prevalence of ST-T Abnormalities and their Association with Adverse Cardiac Events

The prevalence of ST depression $\geq 100\,\mu V$ or T wave inversion $\geq 200\,\mu V$ is very low in community-based populations. Therefore, the focus of the reports in epidemiological literature has been on relatively minor repolarization abnormalities. The first reports on the significance of minor repolarization abnormalities came in the 1960s

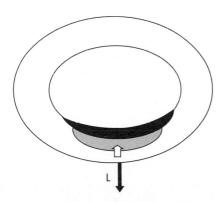

FIGURE 10A.1 Schematic of a possible mechanism for ST depression in old myocardial infarction with chronic ischemia. The residual ischemic layer (*dotted area*) is in between the subendocardial dead infarcted tissue (*black*) and the healthy myocardial zone (*white segments*). Injury current (*block arrow*) during phase 2 of the action potentials flows from the healthy to the ischemic zone across the ischemic boundary, creating ST depression in chest leads with lead vector L in the opposite direction.

from the reports of medical and actuarial departments of large insurance companies,[4] summarized by Blackburn and Parlin.[5]

Electrocardiographic recording and coding procedures were not well standardized in the early studies, generally involving health screening programs, screening of health insurance applicants, or screening for air crew personnel applicants.[6–9] Common to these reports is the finding that even minor ST-T abnormalities were associated with increased mortality risk and the risk of adverse cardiac events. The prevalence of ST-T abnormalities in such relatively young populations and in essentially healthy community-based samples of younger adults is generally low. For instance, the prevalence of isolated "silent" T wave abnormalities in the Tecumseh, Michigan population was 1%.[7] Still, these "silent" T wave abnormalities have been considered in epidemiological literature as markers of subclinical hypertensive or coronary heart disease.

In the Manitoba longitudinal follow-up study of 3,983 Canadian post Second World War pilots,[9] ST-T abnormalities were coded according to the Minnesota Code. Age-specific sudden death rates were calculated per person-years of exposure from the onset of ST-T abnormality at regular periodic examination. The prevalence of ST depression (Minnesota Code 4.1–4.3) was very high among the men who later died of sudden death (31.4%), and the relative risk was 4.8 (men with no ST-T code as the reference group).

Early epidemiological studies excluded women from their cohorts because it was thought that the risk of CHD morbidity and mortality was too low in women for an adequate power for risk analysis. It was also thought that recording ECGs of women in a field operation would pose more difficult logistic problems. Many of the cohorts were selected by excluding persons with clinically overt CHD, or at least evaluating the risk separately for nonsymptomatic and symptomatic subgroups. The exclusion and selection criteria varied considerably from study to study so that the inter-study comparability is limited.

Most epidemiological reports have used ST-T classification criteria of the Minnesota Code since its publication in 1960.[10] ST and T wave abnormalities have been commonly grouped together for risk analysis (Minnesota Codes 4.1–4.3 or 4.4,

5.1–5.3 or 5.4, or some combination of both). Very few studies have evaluated isolated T wave abnormalities separately from the ST codes.

10A.2.1 Age-dependence of the Prevalence of ST and T Wave Abnormalities and their Association with Mortality Risk

10A.2.1.1 Finland's Social Insurance Institution's Coronary Heart Disease Study

The total population sample of the CHD survey of Finland's Social Insurance Institution comprised 5,738 men and 5,224 women aged 30–59 years.[11] As in other similar populations, there was a progressive increase with age both in men and in women in the prevalence of ST abnormalities (Figure 10A.2) as well as for T wave abnormalities (Figure 10A.3).

The study reported the risk for the combined category of "other ischemic ECG" in their hierarchic coding scheme (Minnesota Code 1.1, 1.2 Q waves, code 5.1–5.2 ST-T abnormalities, major atrioventricular and ventricular conduction defects, and atrial fibrillation). The risk was quite high in men 40–59 years old: the relative risk was 7.2 for CHD mortality and 6.4 for cardiovascular disease (CVD) mortality. It was also increased in women for CVD mortality: relative risk was 3.0.

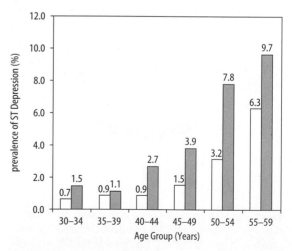

FIGURE 10A.2 Increasing trend by age in the prevalence of ST depression (Minnesota Code 4.1–4.3) in men (open bars) and women (shaded bars). Note the higher prevalence of ST depression in women than in men. (Source: Reunanen et al.[11] Acta Med Scand 1983;673(Suppl):1–120.)

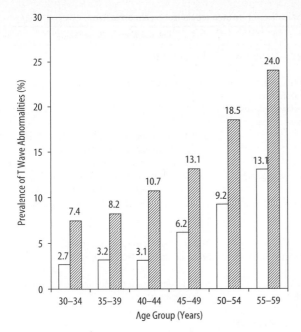

FIGURE 10A.3 Increasing trend by age in the prevalence of T wave abnormalities (Minnesota Code 5.1–5.3) in men (*open bars*) and women (*shaded bars*). Like ST depression, the prevalence of T wave abnormalities is substantially higher in women than in men. (Source: Reunanen et al.[11] Acta Med Scand 1983;673(Suppl): 1–120.)

The report also listed age-standardized mortality risk ratios for "other ischemic ECG" category in the absence of history of chest pain symptoms typical of MI. The age-standardized risk of CHD and CVD mortality was significantly increased in men, with risk ratios 4.4 and 3.9, respectively. The number of women in this category was too small for cause-specific mortality risk estimation.

10A.2.2 ST-T Abnormalities and Mortality Risk in Ostensibly Healthy Male Populations

First, results with mortality data from male cohorts will be considered here. The first set of data in Table 10A.1 comes from the Seven Countries Study[12,13] and the second set from the Chicago Western Electric Study.[14] The first set in Table 10A.2 comes from the Whitehall study[15] and the second set from the Reykjavik study cohort.[16] In these studies, men with a history of CHD were excluded. In addition, the Chicago Western Elec-

tric Study used ECG findings for exclusions (MI, left ventricular hypertrophy [LVH], major ST-T codes) so that this study report deals with minor ST-T abnormalities only. Men with major Q waves (Minnesota Code 1.1 and 1.2) were excluded in the Reykjavik study.

10A.2.2.1 The Seven Countries Study

In the Seven Countries Study, the overall prevalence of any ST-T codes (with or without other ECG abnormalities) was 4.4%. It was 5.7% in the pooled Northern European and US cohorts, 3.4% in Southern European cohorts and 3.5% in Japanese men. Among CVD-free men, the prevalence of ST-T abnormalities (Minnesota Code 4.1–4.4, 5.1–5.3) without Q waves (Minnesota Code 1.1–1.3) was 3.5%. The prevalence among those who died within the first 5 years of follow-up was 13.1%. The prevalence of ST-T findings in the four cohorts of ostensibly healthy middle-aged men cited above varied considerably.

The Seven Countries Study investigators evaluated risk data from the short-term (initial 5 years after baseline) and long-term follow-up (subsequent 6–25 years).[13] Excluded from the study group were men with a history of any heart disease, peripheral arterial or cerebrovascular disease. Electrocardiographic findings were not used as exclusion criteria. The endpoint evaluated for ST-T abnormalities was CHD death. The short-term risk of CHD death for any ST-T codes without Q waves was substantially increased, with hazard ratio 8.29 (2.94, 23.10). The long-term risk was considerably lower and not statistically significant, with hazard ratio 1.39 (0.69, 2.80).

The Seven Countries Study also evaluated the risk for ST and T codes categorized at an individual level of severity regardless of possible presence of other ECG abnormalities (it is not clear whether both codes were entered simultaneously for multivariable adjustment). Hazard ratios for ST depression indicated a significant, fourfold excess short-term risk for ST depression $50\,\mu V$ or more (Minnesota Code 4.2 and 4.1). The long-term risk of CHD death was not significant for any of the ST codes. The highest short-term as well as long-term risk of CHD death was associated with Minnesota Code 5.1, inverted T

TABLE 10A.1 Two prospective studies on male cohorts with risk evaluation for isolated repolarization abnormalities.

	Seven Countries Study[12,13]		Chicago Western Electric Study[14]
Geographic location	Finland, Greece, Italy, the Netherlands, former Yugoslavia, Japan, USA; a total of 16 cohorts		Chicago, IL, USA
Source population	12,763 men (11 cohorts from rural areas of Finland, Greece, Japan and Yugoslavia; three other more diverse cohorts from Yugoslavia; the town of Zutphen, the Netherlands; and cohorts of railroad employees from the USA and Italy)		2,107 male electric company employees
Baseline	1958–1964		Pooled cross-sectional data from baseline (at 1957) and first four annual examinations; multiple observations from each person
Selection/exclusions	Sampling goal: total male population from selected geographic areas. Participation rate ≥60%. Excluded: 854 with prevalent CHD at baseline; no ECG exclusions		Excluded: history of CHD at entry or incident CHD at first four biennial examinations; MI by ECG, LVH (MC 3.1 and 4.1–4.3, 5.1–5.3), MC 4.1, 4.2, 5.1, 5.2
CHD-free sample	11,860		1,673
Age range	40–59 years		40–55 years
Follow-up	Initial 5 years and subsequent 6–25 years		29 years after first five annual examinations
ECG findings evaluated for risk	Graded levels of ST and T findings (4.1–4.4 and 5.1–5.3)		Isolated minor ST-T: MC 4.3, 4.4, 5.3, 5.4
Baseline prevalence	MC 4.1 0.3% MC 4.2 0.8% MC 4.3 0.3% Any ST-T codes: 4.2% in Northern European and US cohorts, 3.8% in Southern Europe and 3.5% in Japan	MC 5.1 0.06% MC 5.2 0.9% MC 5.3 2.3%	10.3% (occurring once or more times in five annual examinations)
Associated risk in CVD-free group	Short-term (0–5 years) risk for CHD death Code 4.1: HR 4.0 (1.21, 13.12) Code 4.2: HR 4.0 (1.57, 9.88) (No CHD deaths in the group with MC 4.3) Code 5.1: HR (too few events) Code 5.2: HR 7.6 (3.66, 15.75) Code 5.3: HR 2.2 (1.02, 4.84)	Long-term (6– 25 years) risk for CHD death Code 4.1: HR 1.7 (0.90, 3.18) Code 4.2: HR 1.2 (0.79, 1.93) Code 4.3 HR 1.6 (0.82, 3.09) Code 5.1: HR (too few events) Code 5.2: HR 1.6 (1.05, 2.39) Code 5.3: HR 1.4 (1.05, 1.79)	CHD mortality: HR 1.67 (1.25, 2.25) CVD mortality: HR 1.38 (1.05, 1.80) All-cause mortality: HR 1.28 (1.04, 1.58)
Multivariate adjustment	Age, no. of cigarettes currently smoked, serum cholesterol, SBP and cohort as indicator variable		Age at year 5, education level, family history of CVD, SBP, cigarette smoking, serum cholesterol, BMI, BMI-squared (not for medications, electrolytes)
Comments	For any ST code in the absence of Q waves: for short-term risk HR 2.9 (1.56, 5.22) and HR 1..4 (1.10, 1.72) for long-term risk		Risk higher for men with minor ST-T abnormalities in >1 examination or in >1 lead group and for codes 4.3, 5.3

CHD coronary heart disease, *CVD* cardiovascular disease, *BMI* body mass index, *HR* hazards ratio, *LVH* left ventricular hypertrophy, *MC* Minnesota Code, *SBP* systolic blood pressure.

waves ≥500 µV in amplitude, with a hazard ratio approximately 17. However, only seven of the 11,860 men had such deep negative T waves.

The prevalence was increased for Minnesota Codes 5.2 and 5.3, ≥100 µV negative or flat T waves, respectively. The associated hazard ratio for 100 µV negative T wave was 7.6 for short-term risk and 1.6 for long-term risk (both significantly increased). The long-term risk of CHD death was significantly increased for flat T waves, with a hazard ratio 1.4 (1.03, 1.77). There was also an over twofold but nonsignificant excess risk for short-term death for flat T waves, with a hazard ratio 2.2 (1.02, 4.84). As mentioned above, these ST and T findings were not necessarily isolated.

TABLE 10A.2 Two additional prospective studies on male populations.

	Whitehall[15]	Reykjavik[16]
Geographic location	London, UK	Male residents of Reykjavik area, Iceland
Source population	18,403 male civil servants	WHI MONICA Center
		9,139 participants
Baseline	Early 1970s	Five stages between 1967 and 1987
Exclusions	Evaluated separately, nonsymptomatic (no history of angina or MI and not under medical care for heart disease or hypertension) and symptomatic subgroups	History of MI or angina pectoris MC 1.1–1.2
CHD-free sample	15,974	8,340
Age range	40–60 years	33–80 years
Follow-up	5-year mortality follow-up	4–24 years (in five stages, 2–5 years between visits)
ECG findings evaluated for risk	Negative T (MC 5.2) and flat T (MC 5.3)	Silent ischemic ST-T: MC 4.1–4.4 or 5.1–5.4 In CHD-free group
Baseline prevalence	0.5% for MC 5.2, 2.8% for MC 5.3 in nonsymptomatic subgroup As isolated ECG finding: 0.1% for 5.2, 2.5% for 5.3	2%, 4%, 9%, 17% and 30% at ages 40, 50, 60, 70 and 80 years, respectively
Associated risk in CHD-free group	CHD mortality: HR 2.7 for isolated MC 5.2 and HR 2.5 for isolated MC 5.3	CHD mortality: HR 2.0 (1.6, 2.6)
Multivariate adjustment	Age, height, weight, BMI, SBP, DBP, hypertension, use of antihypertensive medication, diuretics, digoxin, total cholesterol, triglycerides, fasting and 90- min blood glucose, hematocrit, uric acid, sedimentation rate, smoking, LVH by ECG	Demographic factors and clinical risk factors for CHD.

BMI body mass index, *DBP* diastolic blood pressure, *CHD* coronary heart disease, *HR* hazards ratio, *LVH* left ventricular hypertrophy, *MC* Minnesota Code, *MI* myocardial infarction, *SBP* systolic blood pressure, *WHI* World Health Organization.

10A.2.2.2 The Chicago Study

The prevalence of isolated minor repolarization abnormalities was high, 10.3%, in the Chicago Western Electric Study of 2,107 men aged 40–55 years.[14] This was at least in part because multiple pooled observations from five successive annual examinations were included in the prevalence count. The study also included J-point depression 100 µV or more with upsloping ST (Minnesota Code 4.4) and low-amplitude T wave findings (Minnesota Code 5.4) among minor ST-T abnormalities.

There was a 67% excess long-term risk of CHD death associated with isolated minor ST-T findings in the Chicago study, with multivariable-adjusted hazard ratio 1.67 (1.25, 2.25).

10A.2.2.3 The Whitehall Study

This study described in Table 10A.2 evaluated the prevalence and the risk of 5-year CHD mortality in 15,974 civil servants who were 40–60 years old.[15] The prevalence of negative T waves (Minnesota Code 5.2) was 2.8% and of Minnesota Code 5.3 "flat" T waves 2.8%. As an isolated finding, the prevalence of these T wave abnormalities was low, 5.2% for code 5.2 and 2.5% for code 5.3. The reported multivariable-adjusted hazard ratio for CHD mortality risk was 2.7 for isolated Minnesota Code 5.2, and 2.5 for isolated Minnesota Code 5.3.

10A.2.2.4 The Reykjavik Study

The 9,139 Reykjavik study men came from the WHI MONICA Center.[16] The age range of the men in this study was wider, from 33 to 80 years. Like the Chicago Western Electric Study, the Reykjavik Study also included J-point depression 100 µV or more with upsloping ST (Minnesota Code 4.4) and low-amplitude T wave (Minnesota Code 5.4) among minor ST-T abnormalities evaluated. In the 4- to 24-year follow-up, the excess risk of CHD death for any abnormal ST-T codes was twofold, with multivariable-adjusted hazard ratio 2.0 (1.6, 2.6).

10A.2.3 Prevalence of ST-T Abnormalities and Mortality Risk in CHD-free Men and Women

Baseline prevalence data from three studies in CHD-free male and female subgroups are included here for comparison (Table 10A.3). The first study,

TABLE 10A.3 Three cohorts of men and women with CHD-free subgroups with prospective risk evaluation for primary repolarization abnormalities.

	Belgian Interuniversity Research on Nutrition and Health (BIRNH)[17]	Framingham Study[18]	Amsterdam Health Survey[19]
Geographic location	Random sample from 42 of the 43 Belgian districts	Framingham, Massachusetts, USA	Amsterdam, the Netherlands
Source population	30,000 eligible, 36.5% respondents	Town's representative adult population, 2,336 men, 2,873 women	11,700 civil servants of the city and their spouses; 54% volunteered
Baseline	1981–1984	Pooled cross-sectional, multiple observations from each person	1953–1954
Exclusions	History of MI or angina pectoris MC 1.1–1.2	Overt CHD in medical examination	Case-cohort sampling design (cases compared with random sample from the cohort)
CHD-free sample	4,797 men, 4,320 women	5,127 men and women	Apparently healthy sample of 1,583 men, 1,568 women
Age range	25–74 years	35–69 years (first four biennials)	40–65 years
Follow-up	10 years	30 years	28 years (risk report for 15-year follow-up)
ECG findings evaluated for risk in CHD-free sample	Major ischemic: MC 4.1, 4.2, 5.1 or 5.2 or MC 7.1 (LBBB) Minor ischemic: MC 4.3, 5.3, and/or MC 1.3 (minor Q waves)	Flat or inverted T or ST segment depression >100 μV. Highest graded ST-T abnormality from first four biennials used for long-term risk evaluation	ST depression $\geq$25 μV, ST elevation $\geq$25 μV in lead I at J + 80 ms
Baseline prevalence	Major ischemic, 1.9% in men, 1.8% in women (age-standardized) Minor: 6.5% in men, 8.8% in women	Prevalence (first four biennial examinations): Men 14.1% Women 13.1%	ST depression: 3.3% in men 8.9% in women ST elevation: 20.8% in men 13.0% in women
Associated risk in CHD-free group	CVD mortality Minor ischemic:* HR 1.26 (0.82, 1.93) for men HR 1.46 (0.85, 2.52) for women Major ischemic:[†] HR 4.21 (2.60, 6.82) for men HR 4.72 (2.49, 8.96) for women	Long-term risk for incident CHD during 22-year follow-up after examination 4: HR 1.4 (chi square 10.0; $p < 0.002$), men and women combined	ST depression, CHD mortality: HR 2.2 (1.2, 3.9) for men HR 1.9 (0.6, 6.3) for women All-cause mortality: HR 1.2 (0.8, 1.8) for men HR 1.7 (1.2, 2.5) for women ST elevation $\geq$25 μV, CHD mortality: HR 0.4 (0.2, 0.8) for men HR 0.4 (0.0, 4.0) for women
Multivariate adjustment	*Age, BMI, SBP, use of antihypertensive drugs, total cholesterol, smoking, uric acid, diabetes, LVH by ECG, major ST-T [†]Additional adjustment for minor ST-T	Age, sex, SBP, total serum cholesterol, glucose tolerance, cigarettes per day, event rates age-adjusted, standardized to whole cohort	Age, BMI, total serum cholesterol, diastolic blood pressure, smoking
Comments	Excluding LBBB and minor Q waves, HR 5.11 (3.40, 7.69) for combined ST-T abnormalities, not significant for isolated T pooling men and women		If ST80 $\geq$25 μV (normal pattern) had been taken as the reference group, HR for CHD mortality would be 5.5 for men and 4.8 for women

CHD coronary heart disease, *CVD* cardiovascular disease, *HR* hazard ratio, *LBBB* left bundle branch block, *LVH* left ventricular hypertrophy, *MI* myocardial infarction, *MC* Minnesota Code, *SBP* systolic blood pressure.

the Belgian Interuniversity Research on Nutrition and Health (BIRNH) had 4,797 men and 4,323 women aged 25–74 years.[17] The second cohort was from the Framingham population.[18] It included 5,127 CHD-free men and women aged 35–69 years. The third study, the Amsterdam Health Survey, had an apparently healthy sample of 1,209 men and 848 women 40–60 years old.[19] These three studies used rather diverse criteria for defining ST-T abnormalities as well as for sampling periods, so that the interstudy comparability is not straightforward. However, the data are valid for comparing gender differences within each study. In two of the reports, from the BIRNH and the Framingham study, there was no notable gender difference in the prevalence of ischemic abnormalities.

10A.2.3.1 The BIRNH Study

The prevalence of the major ischemic category was 1.9% in the BIRNH study men and 1.8% in the women. Major Q waves were excluded as were men and women with a history of MI or angina pectoris. The major ischemic category consisted largely of Minnesota Codes 4.1, 4.2, 5.1, and 5.2. The prevalence of the minor ischemic category consisting nearly entirely of minor T wave codes (Minnesota Code 5.3) was 6.5% in men and 8.8% in women.

The follow-up period was 10 years. Main risk evaluation was done for major ischemic findings, which included left bundle branch block (LBBB) in addition to major ST-T codes, and minor ischemic findings, which included minor Q waves in addition to minor ST-T codes. However, there were very few men and women with minor Q waves combined with ST-T codes (four men and 12 women, respectively) so that minor ischemic category consisted nearly entirely of codes 4.3 and 5.3. There were also relatively few subjects with LBBB (28 men and 15 women) in this quite large study group.

The risk of CVD mortality was over fourfold for major ischemic codes in men as well as in women. It was not significant for minor ischemic codes. The results differed when LBBB and minor Q waves were excluded. Interaction testing failed to detect a significant sex difference, and pooling men and women, excess risk for CVD mortality was over fivefold for T wave abnormalities if they occurred in combination with ST abnormalities. The risk was not significant for isolated T wave abnormalities occurring without ST depression.

10A.2.3.2 The Framingham Study

In the 1987 report from the Framingham study, the prevalence of ST-T abnormalities (largely flat or negative T waves) during the first four biennial examinations when the participants were 35–69 years old was 14.1% in men and 13.1% in women, with an approximately equal fraction of possible

and definite categories.[18] The incidence of ST-T abnormalities during the subsequent biennial examinations was 2.9% in men as well as in women.

Electrocardiographic criteria for ST and T wave abnormalities and the sampling procedure for prevalence estimation used in the Framingham study differed from those in other studies. Before the eighth biennial examination, ST-T abnormalities were categorized as "nonspecific" in the absence of LVH, MI or ventricular conduction defects. ST segment depression exceeding $100\,\mu V$ and T wave flattening or inversion (not defined in more detail) were coded as abnormal. Beginning at the eighth biennial examination, these nonspecific ST-T abnormalities were stratified as abnormal ST, abnormal T, or the combination of both, and T wave abnormalities were further categorized as definite or possible. The investigators comment that the variability of the prevalence data from biennial to biennial was either due to observer variation or the transient nature of the abnormality.

The prevalence of isolated T wave abnormalities over biennial examinations 8–12 (when the participants were 44–74 years old) was 7.3% in men and 5.4% in women. The corresponding prevalence of ST abnormalities with or without abnormal T waves was 6.9% in men and 7.7% in women. The prevalence of total ST and T abnormalities over examinations 8–12 was thus 14.1% in men and 13.1% in women. Each subject contributed multiple observations in counting the prevalence over several examinations, which apparently accounted for the reported relatively high prevalence of ST-T abnormalities.

The long-term risk was evaluated for the highest graded ST and T abnormality during the first four biennials. The risk in the model that adjusted for age, gender, smoking, systolic blood pressure, total serum cholesterol and glucose intolerance was significantly increased in the combined male–female group, with hazard ratio 1.4 (chi square 10.0; $p < 0.002$).

10A.2.3.3 The Amsterdam Health Survey

In the Amsterdam Health Survey, ST depression prevalence was substantially higher in women than in men, 8.9% versus 3.3%, respectively, and

ST elevation prevalence substantially higher in men than in women, 20.8% versus 13.0%, respectively.[19] In this study, ST depression and elevation were measured in lead I (for ST elevation at J + 80 ms), with 25 µV as the threshold for abnormal. In the Amsterdam Health Survey, ST depression 25 µV or more was associated with a risk for CHD mortality in men with a hazard ratio 2.2 (1.2, 3.9). The risk in women was also increased, with a nonsignificant hazard ratio 1.9 (0.6. 6.3). For all-cause mortality, the risk was significantly increased in women only. Subjects with ST amplitude between 25 and –25 µV were used as the reference group. The risk of CHD mortality for mild ST elevation (25 µV at J + 80 ms, mostly a normal ST pattern) was reduced by 60% in men and in women (significant in men only).

10A.2.4 Mortality Risk for Diverse Q Wave and ST-T Abnormalities in Two Older Cohorts

The event rates will increase with the age of the study population. Mortality risk predictors in older cohorts can also be expected to differ from those in younger populations. Mortality risk data from two older cohorts, one of them 85 years old and older, are summarized in Table 10A.4.

10A.2.4.1 An Older Finnish Cohort from the Seven Countries Study

A report with a clear hierarchic separation of ST and T wave abnormalities and various other ECG coding categories for risk analysis in older men comes from the Finnish cohort of the Seven Countries Study subsequent to the 25-year examination.[20] The surviving men in the East-West Finland Study cohort were 65–84 years old at the time of the 25-year examination. The 5-year follow-up report of 697 survivors first considered the risk for various ECG coding categories separately for each abnormality and then according to a hierarchic scheme. This hierarchic scheme included ST-T codes with Q waves (Minnesota Code 1.1–1.3 with Minnesota Code 4.1–4.3), ST depression (without T wave codes) and isolated T wave codes (Minnesota Code 5.1–5.3). The risk

TABLE 10A.4 Two older cohorts with risk evaluation for diverse Q wave and ST-T categories.

	East-West Finland, older men[20]	Tampere Health Survey[21]
Geographic location	Older men from Finnish cohort of Seven Countries Study	City of Tampere, Finland
Source population/respondents	697 survivors at 25-year follow-up	674 residents of the city who were 85 years old or older in 1977, 12-lead ECG in 559 (83%)
Baseline for prevalence estimation	1984	1977–1978
Gender	Men	99 men, 460 women
Age range at baseline	60–79 years	85 years and older
Follow-up	5 years	5 years
ECG findings evaluated for risk	Hierarchic categories: (1) Q codes with ST-T; (2) isolated Q; (3) isolated ST; (4) isolated T	Ischemic category: MC 1.1, 1.2, 4.1, 5.1, 6.1, 6.2, 7.1, 7.2, 8.3 Major abnormalities: MC 1.1–1.3, 3.1, 4.1–4.4, 5.1–5.3, 6.3, 7.1, 7.2, 7.7, 8.1, 8.3
Baseline prevalence for categories of interest	For categories above: (1) 5.2%; (2) 8.9%; (3) 13.2%; (4)12.2%	Major abnormalities: 89.5% Ischemic category: 45.3%
Associated risk	Significantly increased for total mortality and fatal MI for Q waves with ST codes (category 1) and for ST codes without Q codes (category 3), not significant for isolated T	Significantly increased ($p > 0.001$) mortality rate (78%) in the group with ischemic abnormalities compared with those without (63%)
Multivariate adjustment	Age- and area-adjusted	Survival rates corrected for heterogeneity of the study group using Finland's population aged 85 years and over during the follow-up period as a normal population
Comments		Lowest 5-year survival rates in MC 8.3 (atrial fibrillation) and 6.3 (first-degree atrioventricular block)

MC Minnesota Code, *MI* myocardial infarction.

was evaluated separately for each category using logistic regression models that also adjusted for major CHD risk factors.

Considering first each coding category separately, major ST and T wave codes as well as high QRS amplitude codes 3.1, 3.3 were associated with an increased risk of total mortality, fatal and nonfatal MI, and the risk was independent from the history of previous CHD. More importantly, in the hierarchic scheme, the risk for ST depression with or without Q waves was the only abnormality with a significant independent excess risk of fatal or any MI and of total mortality. Isolated ST abnormalities as well as ST abnormalities combined with Q waves were associated with an approximately fourfold excess risk of total mortality. For fatal MI, excess risk for ST combined with Q waves was twice as high, approximately eightfold.

10A.2.4.2 The Tampere Health Survey

The Tampere Health Survey report data in Table 10A.4 included 559 residents of the city who were 85 years old and older.[21] In this group of 559 survivors, 460 (82%) were women. The ischemic category (prevalence 45%) considered for the 5-year follow-up risk evaluation included all major Q and ST-T codes, advanced atrioventricular (AV) blocks, LBBB, right bundle branch block (RBBB), and atrial fibrillation. The 78% 5-year mortality rate was significantly higher than in the group without ischemic abnormalities (63%, $p < 0.001$). It was noted that the lowest 5-year survival rate in this very old cohort was for atrial fibrillation and first-degree AV block.

10A.2.5 T Axis Deviation as a Predictor of Mortality

The investigators of the Rotterdam Heart Study reported in the *Lancet* in 1998 that a simple indicator of T wave abnormality, the T axis, was a stronger predictor of fatal and nonfatal cardiac events than any other ECG abnormality or established cardiovascular risk indicator.[22] T axis deviation qualifies to be categorized as one of the "nonspecific" repolarization abnormalities that are in general clinically considered to be nonsignificant or at most of borderline significance. A letter to

the editor of the *Lancet* perhaps reflects a typical response from clinical cardiologists to the claim of T axis deviation being the strongest predictor of adverse cardiovascular events: "What is the poor clinician to do with this information?"[23]

The intriguing results of the Rotterdam study prompted the research group of the Cardiovascular Health Study (CHS) to undertake an evaluation of the T axis in relation to the mortality and morbidity risk in the CHD-free subgroup of the CHS population.[24] These two studies are evaluated here in some detail because of the implied importance of the T wave axis. The secondary focus will be in the interpretation of a possible mechanism of the adverse outcome among those with abnormal T axis deviation as the primary repolarization abnormality.

Both studies used T axis deviation from the normal T axis direction as the primary independent variable. The Rotterdam study used T axis deviation in the frontal plane and the CHS spatial T axis deviation. Although these two measurements of T axis differ when the T wave spatial axis deviates from the frontal plane, an abnormal T axis reflecting a deviation exceeding 45° is in general detected by both definitions. Both studies defined deviation from 30° to 45° as borderline and deviation ≥45° as abnormal.

Risk evaluation in both studies was performed in multivariate models with an extensive adjustment for a host of CHD risk factors and some ECG abnormalities (Table 10A.5). In the Rotterdam study, abnormal T axis was associated with a nearly threefold increased risk of cardiac death (relative risk 2.9 [2.0, 4.3]). The relative risk of cardiac death for borderline T axis was 1.7 (1.0, 2.8). The risk associated with abnormal T axis in the multivariate model was substantially increased also for other endpoints: 3.1 (1.7, 5.5) for sudden death, 1.8 (1.3, 2.7) for nonfatal cardiac events), and 2.2 (1.7, 3.0) for fatal and nonfatal cardiac events combined. Borderline T axis was not significantly associated with other endpoints than cardiac death.

In the CHD-free group of the CHS, the hazard ratio remained significant for marked T axis deviation in the fully adjusted model for incident CHD (1.58 [1.25, 1.99]), and for CHD death (1.98 [1.28, 3.08]). In the fully adjusted model, ECG variables included were MI by ECG,

TABLE 10A.5 Two population-based cohorts with risk evaluation for T wave axis.

	Rotterdam Study[22]	Cardiovascular Health Study[24]
Geographic location	Ommoord District of Rotterdam, the Netherlands	Forcyth County, NC, Sacramento County, CA, Washington County, MD, Pittsburgh County, PA, USA
Source population/ respondents	7,129 residents/78% ECG available in 6,160 (86%)	Random sample from Medicare eligibility lists/57.3% of those contacted and eligible
Baseline for prevalence estimation	1990–1993	Recruitment of 5,201 completed 1990; minority sample of 687 in 1992–1993
Gender	Male, female	Male, female
Age range at baseline	55 years and older	65 years and older
Follow-up	3–6 years (mean 4 years)	8+ years, annual examination
ECG findings evaluated for risk	T axis, QTc, QT dispersion MI by ECG, T wave inversion, LVH by ECG, ST depression	T axis, QTI, MI, LVH, ST depression
Baseline prevalence for categories of interest	Borderline T axis 8.3%, abnormal T axis 10.5%	(A) Marginal T axis deviation: 24% (B) Marked T axis deviation 12%
Associated risk for cardiac death	HR 1.7 (1.1, 2.9) for borderline axis* HR 2.9 (2.0, 4.3) for abnormal axis* HR 1.8 (1.1, 2.8) for borderline axis† HR 2.8 (1.8, 4.5) for abnormal axis†	(A) Marginal T axis deviation: HR 1.2 (0.82, 1.78) (B) Marked T axis deviation: HR 2.0 (1.28, 3.08)
Multivariate adjustment	*Age, gender, history of MI, angina, diabetes, BMI, hypertension, current smoking, total cholesterol/ HDL ratio †Age, gender; ECG abnormalities simultaneously	Age, gender, race, BMI, SBP, DBP, hypertensive status, diabetes, current smoker, total cholesterol/HDL ratio, internal carotid thickness, MI and LVH by ECG, QRS axis, QT index
Comments	Significant independent risk for MI by ECG and QTc dispersion, not significant for inverted T, LVH, ST depression or QTc	

BMI body mass index, *DBP* diastolic blood pressure, *HDL* high density lipoproteins, *HR* hazard ratio, *LVH* left ventricular hypertrophy, *MI* myocardial infarction, *SBP* systolic blood pressure.

rate-adjusted QT, ST depression, left ventricular mass estimated from an ECG model (ECG-LVM), and frontal plane QRS axis. In separate risk analyses in the group with prior CHD, the hazard ratios for marked T axis deviation were 2.35 (1.53, 3.61) for CHD death and 1.93 (1.46, 2.54) for all-cause death, with the adjustment for age, gender and race alone. With an additional adjustment for demographic and clinical factors and for the same ECG variables as in the CHD-free group above, the hazard ratio remained significant for all-cause mortality, 1.48 (1.08, 2.04). The hazard ratio for CHD death was 1.58 (0.97, 2.60).

The results from CHS support the conclusions from the Rotterdam Heart Study, suggesting that abnormal T axis is an independent predictor of adverse cardiac events in community-based older adult populations. However, the reported excess risk associated with abnormal T axis in the Rotterdam study was in general substantially higher than that in the CHS.

Observations in the CHD-free group of CHS indicated that when spatial T axis deviation

increased, the spatial T axis shifted progressively closer to the horizontal plane, and with marked T axis deviation the T axis elevation angle reached 85° (Figure 10A.4). QRS axis orientation differences between the T axis groups were minor. The QRS axis remained approximately 30° posteriorly, and its orientation in the frontal plane shifted slightly to the left (more horizontal) with increasing T axis deviation. In comparison with the pronounced spatial T axis orientation differences, the relatively unchanged QRS axis even with marked T axis deviation supports the assertion that the repolarization changes with T axis deviation were to a large extent primary repolarization abnormalities. Marked T axis deviation in older men and women without overt clinical signs of CHD apparently represents manifestations of subclinical disease with adverse prognostic implications.

A potential problem overlooked in the above T axis report is that a common normal reference direction was used for men and women. In women, T axis is oriented 17 degrees more posteriorly in the horizontal plane than in men. Thus, there may

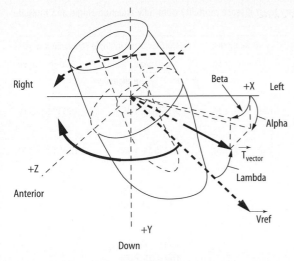

FIGURE 10A.4 Schematic of reference angles for T axis deviations: (1) frontal (XY) plane axis α (*Alpha*) (0° left, +90° down, −90° up, ± 180° right); (2) horizontal (XZ) plane axis or azimuth β (*Beta*) (0° left, +90° back, ± 180° right); and spatial angle λ (*Lambda* – deviation from the reference direction Vref, α 45°, β 45°). Normal apicobasal repolarization sequence is opposite to the Vref direction. Anterior shift of T axis (*solid arrow*) took place in two-thirds of marked axis deviation, and the remaining one-third were posterior shifts (*broken arrow*). (Source: Rautaharju et al.[24] *Am J Cardiol* 2001;88:118–23. Copyright © 2001. Reproduced with permission from Elsevier.)

have been more women than men in the normal T axis group, with a lower risk in women than men in the normal reference group for risk evaluation.

Spatial T axis deviation with a normal sequence of ventricular repolarization can be expected to be closely associated with the spatial QRS/T angle. Risk data for the latter variable will be discussed at the end of this chapter in connection with new data from the Women's Health Initiative (WHI) and CHS.

10A.2.6 New Reports on Repolarization Abnormalities as Mortality Predictors from Large Population-based Cohorts

Some other older and some recent reports have brought new information on the risk associated with repolarization abnormalities, including the relative importance of ST and T wave abnormalities as mortality predictors.

10A.2.6.1 MRFIT

In a MRFIT report from 2002, long-term (18.5 years) mortality risk for seven sets of T wave criteria was evaluated, including T axis and minor T wave abnormalities (Minnesota Code 5.3, 5.4).[25] All major ECG abnormalities were excluded, and adjustment was performed for all known CHD risk factors. Only minor T wave abnormalities (prevalence 7%) were significantly associated with cause-specific or total mortality in these high-risk men. T axis (upper quintile) was not significantly associated with cause-specific or total mortality. The change in T axis from baseline to year six was significantly associated with CHD mortality but the association with CVD or total mortality was not significant.

10A.2.6.2 Women's Health Initiative

The recently published ECG risk study report from the WHI comes from a very large group of postmenopausal women, nearly 40,000 women aged 50 years and older. The first of the reports evaluated the risk of CHD mortality and all-cause mortality,[26] and the second report the risk of incident CVD and incident congestive heart failure (CHF).[27]

When entered as single ECG variables into a multivariable-adjusted CHD risk model, several repolarization variables were significant CHD mortality predictors (Table 10A.6). Among these, wide QRS/T angle was the strongest predictor, with relative risk 2.70. ST V5 depression and T V1 amplitude were also significant predictors.

Rate-adjusted QT (QTrr) was one of the two variables with a significant interaction with the baseline CVD status (relative risks are listed separately for both groups on top of the table), and the risk was significant in CVD-free women only. When all significant ECG predictors were entered simultaneously into the multivariable-adjusted CHD mortality risk model, QRS/T angle retained its dominant, independent association with CHD mortality risk, with an over twofold increase in risk. QTrr also remained a strong independent CHD mortality risk predictor. Of interest was that QRS nondipolar voltage was one of the dominant CHD mortality risk predictors, together with old ECG-MI.

TABLE 10A.6 Hazard ratios and 95% confidence intervals for coronary heart disease mortality from fully adjusted single and multiple ECG variable risk models in the Women's Health Initiative study.

ECG variables (cutpoints)	Multi-adjusted single ECG variable models		Multi-adjusted multiple ECG variable models	
	CVD group	CVD-free group	CVD group	CVD-free group
Cornell voltage				
Reference (<1,800 μV)	1	1	1	1
High ($\geq$1,800 μV)	0.48 (0.17, 1.37)	1.91* (1.09, 3.36)	0.36 (0.12, 1.05)	1.25 (0.69, 2.26)
QTrr				
Reference (<437 ms)	1	1	1	1
Prolonged ($\geq$437 ms)	0.47 (0.14, 1.54)	2.17* (1.24, 3.73)	0.45 (0.14, 1.50)	1.90* (1.09, 3.33)
QRS/T angle				
Reference (0–56°)	1		1	
Borderline (57–96°)	1.32 (0.85, 2.04)		1.23 (0.79, 1.93)	
High ($\geq$97°)	2.70† (1.66, 4.39)		2.12† (1.25, 3.62)	
ECG-MI/ischemic injury				
No MI	1		1	
MI	2.41† (1.52, 3.81)		1.87* (1.15, 3.03)	
Isolated ST-T abnormalities or minor Q waves	1.50 (0.93, 2.42)		1.24 (0.76, 2.02)	
QRS nondipolar voltage				
Reference (<65 μV)	1		1	
Increased ($\geq$65 μV)	2.18 (1.33, 3.57)		1.85* (1.11, 3.09)	
Heart rate variability				
Reference (8–44 ms)	1		1	
Low (<8 ms)	1.95† (1.24, 3.07)		1.87 (1.19, 2.95)	
High (>44 ms)	1.04 (0.55, 1.97)		0.97 (0.51, 1.83)	
T V5 mean amplitude				
Normal (73–235 μV)	1		RM	
Low (<73 μV)	1.80† (1.16, 2.81)			
(Tpeak <117 μV)				
High (>235 μV)	1.22 (0.61, 2.45)			
ST V5 mean amplitude				
Reference (>0 μV)	1		RM	
Depressed ($\leq$0 μV)	1.63* (1.07, 2.47)			
T V1 mean amplitude				
Reference (−41–80 μV)	1		RM	
Low (<−41 μV)	1.14 (0.62, 2.10)			
High (>80 μV)	1.60 (0.98, 2.59)			
T wave roundness index				
Reference (<31%)	1		RM	
Oblong (31–57%)	1.20 (0.79, 1.80)			
Round (>57%)	1.60 (0.93, 2.73)			
ST V5 gradient				
Reference ($\geq$3 μV)	1		RM	
Downsloping or horizontal (<3 μV)	1.47 (0.83, 2.59)			
T nondipolar voltage				
Reference (<13 μV)	1		RM	
Increased ($\geq$13 μV)	1.12 (0.64, 1.98)			

Values are hazard ratios and confidence limits. *CVD* cardiovascular disease, *MI* myocardial infarction, *RM* removed in backwards selection procedure. There were 112 CHD mortality events.

* $p < 0.05$, † $p < 0.01$, ‡ $p < 0.001$.

Source: Rautaharju et al.[26] Circulation 2006;113:473–80. © 2006 American Heart Association, Inc. Reproduced with permission from Lippincott Williams & Wilkins.

The accompanying WHI report evaluated repolarization abnormalities as predictors of incident CHF (Table 10A.7).[27] In women with and without prior CVD combined, dominant among these potentially important subclinical indicators of pending evolution of this serious condition were wide QRS/T angle, ST V5 depression, high T V1 amplitude and prolonged QT. All these repolar-

TABLE 10A.7 Hazard ratios and 95% confidence intervals for incident congestive heart failure from multi-adjusted single and multiple ECG variable models in the Women's Health Initiative study.

ECG variables/(cutpoints)	Multi-adjusted single ECG variable models	Multi-adjusted multiple ECG variable models
QRS/T angle		
Reference (0–56°)	1	1
Increased (57–96°)	$1.59^{\ddagger}$ (1.26, 2.02)	$1.51^{\ddagger}$ (1.17, 1.94)
Wide (≥97°)	$2.73^{\ddagger}$ (2.06, 3.60)	$1.95^{\ddagger}$ (1.41, 2.70)
ECG-MI/ischemic injury		
No MI	1	RM
MI	$1.99^{\ddagger}$ (1.53, 2.59)	
Isolated ST-T abnormalities or minor	$1.55^{\ddagger}$ (1.21, 1.99)	
Q waves		
ST V5 mean amplitude		
Reference (>0 μV)	1	1
Depressed (≤0 μV)	$2.11^{\ddagger}$ (1.62, 2.52)	$1.49^{\dagger}$ (1.17, 1.89)
T V1 mean amplitude		
Reference (−41–80 μV)	1	1
Low (<−41 μV)	1.07 (0.75, 1.51)	1.31 (0.91, 1.90)
High (>80 μV)	$2.16^{\ddagger}$ (1.68, 2.78)	$1.56^{\dagger}$ (1.19, 2.05)
QRS nondipolar voltage		
Reference (<65 μV)	1	1
Increased (≥65 μV)	$2.00^{\ddagger}$ (1.51, 2.65)	$1.64^{\ddagger}$ (1.23,2.19)
T V5 mean amplitude		
Reference (73–235 μV)	1	RM
Low (<73 μV or <117 μV))	$1.84^{\ddagger}$ (1.46, 2.35)	
High (>235 μV)	0.86 (0.54, 1.38)	
ST V5 gradient		
Reference (≥3 μV)	1	RM
Low or negative (<3 μV)	$1.72^{\ddagger}$ (1.28, 2.30)	
QTrr		
Reference (<437 ms)	1	1
Prolonged (≥437 ms)	$1.80^{\dagger}$ (1.40, 2.31)	$1.60^{\dagger}$ (1.25, 2.07)
Cornell voltage		
Reference (<1,800 μV)	1	RM
High (≥1,800 μV)	$1.64^{\ddagger}$ (1.28, 2.10)	
T wave roundness index		
Reference (<31%)	1	RM
Oblong (31–57%)	$1.33^{\dagger}$ (1.06, 1.66)	
Round (>57%)	$1.62^{\ddagger}$ (1.20, 2.19)	
Heart rate variability		
Reference (8–44 ms)	1	1
Low (<8 ms)	1.27 (0.96, 1.69)	1.19 (0.89, 1.58)
High (>44 ms)	$1.53^{\dagger}$ (1.15, 2.04)	1.44* (1.08, 1.92)
T nondipolar voltage		
Reference (<13 μV)	1	RM
Increased (≥13 μV)	1.30 (0.97, 1.75)	

Values are hazard ratios and confidence limits. Cutpoints for the continuous variables partition the distributions so that the highest decile is always selected as a comparison group (for T V1 and T V5 both the highest and lowest deciles). There were 375 incident CHF events. Prevalent CHF events at the baseline (233 subjects) were excluded from incident CHF risk models. Data for ECG variables with a significant interaction with baseline CVD status are listed first, separately for both groups. *MI* myocardial infarction, *RM* removed in backwards selection procedure. * $p < 0.05$, † $p < 0.01$, ‡ $p < 0.001$.
Source: Rautaharju et al.[27] Circulation 2006;113:481–9. © American Heart Association, Inc. Reproduced with permission from Lippincott Williams & Wilkins.

izalization abnormalities reflect an altered temporal/spatial sequence of repolarization and abnormal heterogeneity of action potential durations with aberrations of ionic channel function. The investigators concluded that ventricular repolarization abnormalities in postmenopausal women are as important as an old ECG-MI as predictors of incident CHD, incident CHF, and mortality.

10A.2.6.3 Primary Repolarization Abnormalities and Heart Disease Prevention in Women

Do the above observations have possible implications to primary or secondary prevention in women, when the objective is to prevent, or at least to slow down the progression of CHD? It has been increasingly recognized recently that physicians tend to underestimate the risk of adverse CHD events in women.[28] Minor repolarization abnormalities are often considered to be of little consequence, particularly in women. The WHI report evaluated how much difference the presence of repolarization abnormalities and ECG-MI will make in the annual rate of CHD events in comparison with the corresponding reference groups (Table 10A.8). This difference was substantial for wide QRS/T angle and ECG-MI, and considerable also for the other dominant repolarization abnormalities, suggesting that the presence of these abnormalities in women may signal consideration for intensified primary or secondary prevention effort.

10A.2.6.4 Cardiovascular Health Study

How does the risk of adverse events for the ECG abnormalities in women compare to that in men? The CHS evaluated dominant, independent ECG predictors among ECG variables that were significant when entered as single ECG variables into various multivariable-adjusted risk models (Table 10A.9).[29] The source data come from a larger group of men and women with a longer follow-up time than the previous CHS study reports, which evaluated the mortality risk for T axis deviation.[24] The hypothesis for the study was conservatively formulated to state that the mortality risk for ECG abnormalities in women is not less significant than in men.

The relative risk for CHD mortality in men and in women was 60% increased for wide QRS/T angle, and it was increased twofold for ST depression. These risk levels were as strong as that for an old MI by ECG criteria. Relative risks for the variables that had a significant interaction with gender in Table 10A.9 are listed separately for men and for women, and for the other variables they are listed for the combined gender group. The relative risk of CHD mortality for ECG-LVM was significant in women only, with an over twofold risk increase. Of interest is that QRS nondipolar voltage was also a significant predictor of CHD mortality.

When all these significant ECG predictors were entered simultaneously into risk models, ST depression remained as a significant, dominant predictor of CHD mortality, with 74% excess risk in CHD-free men and women (not shown). The relative risk was 2.35 for men and women with prior CHD. In the latter group, ECG-LVM was also retained as a significant independent predictor, with CHD mortality risk increased by 62%. ST depression in V5, old MI by ECG, and ECG-LVM were retained as dominant ECG predictors of all-cause mortality. The investigators concluded that the association of ECG abnormalities with mortality risk in women was consistently as strong as in men, with no significant gender differences.

TABLE 10A.8 Annual rate/10,000 women of coronary heart disease events in women with specified ECG abnormalities and difference in number of events between reference and abnormal groups* in the Women's Health Initiative study.

	QRS/T angle	ECG-MI	ST V5 mean	ST V5 gradient	T V5 mean	QTrr
Age-adjusted relative risk[†]	2.31	1.91	1.65	1.57	1.57	1.49
Multi-adjusted relative risk[†]	1.90	1.62	1.46	1.42	1.37	1.37
Annual events/10,000 women in high risk group	61.1	60.2	49.3	53.5	50.2	44.1
Annual events/10,000 women in reference group	20.8	21.6	24.1	25.8	25.6	25.8
Annual difference/10,000 women	40	39	25	28	25	18

* Total annual event rate was 27.5/10,000 women.

[†] Hazard ratios from the age-adjusted and multi-adjusted single ECG variable models for CHD events. Hazard ratios presented are lower than differences in events due to adjustment in the models and positive correlation between risk factors.

Source: Rautaharju et al.[26] Circulation 2006;113:473–80. © 2006 American Heart Association, Inc. Reproduced with permission from Lippincott Williams & Wilkins.

TABLE 10A.9 Relative risks (95% confidence limits) of coronary heart disease and all-cause mortality from single electrocardiographic variable models in men and women in the Cardiovascular Health Study.*

Category/subgroup	CHD mortality[†] (452 deaths)	All-cause mortality (1,856 deaths)
Old myocardial infarction		
No infarct (No NC 5.1–5.4)	1	1
Infarct (NC 5.1–5.4)	Men and women 1.82 (1.38, 2.40)[¶]	Men and women 1.61 (1.37, 1.88)[¶]
ST depression in V5		
>−20 μV (men and women)	1	1
≤−20 μV[‡] (both gender groups)	Men and women 2.00 (1.60, 2.50)[¶]	Men and women 1.62 (1.43, 1.82)[¶]
QRS/T angle		
<126° in men	1	1
<107° in women		
≥126° in men	Men and women 1.60 (1.26, 2.02)[¶]	Men and women 1.43 (1.26, 1.63)[¶]
≥107° in women		
QRS nondipolar voltage		
<77 μV in men	1	1
<68 μV in women		
≥77 μV in men	Men and women 1.66 (1.29, 2.13)[‖]	Men 1.00 (0.81, 1.24)
≥68 μV in women		Women 1.40 (1.17, 1.68)[¶]
ECG-LVM		
<201 g in men	1	1
<161 g in women		
≥201 g in men	Men 1.24 (0.81, 1.82)	Men 1.32 (1.06, 1.65)[‖]
≥161 g in women	Women 2.14 (1.45, 3.17)[¶]	Women 1.81 (1.48, 2.22)[¶]

CHD coronary heart disease, *NC* Novacode, *ECG-LVM* ECG estimate of left ventricular mass. * Adjusted for age, gender, coronary heart disease status, race, body mass index, hypertension status, diabetes, and drug usage (diuretics, beta-blockers, antiarrhythmics [class 1a, 1b, 1c and 3], calcium channel blockers). Relative risks are listed separately for men and women for ECG variables with a significant gender interaction. [†] Includes coronary heart disease deaths due to reinfarction among those with prior infarction. [‡] Equal to −50 μV at ST segment time point J + 60 ms. [‖] $p < 0.01$, [¶] $p < 0.001$, risk for individual variables. Source: Rautaharju et al.[29] Am J Cardiol 2006;97:309–15. © 2006. Reproduced with permission from Elsevier.

10A.2.7 Primary Repolarization Abnormalities in Women Suspected of Having Myocardial Ischemia

The Women's Ischemia Syndrome Evaluation (WISE) study sponsored by the National Heart, Lung, and Blood Institute reported findings from one of the study centers in 143 women referred to coronary angiography using ECG measures of primary repolarization abnormalities[30] similar to those used in WHI and CHS referred to previously. The key findings from this retrospective study of these symptomatic women (73% post-menopausal) after an average 3.3-year follow-up are consistent with those from the WHI and CHS reports. Significant predictors of adverse outcome (CHF, nonfatal MI or death) as continuous ECG measures were a wider QRS/T angle, a longer QTrr, and ST depression (measured in V5 lead at time point J + 60 ms) ($p = 0.005$ or less for all). Additional significant predictors were a slight degree of QRS prolongation ($p = 0.004$) and a

higher CHD severity score in angiography (borderline significant).

Because of increasing interest in some of these newer and less commonly used ECG risk predictors, QRS/ T angle in particular, a suggested procedure and algorithms for determination of the spatial QRS/T angle from the conventional ECG measurements are described in Chapter 10B.

References

1. Miller WT, Geselowitz DB. Simulation studies of the electrocardiogram. II. Ischemia and infarction. Circ Res 1978;43:315–23.
2. van Oosterom A. Genesis of the T-wave as based on an equivalent surface source model. J Electrocardiol 2002;34:217–27.
3. Yan GX, Antzelevich C. Cellular basis of the electrocardiographic J wave. Circulation 1996;93:372–9.
4. Kiessling CE, Schaaf RS, Lyle AM. A study of T wave changes in the electrocardiograms of normal individuals. Am J Cardiol 1964;13:598–602.

5. Blackburn H, Parlin RW. The antecedents of disease. Insurance mortality experience. Ann NY Acad Sci 1966;134:965–1017.
6. Hiss RG, Lamb LE. Electrocardiographic findings in 122,043 individuals. Circulation 1962;25:947–61.
7. Ostrander LD. The relation of "silent" T wave inversion to cardiovascular disease in an epidemiologic study. Am J Cardiol 1970;35:325–8.
8. Singer RB, Siber FJ, Browne AE, Pitkin FL. Mortality in 4,100 insured applicants with ECG and chest x-ray: relation to cardiovascular and other risk factors, including relative heart diameter. Trans Assoc Life Insur Med Dir Am 1982;65:180–93.
9. Rabkin SW, Mathewson FAL, Tate RB. The electrocardiogram in apparently healthy men and the risk of sudden death. Br Heart J 1982;47:546–52.
10. Blackburn H, Keys A, Simonson E. The electrocardiogram in population studies. A classification system. Circulation 1960;21:1160–75.
11. Reunanen A, Aromaa A, Pyörälä K et al. The Social Insurance Institution's Coronary Heart Disease Study. Acta Med Scand 1983;673(Suppl):1–120.
12. Menotti A, Blackburn H. Electrocardiographic predictors of coronary heart disease in the seven countries study. In: Kromhout D, Menotti A, Blackburn H (eds). Prevention of Coronary Heart Disease. Diet, lifestyle and risk factors in the Seven Countries Study. Norwell, Massachusetts: Kluver Academic Publishers, 2002, pp 199–211.
13. Menotti A, Blackburn H, Jacobs DR et al. The predictive value of resting electrocardiographic findings in cardiovascular disease-free men. Twenty-five-year follow-up in the Seven Countries Study. Internal document, Division of Epidemiology, School of Public Health, University of Minnesota, 2001.
14. Daviglus ML, Liao Y, Greenland P et al. Association of nonspecific minor ST-T abnormalities with cardiovascular mortality. The Chicago Western Electric Study. JAMA 1999;281:530–6.
15. Rose G, Baxter PJ, Reid DD, McCartney P. Prevalence and prognosis of electrocardiographic findings in middle-aged men. Br Heart J 1978;40:636–43.
16. Sigurdson E, Sigfusson M, Sigvaldason H, Thorgeirsson G. Silent ST-T changes in an epidemiologic cohort study – a marker of hypertension or coronary artery disease, or both: the Reykjavik study. J Am Coll Cardiol 1996;27:1140–7.
17. De Bacquer D, De Backer G, Kornitzer M. Prognostic value of ECG findings for cardiovascular mortality in men and women. J Am Coll Cardiol 1998;32:680–5.
18. Kannel WB, Anderson K, McGee DL et al. Nonspecific electrocardiographic abnormality as a predictor of coronary heart disease: the Framingham Study. Am Heart J 1987;113:370–6.
19. Schouten EG, Dekker JM, Pool J et al. Well shaped ST segment and the risk of cardiovascular mortality. Br Med J 1992;304:356–9.
20. Tervahauta M, Pekkanen J, Punsar S, Nissinen A. Resting electrocardiographic abnormalities as predictors of coronary events and total mortality among elderly men. Am J Med 1996;100:641–5.
21. Rajala S, Haavisto M, Kaltiala K, Mattila K. ECG findings and survival in very old people. Eur Heart J 1985;6:247–52.
22. Kors JA, de Bruyne MC, Hoes AW et al. T axis as an independent indicator of risk of cardiac events in elderly people. Lancet 1998;352:601–5.
23. Krikler DM, Meijler FL. T axis and cardiac events in elderly people. Letter to the Editor. Lancet 1999; 353:68.
24. Rautaharju PM, Clark Nelson J, Kronmal RA et al. Usefulness of T axis deviation is an independent risk indicator for incident cardiac events in older men and women free from coronary heart disease (the Cardiovascular Health Study). Am J Cardiol 2001;88:118–23.
25. Prineas RJ, Grandits G, Rautaharju PM et al. Long-term prognostic significance of isolated minor electrocardiographic T-wave abnormalities in middle-aged men free of clinical cardiovascular disease (the Multiple Risk Factor Intervention Trial [MRFIT]). Am J Cardiol 2002;90:1391–5.
26. Rautaharju PM, Kooperberg C, Larson J, LaCroix A. Electrocardiographic abnormalities that predict coronary heart disease events and mortality in postmenopausal women: the Women's Health Initiative. Circulation 2006;113:473–80.
27. Rautaharju PM, Kooperberg C, Larson JC, LaCroix A. Electrocardiographic predictors of incident congestive heart failure and all-cause mortality in postmenopausal women: the Women's Health Initiative. Circulation 2006;113:481–9.
28. Mosca L, Linfante AH, Benjamin EJ et al. National study of physician awareness and adherence to cardiovascular disease prevention guidelines. Circulation 2005;111:499–510.
29. Rautaharju PM, Ge S, Clark Nelson J et al. Comparison of mortality risk for electrocardiographic abnormalities in men and women with and without coronary heart disease (from the Cardiovascular Health Study). Am J Cardiol 2006;97:309–15.
30. Triola B, Olson MB, Reis SE et al. Electrocardiographic predictors of cardiovascular outcome in women: the National Heart, Lung, and Blood Institute-sponsored Women's Ischemia Syndrome Evaluation (WISE) study. J Am Coll Cardiol 2005;46:51–6.

10B
Procedures for Determination of the Spatial QRS/T Angle from Conventional ECG Measurements

The calculation of the spatial QRS/T angle requires availability of the orthogonal or at least quasi-orthogonal X, Y and Z leads. The Z lead polarity in the following derivation differs from the Z lead polarity of the Frank leads in that the posterior–anterior direction is taken as the positive direction. Consequently, the Z lead amplitudes of the Frank lead Z have to be multiplied by -1.

Step 1. Calculate the mean X, Y and Z lead amplitudes for the QRS and T waves in their respective time windows. Let these mean amplitudes be denoted by Rx, Ry and Rz and Tx, Ty and Tz, respectively.

Step 2. Calculate the spatial magnitude between the QRS and the T vectors, denoted by Rsm and Tsm, respectively.

$Rsm = (Rx^2 + Ry^2 + Rz^2)^{0.5}$, and
$Tsm = (Tx^2 + Ty^2 + Tz^2)^{0.5}$.

Step 3. The algorithm for QRS/T angle θ [°] is as follows:

QRS/T angle θ = ACOs(QRSx*Tx + QRSy*Ty + QRSz*Tz)/(Rsm*Tsm)$^{0.5}$, where ACOs = inverse cosine.

If the X, Y and Z leads are not recorded, for instance the median complexes for the 12-lead ECG from the GE-Marquette program can be used for this purpose. The X, Y and Z components can be derived using either the inverse matrix transform from the coefficients of Horáček[1] or Dower. The latter are documented by Edenbrandt and Pahlm.[2]

Finally, a simple method is introduced here for determination of the QRS/T angle. The algorithm was derived in the combined data set of normal men and women used for the normal standards in Part 2 of this book.

Let Rnet = R amplitude − abs (S or QS amplitude, whichever larger), and Tnet = absT − abs (Tprime amplitude), (abs refers to the absolute value of the signed amplitude). Also, let the spatial magnitudes of the Rnet and Tnet vectors (Rsm and Tsm) be defined as follows:

$Rsm = (RV6net^2 + RaVFnet^2 + RV2net^2)^{0.5}$, and
$Tsm = (TV5net^2 + TaVFnet^2 + TV2net^2)^{0.5}$

The QRS/T angle θ can now be calculated using the following formula, analogous to the formula in Step 3 above:

QRS/T angle θ = 0.76*ACOS(RV6net*TV5net + RaVFnet*TaVFnet + RV2net*TV2net)$^{0.5}$/ (Rsm*Tsm)$^{0.5}$ + 7

This simplified method produced an estimate for the QRS/T angle which correlated at quite high level with the QRS/T angle from the matrix method (r = 0.88).

References

1. Horáček BM, Warren JW, Field DQ, Feldman CL. Statistical and deterministic approaches to designing transformations of electrocardiographic leads. J Electrocardiol 2002;35(Suppl):41–52.
2. Edenbrandt L, Pahlm O. Vectorcardiogram synthesized from a 12-lead ECG: superiority of the inverse Dower matrix. J Electrocardiol 1988;21:361–7.

11
QT Prolongation and QT Dispersion – a Critical Evaluation

Synopsis

Significance

QT prolongation may facilitate initiation of malignant arrhythmic events, and it is used in clinical trials in evaluation of new cardioactive drugs as a marker of adverse response.

Mechanism

The QT interval is the sum of excitation time and action potential duration (APD) of the myocytes in the myocardial region where the repolarization occurs last.

With normal ventricular conduction, APD prolongation can be detected from QT measurements only if the prolongation is spatially uniform, nonuniform with prolongation in the region normally repolarizing last, or if the prolongation in some other region is large enough so that the sum of excitation time and APD in that region becomes longer than that in the region normally repolarizing last. Action potential duration shortening from QT measurement can be detected only if it occurs in the region normally repolarizing last or if it is spatially uniform. Detection of localized APD changes or dispersion of ventricular repolarization from QT measurement differences in individual ECG leads or QT dispersion (QTD) requires: (1) the presence of nondipolar components in T wave originating from the region that is repolarizing last that are above the threshold of Tend detection criteria; or (2), the presence of nondipolar components in T wave originating from some other local region that are sufficiently strong to modify the effect of the stronger dipolar components and thus to influence the end of T wave detection. The presence of such nondipolar T wave components large enough in magnitude has not been demonstrated, and the QTD concept remains an unproven hypothesis.

Risk Factors and Confounding Factors

These include: advancing age, female gender (strong female predominance), prolonged QRS for any reason, prolonged excitation time in left ventricular hypertrophy and in other conditions, systolic and diastolic blood pressure, class 1A and class III antiarrhythmic drugs, diuretics, and ECG evidence of old myocardial infarction (MI) or injury. Among other conditions, QT is prolonged in type 2 diabetes and in patients on maintenance hemodialysis.

Classification Problems

There are two sources of major problems in detection of QT prolongation: QT measurement procedures and incorrect use of the Bazett's formula and other power functions for adjusting QT to ventricular rate. Valid normal limits to be used for QT evaluation need to come from data that have used actual percentile adjusted QT distributions at various ranges of heart rate because QT distributions are non-Gaussian, variably skewed, and normal limits established as (mean + 2*SD) are misleading at heart rates deviating from 60 cpm.

Prevalence and Mortality Risk

The prevalence and reported risks of QT prolongation vary widely because of differences in QT measurement procedures and the thresholds used for QT prolongation. In community-based populations at a 4–6% level of relative QT prolongation, the reported prevalence levels in total male and female populations range from 12 to 25%. The corresponding reported mortality risks in men range from fourfold for coronary heart disease (CHD) mortality to nonsignificant for cardiovascular disease (CVD) and all-cause mortality. In women, the reported mortality risk ranges from nonsignificant to a twofold risk increase. In CHD-free subgroups of male populations at a 10% level of QT prolongation and 4% prevalence, the reported CHD and total mortality risk (one study) was approximately twofold, and in most studies nonsignificant in total CHD-free female populations. In CHD-free combined male and female populations at the levels 7–9% QT prolongation and 3–5% prevalence, the reported CHD and total mortality risk was nonsignificant in one study and threefold for CHD and twofold for total mortality in another study. Women are at a higher risk for malignant arrhythmias caused by antiarrhythmic drugs. Several clinical studies have documented excess mortality risk associated with QT prolongation in survivors of acute MI. QT prolongation in hypertensive patients has been reported to be associated with excess risk of primary cardiac arrest. In nephropathic insulin-dependent diabetes mellitus, QT prolongation has been associated with increased mortality risk, which is independent of the presence of autonomic neuropathy.

Abbreviations and Acronyms

APD – action potential duration
ARIC – Atherosclerosis in Communities study
BMI – body mass index
CHD – coronary heart disease
CHS – Cardiovascular Health Study
cpm – cycles per minute, referring to heart rate
CVD – cardiovascular disease
DESIR – Data from an Epidemiological Study on the Insulin Resistance syndrome

DRT – dispersion of repolarization time
ECG-LVM – left ventricular mass estimated by an ECG model
ET – excitation time
IRAS – Insulin Resistance Atherosclerosis Study
LBBB – left bundle branch block
LQTS – long QT syndrome
LQT1 – long QT1 family of LQTS
LQT2 – long QT2 family of LQTS
LVH – left ventricular hypertrophy
MI – myocardial infarction
NDPV – nondipolar voltage
QTI – QT prolongation index
QTD – QT dispersion
QTbz – QT adjusted to heart rate by Bazett's square root formula
QTfr – QT adjusted to heart rate by Fridericia's cubic root formula
QT0.42 – QT adjusted to heart rate by regressing $RR^{0.42}$ on measured QT
QT0.5 – QT adjusted to heart rate by regressing $RR^{0.5}$ on measured QT
QTrr – QT adjusted to heart rate as a linear function of RR
QTrr,qrs – QT adjusted heart rate with RR and QRS duration as covariates
RBW – relative body weight
RT – repolarization time
T_{peak} – time point of maximum of T spatial magnitude curve
T_{Infl1} – inflection point at the upstroke of the T spatial magnitude curve
T_{Infl2} – inflection point at the downstroke of the T wave
WHI – Women's Health Initiative

11.1 Introduction

This chapter covers multiple facets involved in QT prolongation. Special focus is on the utility and limitations of using QT prolongation for detecting abnormal dispersion of myocardial repolarization due to adverse drug effects. Inherited long QT syndrome (LQTS) will not be covered in any detail because of the relative rarity of the condition. At the end of the chapter, there is a brief summary note emphasizing that the basic prerequisites for the validity of the QT dispersion concept as a measure of dispersion of myocardial repolarization remains largely unsubstantiated.

11.2 Cellular Level Events at Cardiac Source in Relation to Body Surface ECG

Figure 11.1 shows the sequential repolarization process at three instants of time in an oblique trans-section of a model heart along the long axis of the left ventricle. Time point A corresponds to the onset of the fast phase of repolarization at the subepicardial region of the lateral left ventricular lateral wall, coinciding with the onset of the global T wave (spatial T wave magnitude) of the ECG. At

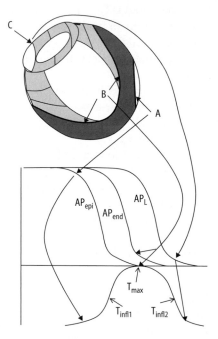

FIGURE 11.1 Schematic of the repolarization process in a model of the left ventricle (*top*). Repolarization front *A* corresponds to the onset of repolarization, front *B* the time point when the maximal number of ventricular cells are at fast repolarization phase, and front *C* the end of repolarization in basal regions. Below are the spatial magnitude curve of the T wave and the action potentials of the epicardial (AP_{epi}), endocardial (AP_{endo}), and basal regions (AP_L), with the latter region repolarizing last. T_{max} corresponds to time point B. The time interval between the inflection points at the upstroke and downstroke of the T wave ($T_{infl2}-T_{infl1}$) is an approximate index of the average dispersion of repolarization times.

time point B, the lateral wall repolarization is completed and the repolarization dipole of the cardiac source has reached its maximal magnitude. The line at time point C corresponds to the repolarization of the base of the heart.

Repolarization between lines A and B is reverse to the sequence of excitation, provided that the action potential duration (APD) shortening from B to A exceeds the excitation time (ET) difference between A and B. In other myocardial regions like the septum, repolarization is not reverse because the APD shortening with ET is less than the delay in excitation. The spatial angle between QRS and T vectors is normally over 60°, indicating that the overall repolarization sequence is semireverse rather than reverse with respect to the sequence of excitation.

Referring again to Figure 11.1:

- Time point C corresponds to the end of the T wave using the global T wave as the common time reference. At this point, the action potential in the region repolarizing last approaches its repolarized level.
- Time point A corresponds to the onset of the T wave when the fast phase of repolarization starts in the subepicardial cells, normally at the free lateral wall of the left ventricle.
- The number of ventricular cells entering the fast phase of repolarization increases from T onset to the peak of the T wave (T_{peak}). T_{peak} corresponds to time point B when the repolarization front reaches its maximal value. It is intuitively the time point when the largest number of repolarizing ventricular cells is at some phase of the rapid repolarization process (action potential phase 3).
- T_{Infl1}, the inflection point at the upstroke of the T spatial magnitude curve, can be conceived as the time point when the rate of increase in the repolarization front has reached its maximal value, when the increase in the number of ventricular cells that are in phase 3 has reached its maximum.
- T_{Infl2}, the inflection point at the downstroke of the T wave, is the time point when the rate of decrease of the uncancelled repolarization front has reached its maximal value. It can be conceived as the time point when the rate of decrease in the number of ventricular cells in phase 3 has

reached its maximum. T_{Infl1} and T_{Infl2} can be identified from the maximum and minimum values of the first time derivative of the spatial T magnitude curve.

- The $T_{end}-T_{peak}$ interval merely reflects the duration of the second phase of repolarization.
- The time interval between T onset and T_{Infl1} is conceptually related to the regional dispersion of lateral wall transmural repolarization.
- The time interval between the inflection points at the upstroke and downstroke of the T wave ($T_{infl2}-T_{infl1}$) can be conceived as a convenient approximate index of the average dispersion of repolarization times (DRT). This measure is similar to the T wave width that Lux et al. have identified as a measure of the range of repolarization times based on their experimental data with Langendorf perfused isolated canine hearts immersed in a torso-shaped electrolytic tank.[1]

It has been claimed recently that the $T_{peak}-T_{end}$ interval is a measure of transmural dispersion of the left ventricle.[2] The logic of such claims is difficult to comprehend.[3] The last of the assertions above suggests that the T onset to T_{Infl1} interval rather than the $T_{peak}-T_{end}$ interval is related to the regional transmural dispersion of repolarization of the free lateral wall of the left ventricle.

It should be recognized that transmural repolarization in apical wall and septum will take place within the same time window as the free wall repolarization. It is likely that there is a significant degree of internal cancellation of the repolarization fronts progressing in opposite directions. Another problem is that the estimation of the time point of T onset is often difficult because of the ill-defined transition between the slow and fast phase of repolarization.

To summarize conceptually reasonably rational expressions of the relationships between the quantities in question and the consequences of the assertions:

- Abnormal dispersion (increased or decreased) of ventricular repolarization can be local (for instance between Purkinje fibers and subendocardial cells or between M cells and subendocardial or subepicardial cells), regional (transmural in a wall section) or global (between myocardial regions). Normal repolarization is always dispersed regionally and globally, otherwise there will be no T wave. Critical arrhythmogenic dispersions are likely to be local or regional
- Measuring the local or regional end of repolarization time (RT) from the onset of excitation, dispersion of repolarization can be expressed as dispersion of repolarization time.
- Increase in APD increases local or regional DRT only if the temporal gradient of DRT in these regions increases. This occurs for instance if the agent increases APD of the cells in a region repolarizing later more than in the cells repolarizing earlier, or if the agent decreases APD of the cells in a region repolarizing earlier more than in cells repolarizing later in that region.
- Change in APD decreases local or regional DRT only if the temporal gradient of DRT decreases. This occurs for instance if the agent decreases APD of the cells in a region repolarizing later more than in the cells repolarizing earlier, or if the agent increases APD of the cells in a region repolarizing earlier more than in cells repolarizing later in that region. In the latter condition, DRT may decrease initially and then increase again.

11.2.1 Prerequisites for Detection of Regional Dispersion of Repolarization Time

Changes in local or regional repolarization time or DRT will influence body surface ECG QT measurements only if certain special prerequisites are met. Otherwise, they will have no notable effect on QT although they can always be expected to influence ST-T waveform to variable degrees. Prolonged repolarization as a response to the action of an agent can be detected from QT measurement in body surface ECG only if APD prolongation involves the cells in the region that repolarized last before the action of the agent, or if APD prolongation in some other region is so pronounced that this region now repolarizes last. A uniform spatial global increase or decrease of APD increases and decreases QT without a change in DRT.

The necessary conditions for detection of local prolonged or shortened DRT from a body surface ECG can be summarized as follows: (1) the presence of nondipolar components in T wave originating from the region that is repolarizing last that are above the threshold of T_{end} detection criteria; or (2), the presence of nondipolar components in T wave originating from some other local region that are sufficiently strong to modify the effect of the stronger dipolar components and thus to influence the end of T wave detection. The presence of nondipolar components of sufficient magnitude in the T wave for detection of changes in local or regional DRT has not been demonstrated.

Differences in the QT intervals measured from various ECG leads have little to do with dispersion of relative refractory periods or DRT of ventricular myocardium. A summary of the QT dispersion (QTD) question is included at the end of this chapter. Dispersed repolarization always changes T wave waveform and spatial direction of the terminal T wave. This increases interval measurement difficulties with abnormal waveforms and measurement variation at the end of the T wave due to changed spatial projection of terminal T waves on different leads and increased problems in identification of the end of T.

Among other factors influencing the shape of the T wave is the shape of the ventricle, and the shape changes during contraction. It becomes rounder, with the apex approaching the base of the ventricle. More than 40% of blood is normally ejected into the aorta during contraction.

Dispersion of repolarization time depends on the RT differences between various myocardial zones. With a gradual increase of epicardial RT (RT_{epi}) in a location at the free wall of the left ventricle, the regional DRT ordinarily first decreases and then increases when RT_{epi} becomes longer than endocardial RT (RT_{endo}). In general, global QT that can be measured from body surface ECGs does not start increasing until RT_{epi} becomes longer than RT_L, the repolarization time in the region repolarizing last (Figure 11.2).

It is not sufficient to consider repolarization in one transmural segmental preparation and the corresponding transmural electrograms to deduce the sequence of global repolarization in terms of the discordance or concordance of the process in the whole heart.

Effective refractory period in ventricular myocardium is linked to APD. Both maintain in physiological conditions a closely similar fixed relationship to cycle length. Compared to APD

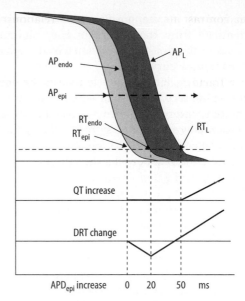

FIGURE 11.2 Schematic demonstrating the effect of gradually increasing repolarization time in subepicardial layers (RT_{epi}) on dispersion of repolarization time (DRT) and QT. DRT initially shortens until epicardial repolarization time (RT_{epi}) becomes longer than subendocardial repolarization time (RT_{endo}). There is no increase above the initial values of QT or DRT until RT_{epi} becomes longer than RT_L, repolarization time in the region that initially repolarized last. AP_{epi}, AP_{endo} and AP_L are action potentials at subepicardial, subendocardial, and the region corresponding to RT_L.

measured as the interval from the upstroke to the time point where repolarization has reached 90% level, the effective refractory period is 11–15 ms shorter than APD.[4] Increased temporal dispersion of refractory periods is conceived to be an inherent ingredient, a substrate, to tachyarrhythmias, with triggered activity, enhanced automaticity, and re-entry as potential associated mechanisms.[5–8]

Drugs that prolong the effective refractory period can be expected to be, in principle, antiarrhythmic if at the same time they reduce dispersion of repolarization recovery time. Drugs that selectively prolong epicardial APD more than endocardial APD initially decrease transmural DRT and then start increasing it. QT prolongation does not start until the local epicardial APD becomes longer than that in the region where the APD was longest before the drug's action.

In contrast to the normal fixed relationship between APD and relative refractory period, their response to some QT prolonging drugs may differ. For instance procainamid prolongs the effective refractory period more than APD at short cycle lengths ($\leq$400 ms).[4] (Voltage-independent but time-dependent suppression of excitability – drug's rate-dependence of sodium channel blockade.) Type 1C antiarrhythmic drugs prolong the effective refractory period in relation to APD at tolerable pacing rates.

Concerning the "vulnerable period", it should not be taken for granted that a global measure of the dispersion of local recovery times signals predisposition to arrhythmic episodes. Consider, for instance, complete left bundle branch block (LBBB). Global dispersion of ET can be expected to range from 120 ms to as long as 180 ms or even 200 ms. In this condition, repolarization is closely concordant to depolarization (T wave of opposite polarity to QRS in all leads). The onset of excitation and the onset of repolarization occur in the same spatial sequence. Gobal DRTs can be expected to be substantially increased, in spite of shortening of APD as a function of ET. Left bundle branch block is not generally associated with ventricular tachycardias unless there are other aggravating conditions such as myocardial infarction (MI). This is probably because the local gradients in recovery time from refractoriness are relatively small in isolated LBBB in comparison with global dispersion of refractory period or global dispersion of recovery time. Thus, more attention should be paid to local heterogeneity on the recovery time and local dispersion of repolarization than just considering the global measures of dispersion of repolarization.

In patients with LQTS, global dispersion of the end of the recovery from refractoriness is due to wide dispersion of refractory periods. Dispersion of local excitation time also occurs in patients with previous MI and vulnerability to ventricular tachycardia.[8] The exact pathophysiological mechanism for the association between moderate QT prolongation and mortality risk in clinically normal subjects with normal ventricular conduction is not as clear-cut, and even in patients with LQTS, a multitude of mechanisms are involved in producing a variety of aberrations in QT and T wave morphology.

11.3 Basic Determinants of QT Interval and QT Prolongation

While the QT interval is influenced by numerous factors, there are only two primary basic factors that determine the length of the QT interval. These are the excitation time and the APD of the myocytes in the region that repolarizes last (ET_L and APD_L). This simple fact is illustrated in Figure 11.3. This relationship holds in all conditions. The end of the T wave coincides with the repolarization in the region repolarizing last. ET_L is not equal to QRS interval because the region that repolarizes last is generally not the last to depolarize. ET_L is some fraction of QRS, and the global $QT = (ET_L + APD_L)$. Recognition of this simple fact would reduce the confusion often prevailing in the literature about the QT interval.

11.3.1 Potential Role of the M Cells

The M cells may be involved in determining the normal QT interval and they may be involved also in some pathophysiological mechanisms producing QT prolongation. As noted above, QT and QT

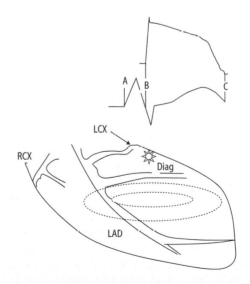

FIGURE 11.3 Schematic of the heart showing region L, which repolarizes last (the sun-like symbol). The excitation time of region L (ET_L) is the fraction of the QRS interval between lines *A* and *B*, and the action potential duration of L (APD_L) is the interval between lines *B* and *C* shown on the ECG below the action potential of region L. The global QT is ($ET_L + APD_L$). *LAD, LCX, Diag* and *RCX* are the main coronary arteries on the cardiac surface.

prolongation is determined by the excitation time and the repolarization time of the myocytes in the ventricular region repolarizing last. QT prolongation will take place in three conditions: (1) there is a uniform prolongation of APD in all ventricular regions; (2) the sum of excitation time and APD of the cells in the region normally repolarizing last is prolonged; (3) the sum of excitation time and APD of the myocytes in some other region is prolonged and becomes longer than the respective sum in the region normally repolarizing last.

The APD response to stimulus rate changes is more pronounced in M cells than in ventricular myocytes in epicardial or endocardial layers, and in M cells themselves, there is a spatial rate sensitivity gradient so that the rate sensitivity is higher in the M cell population in apical than in basal regions.[9] The APD of M cells increases markedly with hypokalemia and also the effect of drugs that increase APD is enhanced. M cells differ from other ventricular myocyte populations in several aspects.[10] The M cell response to digitalis with APD shortening (like in Purkinje fibers) could explain the 41% reduced likelihood of QT prolongation with digitalis administration. The sensitivity to the APD prolonging effect in M cells could explain the over fourfold excess of QT prolongation with class 1A antiarrhythmic drugs. Delayed onset of excitation in the subepicardial layers with M cells is likely to occur in conditions inducing left ventricular hypertrophy (LVH). QRS prolongs when left ventricular mass increases. Myocardial ischemia or injury in MI may also delay the onset of excitation in M cell layers. Shortening of APD may more readily influence M cells in subendocardial than in subepicardial layers.

There are some problems with the concept that M cells determine the QT interval. With the longest repolarization times in the middle layers containing M cells for instance in the left lateral wall of the left ventricle, repolarization should first proceed from subepicardial layers towards the middle layers and then from subendocardial layers towards the middle layers. If this were the case, one would expect biphasic, positive-negative T waves in the lateral leads, and this is normally not the case. This possibly depends on the density of M cells and on how tight their coupling is to other cells.

11.4 QT Adjustment for Physiological Factors

11.4.1 QT Adjustment for Heart Rate

Stimulus rate has a dominating influence on APD and similarly, the QT interval is strongly dependent on the heart rate. In 1920, Bazett graphed QT measurements from 39 young subjects against the length of the RR interval and noted that the measured QT appeared to be proportional to the square root of the RR interval.[11] This relationship was originally derived from the mechanical cycle length[12] from the onset of isovolumic contraction to the opening of the mitral valve. Bazett's introduction of the square root function initiated a persistent error in QT rate adjustment.[13] It also stimulated a popular trend in ECG research, the search for an optimal coefficient for the power function of RR and other functions of RR and heart rate.[14]

11.4.2 Two Fundamental Problems with Bazett-type Rate Adjustment with Power Functions

Bazett was not wrong in deducing that QT is a function of the square root of RR. What is wrong is the way QT rate adjustment is performed. There are two fundamental problems that cause serious errors in rate adjustment.

11.4.2.1 Error 1

Consider that QT is expressed as a reasonable first approximation as some power function of RR:

$$QT = C1 + C2* RR^n, \qquad [11.1]$$

where C1 is the intercept, C2 the slope coefficient of the regression and n the exponent of RR.

The division of QT on the left side of Equation 11.1 and the slope coefficient C2 on the right side by RR^n yields Equation 11.2:

$$QT/RR^n = C1/RR^n + C2. \qquad [11.2]$$

Equation 11.2 shows the first error in Bazett's and Fridericia's formulas. The ratio QT/RR is not constant unless the intercept C1 is 0; otherwise, there remains an uncorrected nonlinear error

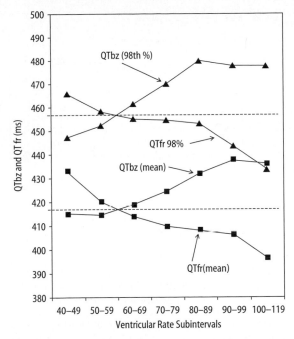

FIGURE 11.4 Mean values (*squares*) and 98th percentiles (*triangles*) for QT adjusted by the formulas of Bazett (*QTbz*) and Fridericia (*QTfr*) by ventricular rate. The omission of the QT versus RR regression intercept creates a strong systematic bias with a residual positive correlation with ventricular rate for QTbz ($r = 0.32$) and a negative correlation for QTfr ($r = -0.30$), making these formulas unusable for QT analysis. (Source: Rautaharju et al.[15] J Cardiovasc Electrophysiol 2002;13:1211–18. Copyright © 2002. Reproduced with permission from Blackwell Futura Publishing, Inc.)

term equal to $C1/RR^n$, where $n = 1/2$ for Bazett's formula and $n = 1/3$ for Fridericia's formula. The magnitude of the error depends on the magnitude of the regression intercept. The residual correlation between Bazett's QTc and heart rate in normal subjects is $r = 0.32$ (a positive correlation) and $r = -0.29$ for Fridericia's formula (indicating a negative residual correlation) (Figure 11.4).[15]

11.4.2.2 *Error 2*

The second problem with these QT adjustment formulas whereby QT is divided by the prediction function is that they correct the mean adjusted QT making it independent of heart rate but they do not properly correct deviations above or below the mean predicted QT at any range of RR. This error causes serious problems in deriving normal limits.

There is a simple algebraic reason behind this anomaly.[15] As well known, QT increases strongly with increasing RR, thus requiring rate adjustment. However, QT variance (and thus the standard deviation [SD]) remains relatively constant at all ranges of RR. Consider ($QT_{50\%} + L$) as an upper normal limit of the QT distribution at a given value of RR, with $L = 2*SD$ and $QT_{50\%}$ the median QT. When the adjustment is made as:

$$(QT_{50\%} + L)/RR^{1/2} = (QT_{50\%}/RR^{1/2}) + L/RR^{1/2} \quad [11.3]$$

the division of $QT_{50\%}$ by $RR^{1/2}$ properly adjusts the median (and the mean) QT. However, L no longer remains constant. It decreases in a nonlinear fashion with increasing RR, producing an error similar to error type 1. Error type 2 is independent of the value of the regression coefficient. Collectively, errors 1 and 2 distort the upper as well as the lower normal limits whereby the normal range becomes narrower for heart rates below 60 cpm and widens at heart rates above 60 cpm, as seen from Figure 11.5.

11.4.3 Commonly Used Normal Limits – an Additional Error

This third error is inherent to all normal limits even if appropriately derived adjustment functions are applied. QT distributions at different heart rate ranges deviate considerably from Gaussian normal distributions (rate-variant skew and kurtosis). This problem invalidates nearly all normal limits established, including normal limits derived for the otherwise reasonable so-called bin methods.[16,17] Normal limits have to be established from actual percentile distributions of adjusted QT values at each HR range of interest rather than assuming normal distributions and using (mean ± 2*SD). Properly established rate-specific QT adjustment functions and the corresponding normal standards for QT and QT subintervals are listed in Table 11.1, reproduced from Table A3 in Section A of Part 2 of this book.

Equation 11.4 shows the proper format for using the power functions for QT rate correction:[15]

$$QTa = QT - C2*RR^n, \quad [11.4]$$

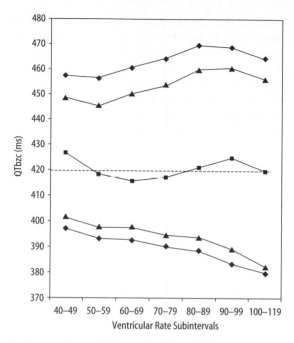

FIGURE 11.5 Median values (*squares*) and upper and lower second and fifth percentiles (*diamonds* and *triangles*, respectively) for QT adjusted by Bazett's formula corrected for intercept and adjusted for gender (*QTbzc*). The corrections make the median relatively trend free but fail to regularize normal limits due to inverse proportional scaling of the adjusted QT. (Source: Rautaharju et al.[15] J Cardiovasc Electrophysiol 2002;13:1211–18. Copyright © 2002. Reproduced with permission from Blackwell Futura Publishing, Inc.)

where QTa is the adjusted QT and n is the exponent of the power function. Equation 11.5 is an expression equivalent to Equation 11.4, with QT adjusted to heart rate 60 cpm (RR = 1) so that there is no adjustment at that heart rate:

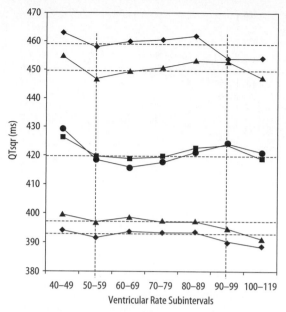

FIGURE 11.6 QT adjusted to square root of RR (*QTsqr*) with a regression function of the type QTa = QT + k*(1 − RRⁿ) where QTa is the adjusted QT and n = 1/2 (or any other exponent between 1/3 and 1). The upper and lower normal limits are rate-invariant in the range of normal heart rates within 1%. (Source: Rautaharju et al.[15] J Cardiovasc Electrophysiol 2002;13:1211–18. Copyright © 2002. Reproduced with permission from Blackwell Futura Publishing, Inc.)

$$QTa = QT + (C2*(1 − RR)). \qquad [11.5]$$

With an appropriate format of the adjustment function, any power function with an exponent between 1/3 and 1 (linear function of RR) can be used for QT rate adjustment, including the square root function, as demonstrated by Figure 11.6. A

TABLE 11.1 Race-specific QT adjustment functions, R-square values for the corresponding prediction function, mean values, standard deviations, and upper and lower second and fifth percentile normal limits.

Ethnicity	Adjustment function	R^2	Mean; SD	2% → 98%	5% → 95%
White	QTrr = QT + 183 * [1 − RR]	0.73	415; 14.1	388 → 449	394 → 439
Black	QTrr = QT + 186 * [1 − RR]	0.72	414; 15.2	383 → 453	392 → 442
Hispanic	QTrr = QT + 193 * [1 − RR]	0.60	413; 19.6	389 → 451	393 → 440
American–Indian	QTrr = QT + 186 * [1 − RR]	0.73	413; 13.6	†	395 → 443
Asian	QTrr = QT + 180 * [1 − RR]	0.66	420; 16.2	395 → 460	398 → 451

QTrr QT adjusted as a linear function of RR, *RR* RR interval(s). Adjusted intervals are in ms; *SD* standard deviation. † Upper and lower second percentile limits for American–Indian women were not determined because of too small sample size. Source: Rautaharju et al.[19] Am J Cardiol 2006;97:309–15. Copyright © 2006 Elsevier. Reproduced with permission from Elsevier.

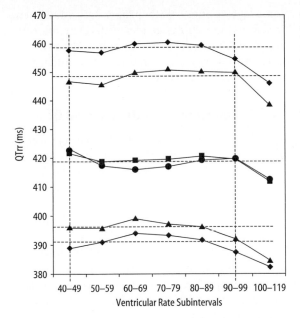

FIGURE 11.7 Mean values (*squares*) and medians (*spheres*) with upper and lower second and fifth percentiles (*diamonds* and *tri angles*, respectively) for QT adjusted by linear function of RR (*QTrr*). Although small but notable nonlinear higher order (quadratic) trends are seen in the upper and lower limits for QTrr, regularized normal limits are obtained within 5 ms (1%) in the range of normal sinus rate. (Source: Rautaharju et al.[15] J Cardiovasc Electrophysiol 2002;13:1211–18. Copyright © 2002. Reproduced with permission from Blackwell Futura Publishing, Inc.)

more extensive experience in diverse populations has revealed, however, that the simple adjustment with QT as a linear function of RR of the form QTrr = QT + k*(1 − RR) produces a stable QT adjustment within normal heart rates and generally avoids residual nonlinear trends in the adjusted QT distributions with heart rate (Figure 11.7).

11.4.4 QT Adjustment for QRS Duration

The QRS duration potentially influences the QT interval even with normal ventricular conduction. This is so because the QT interval in any ventricular myocardial region is the sum of the excitation time and the APD, as noted repeatedly previously. This would seem to suggest that QT is strongly dependent on the QRS interval. However, APD tends to shorten with excitation time, in most myocardial regions more than the delay in excita-

tion time. For these reasons, QRS duration has practically a negligible effect on the mean rate-adjusted QT and the normal limits as long as ventricular conduction remains normal.[23] The JT interval is much more strongly dependent on QRS duration than the QT interval. The QRS interval has to be incorporated as a covariate with the RR interval in JT adjustment functions.

The fact that QRS duration does not notably influence the mean QT interval or normal limits established in carefully selected healthy subjects does not imply that QRS duration is not associated with prolonged QT interval in total community-based or clinical populations because these populations include normal as well as clinically abnormal subgroups.

The QRS duration becomes an important determinant of the QT interval in ventricular conduction defects, and it has to be incorporated with proper weight as a covariate with RR in QT adjustment.[23] Just subtracting QRS duration from QTbz as proposed by some investigators[24,25] inherits the problems associated with QTbz, and normal standards for QT prolongation in bundle branch blocks are not valid with this approach.

11.5 Demographic Determinants of Rate-adjusted QT

11.5.1 Racial Differences in Rate-adjusted QT

A recent publication from the Atherosclerosis in Communities (ARIC) study reported that in a subgroup of healthy 45- to 64-year-old men and women, the rate-adjusted QT (Bazett's formula) was 6 ms shorter in African–American men than in white men and 2 ms shorter in African–American women than in white women.[18] The healthy subgroup of the ARIC study had a relatively small sample of African–Americans (116 men and 377 women).

In our standard normal adult population (in Part 2 of this book) stratified by age, QTrr was equal in African–American and white men (422 ms) and again equal (418 ms) in African–American and white women in age groups 60 years old and older. In age group 40–59 years,

QTrr was 1ms longer in African–American than in white men and 2ms shorter in African–American than in white women.

In a large population of racially diverse postmenopausal women, QTrr mean differences comparing other racial groups with white women were practically negligible, except that the median QTrr was 6ms longer and the upper second and fifth percentile limits 10ms longer in Asian women than in white women.[19] The factors associated with the longer QTrr in Asian women remain to be investigated in future studies. Otherwise, racial differences in rate-adjusted QT can be considered small and of little practical significance. It is obvious that in general, gender and age have a more pronounced influence on the rate-adjusted QT than ethnicity.

11.5.2 Gender Differences in Rate-adjusted QT

Early electrocardiographers already recognized that the QT interval tends to be longer in women than in men. The reported magnitude of the gender difference varies. A gender adjustment of 15ms in younger adults and approximately 10ms in adults 40 years old and older has been recommended.[20] Commonly used limits for QT prolongation in drug evaluation for Bazett's QTc are 20ms longer in women than in men (470ms versus 450ms).[21] Gender difference in QT has been documented to arise because the rate-adjusted QT shortens in adolescent boys.[22] In adults, the gender difference after adolescence gradually decreases, and at age 60 and older, the normal rate-adjusted QT may actually become longer in men than in women, as seen also from Table 11.2. The often-used 20-ms higher limit for QT in women is in part due to erratic rate adjustment with Bazett's formula and the gender difference in heart rate in

some age groups. With proper QT adjustment functions, the 20-ms gender difference for rate-adjusted QT is misleading in adults 50 years and older, and it may result in erroneous conclusions about QT prolongation.

11.5.3 Age Trends in Rate-adjusted QT

The observations above indicate that age trends differ between adult men and in women. In women, the age trend remains small or negligible in comparison with other determinants of QT. In younger men, it is essential to adjust QT prolongation limits, or to use age-specific QT adjustment functions.[13] After the age of 50 years, it seems unnecessary to use QT adjustment formulas for age in men. The apparent trend towards increasing adjusted QT after age 50 may merely reflect the presence of subclinical disease rather than a normal aging pattern.

11.5.4 Overweight and QT Prolongation

Several studies have reported progressively increasing QTbz with increasing relative body weight or body mass index (BMI). QT >440ms (QTbz) was present in approximately 26% of the subjects with BMI >40 mg/m^2 (morbid obesity).[30] Frank et al. performed statistical evaluation of the association of obesity with QT interval in a group of 1,029 subjects with overweight ranging from minimal to severe obesity.[31] None of the patients were on cardioactive drugs. QTbz was prolonged ≥420ms in 28% of the study group. Relative body weight was determined as a percentage of the midpoint of the ideal weight for each height category according to the Metropolitan Life Insurance Company table. There was a modest but significant association in cross-sectional data between relative body weight and QTbz ($r = 0.10$, $p =$

TABLE 11.2 Mean values and standard deviations of rate-adjusted QT (QTrr) by race- and gender-specific adjustment functions[†] in normal adults 40–94 years old by age and race.

Age group (years)	White men		Black men		White women		Black women	
	n	Mean (SD)	n	Mean (SD)	n	Mean (SD)	n	Mean (SD)
40–59	1,478	414.0 (13.3)	452	415.0 (16.2)[‡]	2,252	419.6 (16.1)	778	419.3 (15.0)[‡]
60–94	2,337	422.4 (15.2)	459	421.7 (15.9)	2,312	418.2 (16.7)	639	418.0 (17.0)

[†] QTrr = QT + 185 * (1 − RR) + 6ms in white men, QTrr = QT + 182 * (1 − RR) in white women, QTrr = QT + 181 * (1 − RR) + 6ms in black men and QTrr = QT + 188 * (1 − RR) in black women; SD standard deviation; [‡] $P < 0.001$.

0.0008). The linear regression equation revealed that there was a 1-ms increase in QTbz for each 10% increment in relative body weight. This can be compared with an approximately 3-ms increase in QRS duration and a 5-ms increase in PR interval with 100% increase in relative body weight. The increase in QTbz with overweight was independent of age, gender and blood pressure.

Peiris et al. determined obesity by hydrostatic weighing and intra-abdominal fat distribution by computerized tomography in 27 obese premenopausal women.[32] These investigators found that intra-abdominal fat was significantly associated with prolongation of QTbz independent of obesity per se and other cardiovascular risk factors.

11.5.5 Weight Loss and QT Prolongation

Rapid weight loss on unbalanced low calorie diets has been suspected to be associated with fatal cardiac events, occasionally possibly due to QT prolongation.[33] Weight loss with a proper low calorie diet has been reported to be associated with QT shortening without adverse cardiac events. Carella et al. observed 522 obese patients in a 26-week intervention program.[34] QT interval was measured visually and also by a computer program (mean QTbz was 420 ms and 410 ms by visual and computer measurement, respectively, with SE 3 ms for both). Although the data pre-

sented are to some extent difficult to reconstruct, there appeared to be a significant association between QTbz and body fat mass evaluated in a smaller subgroup with hydrodensitometry. Furthermore, there was an approximately 20-ms decrease in QTbz after the initial 6- to 10-week very low calorie diet in 46 patients with weight loss more than 23 kg or with pre-diet QTbz ≥440 ms.

11.6 Correlates of QT Prolongation in Older Adults

The Cardiovascular Health Study (CHS) investigators evaluated correlates of QT prolongation in their study population of men and women 65 years old and older representing random samples from four US communities.[26] QT prolongation was defined by an older formula for rate adjustment: the QT prolongation index (QTI). QTI >110% is the upper 2.5% limit for a normal rate-corrected QT established in a large, clinically normal, North American population sample.[13] Multivariate logistic regression analysis revealed several electrocardiographic and other subclinical and clinical factors that have an independent association with QT prolongation, as shown in Table 11.3.

TABLE 11.3 Odds ratios (95% confidence intervals) for prolonged QT for variables significantly associated with QT prolongation.

	Entered individually OR (95% CI)	Entered simultaneously OR (95% CI)
Dichotomous variables:		
Female gender	1.81 (1.50, 2.19)	3.01 (2.42, 3.76)
Digitalis use	0.90 (0.64, 1.27)	0.39 (0.26, 0.58)
Diuretic use	2.20 (1.84, 2.65)	1.73 (1.43, 2.11)
Class 1A antiarrhythmic use	4.08 (2.57, 6.46)	4.41 (2.58, 7.54)
Continuous variables (increment):		
Age (8 years)	1.31 (1.16, 1.48)	1.19 (1.04, 1.37)
Systolic blood pressure (28 mmHg)	1.61 (1.45, 1.80)	1.31 (1.13, 1.51)
Diastolic blood pressure (15 mmHg)	1.29 (1.15, 1.46)	1.21 (1.05, 1.39)
QRS duration (14 ms)	1.79 (1.58, 2.03)	1.89 (1.63, 2.18)
ECG-LVM (27 g/m^2)	1.54 (1.41, 1.69)	1.25 (1.13, 1.39)
Cardiac infarction/injury score (14 units)	1.59 (1.43, 1.78)	1.43 (1.26, 1.62)
Serum potassium (0.4 mEq/l)	0.74 (0.67, 0.81)	–

OR odds ratio, *CI* confidence interval, *ECG-LVM* ECG estimate of left ventricular mass. Source: modified from Rautaharju et al.[26] Am J Cardiol 1994;73:999–1002. © 1994 the American Journal of Cardiology. Reproduced with permission from Elsevier.

A 14-ms increment in QRS duration was associated with an 89% increased risk of prolonged QT. Women were three times more likely than men to have prolonged QT. The strongest association with prolonged QT was observed for Class 1A antiarrhythmics, still in clinical use at the time CHS was initiated. Men and women using diuretics had a risk of QT prolongation increased by 73%. Other factors with an independent association with prolonged QT included ECG evidence of myocardial injury as reflected by an increased Cardiac Injury Score,[27] increased left ventricular mass by an ECG model (ECG-LVM),[28,29] systolic and diastolic blood pressure, and age. Digitalis use was associated with a significantly decreased risk of QT prolongation. The likelihood of QT prolongation increased with increasing age.

11.7 Mechanism of QT Prolongation in Women

What could possible explain the threefold excess in prolonged QT in women, after adjustment for a variety of other factors associated with prolonged QT? QRS duration is shorter in women than in men. With a smaller ventricular mass one would expect ECG intervals in general to be shorter in women than in men, assuming that there is no significant difference in ventricular conduction velocity.

As noted before, the gender difference is age-dependent and is due to a QT shortening in males at puberty, rather than QT prolongation in females.[22] After puberty, the rate-adjusted QT interval increases in men linearly and at age 60 years and older, the gender difference practically disappears. The rate-adjusted QT remains remarkably constant in normal adult women.

The total serum calcium levels are lower in women during reproductive years than in men in the corresponding age groups.[35] Low total serum calcium level is associated with prolongation of the QT interval. It is not known how significant is the gender difference in serum calcium level in explaining the gender difference in QT or how the development of osteoporosis in postmenopausal women might influence these trends. In the absence of data about ionized serum calcium levels this question will remain open.

11.7.1 The Role of Hormonal and Genetic Factors

It is tempting to speculate that increased androgen activity following puberty in males is associated with the basic mechanisms producing the gender difference in rate-adjusted QT. The gradually decreasing level of androgen activity (hypogonadal state) in adult men[36] may be associated with the gradually decreasing gender difference in rate-adjusted QT. The continuing age-trend towards longer QT in middle-aged and older men and a similar smaller age-trend in postmenopausal women may also reflect the changing balance in sex hormone levels in addition to abnormal structural/histological changes with evolving coronary heart disease (CHD) and hypertension (ventricular conduction problems, remodeling with LVH and MI, etc.). Androgen deficiency in a variety of diseased conditions such as end-stage liver disease[37] prolongs ventricular repolarization. There is a significant prolongation of repolarization in men following castration and the change is reversed by testosterone. Also, repolarization is shorter in women with virilization than in normal women as shown by Bidoggia et al. in a pair-matched study.[38] These authors also demonstrated a significant gender difference in the ST-T patterns of healthy men and women.[39]

Androgen is known to modulate outward potassium channel currents and rate-dependent QT in rabbits.[40,41] Androgen receptors have been demonstrated to be present in atrial and ventricular myocardial cells of female rhesus monkeys and baboons.[42] Cardiac myocytes of multiple mammalian species, including humans, express the gene encoding an androgen receptor, and androgens produce a hypertrophic response acting directly on cardiac muscle cells.[43] In contrast, equivocal documentation of the existence of estrogen and progesterone receptors in ventricular myocardium is lacking.[44] This may explain the small, clinically nearly negligible effect of hormone replacement therapy on the QT interval in postmenopausal women.[45–47] A Women's Health Initiative (WHI) report concluded that estrogen alone mildly prolongs QT and the effect is reversed by progesterone.[48] Interestingly, another recent study demonstrated that although there was no significant change in QTc, the QT rate sensitivity is nearly doubled with estrogen replacement.[47]

11.7.2 Glucose Tolerance, Diabetes, Autonomic Neuropathy, and QT Prolongation

Several clinical studies have demonstrated that the rate-corrected QT is prolonged in diabetic patients with autonomic neuropathy.[49–53] An Italian study in a random sample of 379 type 1 diabetic patients reported the prevalence of QTc prolongation (>440 ms) to be 31% in the group with autonomic neuropathy, compared to 24% of diabetics without neuropathy and 8% of nondiabetic control subjects.[54]

Not all clinical studies have found a significant association between prolonged QTc and autonomic neuropathy. Kirvelä et al. compared QTc measured from 24-hour ECG recordings of 12 diabetic and 11 nondiabetic uremic patients and 12 control subjects and found no significant differences between the three study groups in the mean 24-hour QTc values or between mean QT measured at comparable heart rates of 70, 80, 90, or 100 cpm.[55] The authors concluded that the QT interval cannot be used as a diagnostic index of cardiac autonomic neuropathy. Similar conclusions were drawn by Bravenboer et al.[56] who found no significant correlation between QTc and various autonomic function tests (five cardiovascular tests and pupillometry).

In another study, lengthening of the QT interval during hypoglycemia induced by hyperinsulinemic glucose clamps was observed in a small group of diabetic patients, and furthermore, QTc prolongation was found to be correlated with the rise of adrenaline both in insulin-dependent and noninsulin-dependent diabetic patients.[57] Plasma potassium decrease was also greater in noninsulin-dependent diabetics during hypoglycemia than during euglycemic periods but not in insulin-dependent diabetics.

Fasting glucose, insulin, C-peptide, and glucose levels 1 and 2 hours after an oral glucose load were significantly associated with QTc in the Zutphen study.[58] After an adjustment for CHD risk factors, C-peptide and the area under the glucose curve remained significant, independently additive predictors of QTc duration. Although no direct measure of insulin sensitivity was available, these indirect markers of insulin resistance suggest that QTc prolongation may be part of the insulin resistance syndrome.

QT adjusted by power function (exponent 0.35 in men and 0.34 in women) had a significant inverse correlation with fasting insulin in men and with fasting plasma glucose in men (r −0.09 and −0.11, respectively) in healthy subjects in DESIR, a study on insulin resistance syndrome.[59]

The Insulin Resistance Atherosclerosis Study (IRAS) evaluated factors associated with QT interval in a large triethnic (white, Hispanic, African–American) population ($n = 1,577$).[60] Multivariate analyses revealed that hypertension and ECG-LVM were the main determinants of the rate-adjusted QT in diabetic as well as in nondiabetic subjects. QTbz increased from 437 ms in normotensive subjects with ECG-LVM below the study group median value to 452 ms in hypertensive subjects with ECG-LVM above the median value.

11.7.3 Other Factors Associated with QT Prolongation

QTc has been reported to be prolonged in patients receiving maintenance hemodialysis, with diabetes mellitus and the presence of complex ectopic ventricular complexes making an additional independent contribution.[61] Liver dysfunction in end-stage liver disease is associated with QT prolongation, considered as a marker of poor prognosis.[62] Drugs and QT prolongation will be discussed later in this chapter.

11.8 Prevalence of QT Prolongation

The prevalence of reported QT prolongation varies profoundly depending on the characteristics of the study population, type of ECG recording, QT measurement procedure, QT rate adjustment formula, and the cutpoint used for defining QT prolongation. The variation is so large that comparison of the prevalence rates of

QT prolongation in various populations is difficult and can be misleading. There is one way to cope in part with the difficulties caused by methodological differences in various studies, and that is to estimate relative QT prolongation in various studies. The relative QT prolongation, introduced as QT prolongation index,[13] expresses the relative rate-adjusted QT prolongation as a percentage ratio of the adjusted QT of the study population.

The prevalence estimates in various study groups representing community-dwelling men and women turn out to be fairly uniform, both in men and in women, at various levels of QT% or QTI. The prevalence is 25% at 4% QT prolongation, 12% at 6% prolongation, and ranges from 4 to 9% at 9% prolongation. The prevalence decreases to 4% at 10% QT prolongation and down to 2% at 12% prolongation.

The QT data from the third National Health and Nutrition Examination Survey (NHANES 3) were reprocessed with the Marquette ECG program and edited using a selective editing logic based on the measurements from two computer programs as described previously.[15] These data are reproduced in Table 11.4. The prevalence of an 8% QT prolongation corresponding to QTrr ≥450 ms was 3.2% in men and 4.1% in women. It was 3.7% in whites and 4.0% in blacks. The prevalence of 10% prolongation (QTrr ≥460 ms) was low in this largely normal community-based population, ranging from 1.3% to 3.2% in various subgroups.

Upper 5 and 2% normal limits derived for rate- and gender-adjusted QT were 450 and 460 ms, respectively.[19]

Using these limits and identical adjustment functions for rate and gender (6-ms adjustment

for male gender), the prevalence of QT prolongation was determined using data from a recent report from CHS.[63] In CHD-free men and women, QT prolongation prevalence was 5% at the upper 5% normal limit, and 3% at the 2% upper normal limit. In men and women with CHD, the prevalence was 7 and 8%, respectively, at the upper 5% limit, and 3% in men and 5% in women at the upper 2% normal limit. Using these upper 5 and 2% normal limits in women from the WHI,[64] QT prolongation prevalence was 5 and 2%, respectively, in CHD-free women. The corresponding prevalence in women with CHD was 7 and 4% at the upper 5 and 2% normal limit, respectively.

11.9 Mortality Risk for QT Prolongation

11.9.1 Mortality Risk for QT Prolongation in Men

Mortality data in men from the Zutphen, Amsterdam, and Rotterdam studies, and from Finland's Social Insurance Institution study are presented here. Descriptive data for these source populations are summarized in Table 11.5 and the mortality data in Table 11.6.

11.9.1.1 The Zutphen Study

The Zutphen study in the Netherlands[65] reported that population-associated risk for even modest QT prolongation (QTc ≥385 ms, two upper tertiles of the population) was very high. The study was initiated in 1960 as a component of the Seven Countries study involving population surveys of middle-aged men. QT intervals were measured visually from paper tracings, and the longest QT from leads V2, V6 and I, II or III was used to determine QTc.

After exclusion of prevalent MI cases, 851 men aged 40–60 years remained in the baseline sample for risk evaluation for the initial 15-year follow-up. QTc < 385 ms was used to define the reference group for determining risk ratios, corresponding approximately to the lowest tertile. Risk data in Table 11.6 are shown for QTbz ≥420 ms. In the initial follow-up period, the multivariate-adjusted risk ratio for CHD mortality was 4.2 (1.6, 11.4) for

TABLE 11.4 The prevalence of prolonged QT in the NHANES 3 study population at 8% and 10% prolongation of the rate- and gender-adjusted QT.

Subgroup	Subroup size*	QTrr ≥450 ms[†] Number (%)	QTrr ≥460 ms[†] Number (%)
Men	2,591	83 (3.2)	33 (1.3)
Women	2,862	122 (4.3)	51 (1.8)
Caucasian whites	4,118	151 (3.7)	62 (1.5)
African–American	1,335	54 (4.0)	22 (1.6)
All	5,453	206 (3.8)	85 (1.6)

* With all measurements available.

[†] QTrr ≥450 and ≥460 ms correspond to an 8% and 10% QT prolongation from the mean population QTrr.

TABLE 11.5 Source populations of men used in Table 11.6 for risk evaluation of QT prolongation.

Study	Baseline year	Follow-up (years)	Age (years)	Leads for QT	Reference group QT (ms)	Comparison group QT (ms)
Zutphen[65] ($n = 851$)	1960	15	40–60	I, II, III Longest QT	QTbz < 385	QTbz ≥ 420
Zutphen Pooled data	1960, 1965 and 1970	5	40–70		QTbz < 385	QTbz ≥ 420
Zutphen Older age group ($n = 720$)	1985	5	65–85		QTbz < 385	QTbz ≥ 420
Amsterdam[66] ($n = 898$) CHD-free subgroup ($n = 736$)	1953–1954	15	40–65	I, II, III Longest QT	QTbz ≤ 420	QTbz > 440
Rotterdam[67] ($n = 2,093$)	1990–1993	3–6	≥55	All 12 Global QT	QTbz < 406 QTlc < 400	QTbz ≥ 437 QTlc# ≥ 424
Finland's Social Insurance Institution[68] ($n = 5,598$)	1966–1977	23	30–59	I, II, III Longest QT	QTbin 372–410	QTbin > 430
CHD-free subgroup ($n = 5,103$)	1966–1977	23	30–59	I, II, III Longest QT	QTbin 372–410	QTbin > 430

QTc ≥420 ms. Age-adjusted risk ratio for CHD death was approximately identical to that from the multivariable-adjusted model.

Pooled data from the three overlapping 15-year follow-up periods were also used to make full use of multiple measurements. This was done using Cox proportional hazards model with time-dependent covariates, with results interpreted as risk ratios. The risk ratio from the multivariate model (with adjustment for age, systolic blood pressure, BMI, total serum cholesterol, and cigarette smoking) for CHD mortality was 4.4 (1.2, 16.4) for the group with QTc ≥420 ms. The risk ratios for incident MI and for sudden death, although larger than one, were not statistically significant. Neither the intermediate nor the long QTc was associated with excess risk in the subsequent two follow-up periods during the 1970–1985 follow-up in multivariate models for any of the endpoints except that for QTc ≥420 there was a considerably increased risk for sudden death (relative risk 3.8 [1.4,10.1]).

TABLE 11.6 Cardiovascular disease and all-cause mortality risk for male population cohorts in Table 11.5.

	QT index (%)*	At risk (%)	RR[†] (95% CI) for CVD[‡] mortality	RR[‡] for total mortality
Zutphen ($n = 851$)	≥106	12	4.2 (1.6, 11.4)	–
Zutphen Pooled data	≥106	–	4.4 (1.2, 16.4)	–
Zutphen Older age group ($n = 720$)	≥106	35	3.0 (1.2, 7.3)	–
Amsterdam ($n = 898$)	–	5	1.8 ($p < 0.05$)	1.7 ($p < 0.05$)
CHD-free subgroup ($n = 739$)		–	1.2 (n.s.)	1.5 (n.s.)
Rotterdam ($n = 2,093$)	≥104	25	1.3 (0.7, 2.4)[§]	1.5 (1.0, 2.3)[§]
	≥103	25	1.6 (0.8, 3.3)[‖]	1.5 (1.0, 2.3)[‖]
Finland's Social Insurance Institution ($n = 5,598$)	>110	4	1.42 (1.09, 1.84)[¶]	1.33 (1.08, 1.63)[¶]
CHD-free subgroup ($n = 5,103$)	>110	4	1.25 (0.92, 1.70)[¶]	1.21 (0.93,1.53)[¶]

RR relative risk, *CHD* coronary heart disease, *CVD* cardiovascular disease, *n.s.* not significant.
* QT index expressing proportional QT prolongation was determined as the per cent ratio (QTa/mean QTa) * 100, where QTa is the.rate-adjusted QT and the mean QTa is the mean (or the median) adjusted QT of the population. Not determined if the rate-adjusted mean value is not available.
[†] From models with multivariable adjustment for confounders (age-adjusted model in the Rotterdam study).
[‡] Relative risk for CHD mortality in the Zutphen study.
[§] Rate adjustment by Bazett's formula.
[‖] Rate adjustment as a linear function of RR (QTlc).
[¶] Rate adjustment by the bin method.
In all other studies, rate adjustment by Bazett's formula.

In 1985 when the initial cohort was 65–85 years old, an additional group of men from the same birth cohort was included with the survivors from the original cohort for risk evaluation. After exclusion of men in the added sample with previous MI, 720 men remained for this final 5-year follow-up of elderly men. The subgroup with QTc < 385 was again used as the reference group (approximately the lowest quartile of this subgroup). The prevalence of QTc ≥420 ms was 35%. (In 19% of the men, QTc was ≥440 ms.) The multivariable-adjusted risk ratio for CHD mortality was 3.0 (1.2–7.3); it was equally high for sudden death and not significant for incident MI. In the subgroup with QTc ≥420 ms, the age-adjusted risk ratio for incident MI was 2.8 (1.0, 7.5) and for CHD death 5.0 (1.4, 18.0).

11.9.1.2 The Amsterdam Civil Servant Study

The Amsterdam study population consisted of civil servants of the City of Amsterdam and their spouses aged 40–65 years who volunteered to participate in a general health survey during 1953–1954.[66] Participation rate was approximately 54% of the civil servants. Case-control sampling design was used to limit the number of ECGs from the "noncase" (survivor) group that had to be analyzed. A random sample from the total study group (approximately twice the number of expected cardiovascular deaths) was used for selection of the referents. With this selection, the death of a given referent may enter as an endpoint both in the referent as well as in the case group. However, in risk analysis, deaths drawn from the sample were used only once as cases to obtain a more unbiased estimate of relative risk. The selection yielded a final study group of 898 men with valid QT data. Smaller samples were available for risk analyses depending on the follow-up time, for instance 736 men from the healthy subgroup for all-cause mortality analysis in the 15-year follow-up. The healthy subgroup was also selected for risk analysis, with 205 men with a history of angina pectoris or resting ECG abnormalities excluded from this study group. The longest QT from leads I, II and III was selected for risk evaluation.

The reference group (for men and for women) for risk evaluation was the subgroup with QTc < 420 ms. In the first 15-year follow-up, the multivariable-adjusted relative risk in men for QTc > 440 ms was 1.8 for CVD deaths and 1.7 for all-cause mortality ($p < 0.05$ for both). Age appeared to be the only significant confounder in this study group. The increased all-cause mortality risk in men was mainly associated with a significant excess risk for cardiovascular and ischemic heart disease mortality, including in the subgroup of ostensibly healthy men.

In the healthy subgroup of men, the 15-year relative risk for CVD mortality was 1.2 and 1.5 for total mortality, neither of them significant probably due to smaller sample size with more pronounced QT prolongation. The 28-year risk ratio was increased by 40% for all-cause and CVD mortality, significant only for all-cause mortality ($p < 0.05$).

11.9.1.3 The Rotterdam Study

The Rotterdam study included men and women aged 55 years and older from the Ommoord district of the city.[67] Response rate was 78%. Baseline data were collected from 1990 to 1993, including a digital ECG recording in 6,160 (86%) of the participants. Excluded were participants with arrhythmias or complete bundle branch blocks. This left 2,093 men and 3,176 women with follow-up data, ECG and other data suitable for risk evaluation. The follow-up of the report covered a 3- to 6-year period (mean 4 years).

Mortality risk was evaluated for the quartiles of QT corrected for ventricular rate by five different formulas, including Bazett's QTc and QT adjusted by linear function of RR (QTlc, which is equivalent to QTrr) derived from the study population. For all-cause mortality and comparing the highest QT quartile with the lowest, there was an increased risk ranging from 50 to 80% for different rate correction formulas. The risk of cardiac mortality (including pulmonary heart disease and pulmonary embolism) was not significant in men with any of the rate correction formulas.

11.9.1.4 Finland's Social Insurance Institution's CHD Study

Risk evaluation for QT prolongation in the Finnish study was done in a representative sample of Finland's male and female population in the age

TABLE 11.7 Source populations of women for mortality risk evaluation for QT prolongation by health status.

Study group	Baseline year	Follow-up (years)	Age (years)	Leads for QT	Reference group QT* (ms)
Total groups					
Amsterdam[66] ($n = 591$)	1953–1954	15	40–65	I, II, III Longest QT	QTbz $\leq$ 420
Rotterdam[67] ($n = 3{,}176$)	1990–1993	3–6	$\geq$55	All 12 Global QT	QTbz $<$ 418
Finland's Social Insurance[69] ($n = 5{,}598$)	1966–1977	23	30–59	I, II, III Longest QT	QTbin 372–410
CHD-free subgroups					
Amsterdam ($n = 508$)	1953–1954	15	40–65	I, II, III Longest QT	QTbz $\leq$ 420
Finland's Social Insurance ($n = 5{,}129$)	1966–1977	23	30–59	I, II, III Longest QT	QTbin 378–417

* Rate adjustment by Bazett's formula (QTbz), linear function of RR (QTlc), or the nomogram (bin) method (QTbin).

range of 30–59 years.[68,69] The follow-up period was 23 years. QT rate adjustment was done in an appropriate manner as a deviation from the study population's mean QT for each range of heart rate at 5-cpm class intervals, separately for men and women. Risk analysis results in various subgroup analyses were diverse. The reference group for calculating relative risk was the group with rate-corrected QT deviation <5% from the predicted value. In the total population of the Finnish study, the relative risk adjusted for age and other risk factors in men was 2.12 (1.25–3.59) for cardiovascular mortality and 1.92 (1.23–3.00) for all-cause mortality. No significant difference was observed for relative mortality risks in the subgroup of healthy men after adjustment for age and other risk factors.

In various subgroup analyses of the Finnish study, the risk increase for prolonged QT in healthy men was significant only for sudden death in the lowest quartile of heart rate, with relative risk 2.75 (1.00–7.40). Interestingly, a shortened rate-corrected QT was associated with smoking. QT shortening over 10% was associated with excess risk of cardiovascular death in men with heart disease who smoked, with a RR 3.72 (1.45–9.54). All nonsmoking men, those with as well as those without signs of cardiovascular disease (CVD), who had a short rate-corrected QT had a low mortality risk.

11.9.2 Mortality Risk for QT Prolongation in Women

Three of the studies described above for men included women. Descriptive data for these female populations are summarized in Table 11.7 and the mortality data in Table 11.8.

TABLE 11.8 Cardiovascular disease and all-cause mortality for female populations from Table 11.7 by health status.

	Comparison group QT* (ms)	QT index[†] (%)	At risk (%)	RR[‡] (95% CI) for CVD mortality	RR[‡] (95% CI) for total mortality
Total groups					
Amsterdam ($n = 591$)	QTbz $>$ 440	–	16	1.4 (n.s.)	1.6 ($p < 0.05$)
Rotterdam ($n = 3{,}176$)	QTbz $\geq$ 446	$\geq$103	25	2.4 (1.1, 5.3)	1.9 (1.3, 2.9)
	QTlc $\geq$ 424	$\geq$103	25	2.1 (1.1, 4.2)	1.7 (1.2, 2.4)
Finland's Social Insurance Institution ($n = 5{,}598$)	QTbin $>$ 437	$>$110	4	1.32 (0.89, 1.97)	0.98 (0.70, 1.37)
CHD-free subgroups					
Amsterdam ($n = 508$)	QTbz $>$ 440	–	–	1.7 (n.s.)	1.6 (n.s.)
Finland's Social Insurance ($n = 5{,}129$)	QTbin $>$ 437	$>$108	3	1.28 (0.80, 2.02)	0.91 (0.62, 1.34)

n.s. not significant, *RR* relative risk.

* Rate adjustment by Bazett's formula (QTbz), linear function of RR (QTlc), or the nomogram (bin) method (QTbin).

† QT index expressing proportional QT prolongation was determined as the per cent ratio (QTa/mean QTa) $*$ 100, where QTa is the rate-adjusted QT and QTa is the mean (or the median) adjusted QT of the population. (Cannot be determined if the rate adjusted mean value is not available.)

‡ From models with multivariable adjustment for confounders (age-adjusted model in the Rotterdam study).

Only the Rotterdam study found a significantly increased CVD mortality risk for QT prolongation in women. In that study, the risk ratios for cardiac mortality ranged from 1.7 to 2.4, and they were significant for three of the five rate-correction formulas, including Bazett's formula and the linear regression formula. For these two formulas, the excess risk for the upper QT quartile compared with the lowest quartile was approximately twofold for CVD and total mortality.

The relative risk in the Amsterdam study was increased by 40% for CHD mortality (not significant) and by 60% for all-cause mortality ($p < 0.05$). In the Finnish study, there was no significant association between QT prolongation and CVD or total mortality risk. In two of the studies in Table 11.8 with risk data reported for women (the Amsterdam study and the Finnish study), none of the risk estimates was significant for CHD or all-cause mortality in CHD-free women.

11.9.3 Mortality Risk Reports from Combined Male and Female Populations

Three of the studies reported risk data for QTbz in combined male and female populations: the Glastrup study,[70] the Framingham Heart Study,[71] and the CHS (Table 11.9).[72] The data from these studies are summarized in Tables 11.9 and 11.10. The Glastrup study reported QT data for the total population and for a CHD-free subgroup, and also the Framingham Heart Study and the CHS had CHD-free subgroups. The CHS reported risk data separately for the subgroup with prior CHD. It should also be noted that the Framingham risk data for baseline QT are for a very long follow-up, 30 years.

11.9.3.1 The Clastrup Study

This Danish population health survey[70] reported risk data from a cohort of 3,455 subjects (1,797 men and 1,658 women). The initial sample was 3,780 (approximately 80% participation rate), approximately 450 subjects in each age and gender stratum 30, 40, 50 or 60 years of age. Excluded were subjects with bundle branch block or arrhythmias or those with less than nine leads with measurable QT. Visual QT measurements were made using a digitizing tablet. QT rate adjustment was with Bazett's formula, determined for the mean QT of all measurable leads. The follow-up time was 13 years.

Separate risk analyses were done in a subgroup of 2,269 clinically normal participants (without circulatory or other disease), who had a normal blood pressure, were not on any medical therapeutic treatment, and who had a normal ECG according to the Minnesota Code. Mean QTc in the total group was 405 (SD 25) ms and in the normal group 400 (SD 23) ms. The reference group for risk evaluation was the subgroup with QTc 380 ms (12.4% of the total group and 15.4% of the normal group). The cutpoint for identification of the long QTc group was 440 ms (prevalence 9.1% in the total group and 5.1% in the normal group). In the total cohort, the relative risk of cardiovascular mortality for QTc ≥440 ms (prevalence 9.1%) was 3.31 (1.04, 9.91) and of all-cause mortality 1.89 (1.04, 3.37). QTc 440 ms corresponds to QTc prolongation by approximately 9%

TABLE 11.9 Characteristics of populations from three studies used for mortality risk evaluation in Table 11.10 in combined gender groups by health status at baseline.

Population	Baseline year	Follow-up (years)	Age (years)	Leads for QT	Reference group QT* (ms)	Comparison group QT* (ms)
Total populations						
Glastrup study[70] ($n = 3,455$)	1982–1984	11[†]	30–60	All 12, mean QT	QTbz < 380	QTbz > 440
CHD-free populations						
Glastrup study[70] ($n = 2,269$)	1982–1984	11[†]	30–60	All 12, mean QT	QTbz < 380	QTbz > 440
Framingham[71] ($n = 5,125$)	1948	30	30–62	All 12, longest QT	QTbz < 360	QTbz ≥ 440
CHS[72] ($n = 4,129$)	1989–1990	9	≥65	Global QT	QTbz ≤ 410	QTbz ≥ 450
Prior CHD CHS[72] ($n = 859$)	1989–1990	9	≥65	Global QT	QTbz ≤ 410	QTbz ≥ 450

CHD coronary heart disease, *CHS* Cardiovascular Health Study.

* Rate adjustment by Bazett's formula (QTbz).

† 13 years for total mortality.

from the mean QTc of the population. In the normal subgroup, QTc had no significant association with CHD or total mortality. There were too few cardiovascular deaths in this subgroup to carry out meaningful risk evaluation.

11.9.3.2 The Framingham Heart Study

The well-known Framingham Heart Study evaluated the risk of total mortality, sudden cardiac death, and coronary artery disease mortality for QTbz in 5,125 men and women of the original cohort of 5,209 persons, between ages 30 and 62 at baseline.[71] Excluded were subjects with CHD or who were taking medications potentially influencing QT. QT and RR intervals were measured manually. The average of two to three complexes from the lead with the longest QT was taken as the representative QT. Risk analysis was done in the pooled group of men and women and separately in men and in women in quintiles covering the following five ranges of QTbz: <0.36 s, $0.36–0.38$ s, $0.39–0.40$ s, $0.41–0.43$ s, and ≥ 0.44 s. The prevalence was 5, 15, 29, 43 and 7% in women and 15, 29, 29, 25, and 2% in men, from the lowest to the highest QTc range, respectively.

Contrary to the results from many other studies with a shorter follow-up, there was no significant association in this long-term study between QTbz prolongation and total mortality, coronary artery disease mortality or sudden death. Separate analyses by gender produced the same result, with no significant associations with any of the outcomes.

11.9.3.3 The Cardiovascular Health Study

A recent report from the CHS evaluated the risk associated with Bazett's QTc for CHD and all-cause mortality during the period up to the end of the 10th annual follow-up visit.[72] The CHS participants were 65 years old and older at the baseline of the study. Excluded from the study group were participants with ventricular conduction defects (QRS ≥ 120 ms) or atrial fibrillation. Relative risks were reported for multivariable-adjusted risk models including a variety of demographic and clinical risk factors. Interactions between gender and other demographic and CVD risk factors tested using nested likelihood ratio tests showed that none of the gender interactions was significant, and the risk data were reported for the combined gender groups. Men and women with QTbz ≤ 410 ms were taken as the reference group for risk evaluation.

Relative risks shown for CHS in Table 11.10 are listed for QTbz > 450 ms in the groups stratified by the CHD status at the baseline. QTbz 450 corresponds to a QTbz prolongation by approximately 7% compared to the average QTbz for the CHD-free subgroup of the study population. Multivariable-adjusted relative risk for CHD mortality was 1.6 (1.0, 2.5) in the CHD-free group (unadjusted risk approximately twice as high), and 2.0 (1.1, 3.7) in the group with prior CHD. The corresponding relative risk for all-cause mortality was 1.3 (1.07, 1.67) for the CHD-free group and 2.3 (1.6, 3.3) in the group with prior CHD.

TABLE 11.10 Mortality risk for QT prolongation for three studies from Table 11.7 in combined gender groups by health status at baseline.

	QT index[†] (%) of the comparison group	At risk (%)	RR[‡] (95% CI) for CHD[‡] mortality	R[‡] (95% CI) for total mortality
Total populations				
Glastrup study ($n = 3,455$)	>109	9	3.31 (1.04, 9.91)	1.89 (1.04, 3.37)
CHD-free populations				
Glastrup study ($n = 2,269$)	>109	5	–	1.17 (0.43, 2.87)
Framingham ($n = 5,125$)	≥ 113	15	0.85 (0.48, 1.50)	1.02 (0.70, 1.49)
CHS ($n = 4,129$)	≥ 107	3	1.6 (1.0, 2.5)	1.3 (1.1, 1.7)
Prior CHD CHS ($n = 859$)	≥ 107	10	2.0 (1.1, 3.7)	2.3 (1.6, 3.3)

CHD coronary heart disease, *CHS* Cardiovascular Health Study, *RR* relative risk.
* QT index expressing proportional QT prolongation was determined as the per cent ratio (QTa/mean QTa) ∗ 100, where QTa is the rate-adjusted QT and mean QTa is the mean (or the median) adjusted QT of the population.
† From models with multivariable adjustment for confounders.
‡ CVD mortality in Glastrup study.

11.9.4 Overall Conclusions about the Mortality Risk for QT Prolongation in Community-based Populations

At a 4–6% level of QT prolongation, the reported prevalence ranges from 12 to 25% in total male and female populations. The corresponding reported mortality risks of all-cause and CHD mortality in men ranges from nonsignificant to fourfold and in women from nonsignificant to twofold. In CHD-free subgroups of male populations at a 10% level of QT prolongation and 4% prevalence, the reported CVD and total mortality risk (one study) was approximately twofold for CHD and total mortality, and nonsignificant in total CHD-free female populations in most studies. In combined CHD-free male and female populations at the level 7–9% QT prolongation and 3–5% prevalence, the reported CHD and total mortality risk was nonsignificant in one study and threefold for CHD and twofold for total mortality in another study. Long-range mortality risk in one large study was nonsignificant for CHD as well as for total mortality.

11.10 Other Conditions with QT Prolongation and Increased Mortality Risk

11.10.1 Survivors of Acute Myocardial Infarction

Reports on the risk associated with QT prolongation in survivors of acute MI are not consistent; they are in fact controversial. Although some clinical reports have associated QT prolongation in survivors of acute MI with a twofold and up to a 13-fold increased mortality risk in often small groups of clinical patients,[73–75] it is not always clear how much independent predictive information is associated with QT prolongation above routine clinical cardiac assessment variables at discharge. In many clinical studies the mortality risk for QT prolongation, although generally increased, has not been significant.[76–78] For instance, Pohjola-Sintonen et al. concluded that rate-adjusted QT (QTbz) is not a useful prognostic tool after acute MI.[77]

The largest of the controlled clinical trials was the Beta Blocker Heart Attack Trial (BHAT).[79] These investigators performed a detailed assessment of the risk of total mortality, sudden and nonsudden death, and nonfatal re-infarction in 3,837 survivors of acute MI. Ten per cent of patients on antiarrhythmic drugs were excluded from risk evaluation. The remaining group was stratified approximately into three tertiles for risk evaluation for the average of 25 months follow-up. The prevalence of QT prolongation $\geq$450 ms (upper tertile) was 31%. The total death rate was significantly higher in the upper tertile group than in the mid and lower tertile groups, with an equal beneficial effect of propranolol in all tertiles of QTc.

11.10.2 QT Prolongation and Sudden Death in Hypertensive Patients

Results from a case-control study in hypertensive patients demonstrated that QT prolongation was associated with excess risk of primary cardiac arrest.[86] The study compared 131 patients who had a primary cardiac arrest with 562 controls. The controls were a stratified random sample of treated hypertensive patients. Both groups received care at a health maintenance organization. In a multivariate model adjusting for clinical characteristics and other ECG abnormalities and comparing the highest with the lowest quintile of QTI, the odds ratio for cardiac arrest was 2.1 (1.2, 2.8). The limits for the highest and the lowest QTI quintile were 111 and 99%, respectively. (The upper normal limit for QTI is 110%.)

11.11 QT Prolonging Drugs

Investigations on a possible association between pharmacological agents and QT play a prominent role in present-day electrocardiography. Ionic channel mechanisms involved in drug-induced QT prolongation were discussed in Chapter 3. The reader is advised to consult an extensive review from 2001 by Bednar et al.,[80] which contains data from no fewer than 81 studies pertaining to drug-induced QT prolongation, including many that were chronically administered at that time. The review comments on the paucity of carefully controlled clinical trials designed to study the peak drug effect on QT interval.

All new drugs, including noncardiovascular agents, must undergo rigorous testing before they will get approval by regulatory agencies. Over 100 antianginal and noncardiovascular drugs have been recognized by regulatory agencies to be associated with "QT liability".[81] A variety of drugs, mainly antiarrhythmics, can prolong QT interval, ranging from moderate to pronounced QT prolongation. Pronounced QT prolongation associated with drug action and severe clinical symptoms is called acquired LQTS. Arrhythmias considered to be associated with QT prolonging drugs (such as the antibiotic erythromycin,[82] which occasionally produces torsades de pointes arrhythmias) often have a strong female predominance for QT prolongation (like in familial inherited LQTS). Class 1A and class III antiarrhythmic drugs produce QT prolongation as their electrophysiological effect.[83] These antiarrhythmic drugs have a tendency to produce ventricular tachyarrhythmias and they have a proarrhythmic effect also in LQTS.

Class IA and class III drugs induce early afterdepolarizations that in turn may induce re-entry and torsade de pointes arrhythmia. Other factors producing increased dispersion of repolarization (due to nonuniform increase in APD, dispersion of ET or DRT) include hypokalemia, bradycardia, LVH, and female gender.

Table 3.5 in Chapter 3 categorized major classes of antiarrhythmic drugs according to the scheme by Vaugham Williams. The categories were largely defined on the basis of QT prolonging effect. Table 3.6 in that chapter in turn categorized arrhythmogenic mechanisms, desired antiarrhythmic effect on the most likely vulnerable parameter, and ionic currents most likely to achieve the desired antiarrhythmic effect.

Several sources provide information on QT prolonging drugs, in particular in relation to torsades de pointes arrhythmia. The Arizona Center for Education and Research on Therapeutics (CERT) of the University of Arizona has a web site that includes a list of drugs that prolong the QT interval and/or induce torsades de pointes (© 2002 Arizona CERT). The July 6, 2004 update contains 117 generic drug names grouped into four categories: (1) drugs generally accepted by regulatory authorities to have a risk of causing torsades de pointes; (2) drugs that in some reports have been associated with torsades de pointes but at this time lack substantial evidence for causing this malignant arrhythmia; (3) drugs that should not be used in patients with diagnosed or suspected congenital LQTS; and (4) drugs that some reports have weakly associated with torsades de pointes but that in usually administered clinical dosages are unlikely to be a risk for torsades de pointes. The lists of QT prolonging agents are extensive.[84]

11.12 ECG Phenotypes and Long QT Syndrome

As noted at the beginning of this chapter and in Chapter 3, APD, ST-T wave morphology, and QT interval depend on a delicate balance between inward and outward currents modulated by the ionic channels during repolarization. Small changes in these individual currents during repolarization can prolong or shorten APD or alter the waveform of APD. QT prolongation is just one of the manifestations of altered ionic flow balance. Earlier ECG research in LQTS focused almost entirely on QT prolongation, mainly because it is the easiest ECG manifestation to measure. The focus has expanded recently beyond QT interval,[87–89] and future research will hopefully cover more comprehensive aspects of the analysis of ST-T morphology in amplitude-time-interval domain.

Moss et al. have documented ECG phenotypes with aberrations in ST-T morphology in family members linked to three distinct forms of LQTS, with affected genes in chromosomes 3, 7 and 11, respectively.[87] A mutation in sodium channel (α-subunit) gene (called SCN5A by gene mappers) with a locus in chromosome 3 produced an ECG phenotype with a late onset of the T wave of normal duration and amplitude. This pattern would seem to suggest a uniformly prolonged action potential plateau throughout the myocardium, with relatively unchanged fast phase of repolarization (phase 3 of the action potential) in various myocardial regions.

A defect in a gene regulating outward current during plateau (delayed rectifier potassium current [I_{Kr}] with a locus in chromosome 7) produced T waves of low amplitude. Mutations in gene KVLQT1 with a locus in chromosome 11 were associated with a broad T wave of normal amplitude. T wave morphology patterns in affected persons with LQTS in a given genotype differed substantially from the patterns in unaffected family members. The authors point out, however, that it is unlikely that an analysis of T wave morphology patterns can be used to identify accurately the genotype in individuals with suspected LQTS because multiple genetic and acquired factors can influence ventricular repolarization. The examples mentioned, however, indicate that in spite of limited specificity in various genotypes, even relatively minor alterations in specific ionic channel mechanisms regulating repolarization can cause pronounced changes in ST-T waveforms.

Lupoglazoff et al.[90] described morphologic changes in T wave patterns in Holter recordings of 32 LQT1 and LQT2 families. These investigators characterized T wave patterns as type G0 (normal), type G1 ("bulged", with a perceptible "hump" after the peak of the T wave), or type G2 (a distinct "protuberance" during the descending limb of the T wave), following the phenotypic description of Lehmann et al.[88] T wave pattern was classified as normal in 96% of the control group of 100 subjects. The majority of the subjects with LQT1 (122 of 133, 92%) had a normal T wave morphology in 92% of their Holter recordings. None had notched type G2 recordings and 11 of 133 (8%) type G1 T waves. However, the authors reported that all but one of the LQT1 subjects had a broad-based T wave. (Type G0 apparently included broad-based T waves.)

The LQT2 group had notches of type G2 in 36 of 57 cases (63%) and type G1 T waves in 10 of 57 cases (18%), suggesting that the majority of the subjects with LQT2 (83%) had aberrations of the T wave. G2 type notches were present in 15 of the 30 Holter recordings of the LQT2 patients who did not have these notches in the conventional ECG recordings. The authors speculate that the notched T waves are possibly related to I_{Kr} decrease, an indicator of genetic defects in HERG. I_{Kr} block increases dispersion of repolarization (at least in part by preferential prolongation of APD of the M cells), prolongs QT interval and produces a tall broad-based T wave with or without a notch in the descending limb when the extracellular potassium ([K^+]o) is normal.[92] Mild hypokalemia can enhance dispersion of repolarization, and severe hypokalemia has the opposite effect. It also reduces the slope of phase 3 of the APD and decreases T wave amplitude by reducing the voltage gradients. Altered voltage gradients from endocardial and epicardial regions to subepicardial M cell region can reduce T wave amplitude and enhance the notching of the T wave.

Swan et al. have documented that QT prolongation as well as clinical criteria are inadequate in distinguishing LQT1 patients from healthy relatives, and the presence of the LQTI1 gene is associated with excess risk of arrhythmic events even with no or marginal prolongation of QT.[92] It seems that analysis of the repolarization patterns will require a more careful quantification than performed in the past. The use of principal component analysis[89] is a step in the right direction, although the use of the ratio of the magnitude of the two first components to describe the complexity of the T wave still reveals only limited information of many aspects of T wave morphology.

11.13 QT Dispersion – a Dead End

There has been a considerable degree of controversy about the meaning of QTD. The basic necessary condition for the validity of the QTD concept is that there are nondipolar components in the 12-lead ECG, particularly in the terminal part of the T wave, that are not present in the first three (dipolar XYZ) components of the signal. Secondly, these nondipolar components have to be of sufficient magnitude before their presence can be identified from the usually more dominant dipolar components. A critical analysis of the ECG data of 3,844 subjects, 966 with CHD and 3,844 considered CHD-free, revealed that the mean value of the nondipolar voltage (NDPV) in T wave was 11 μV (SD 3.9), with 6 μV (SD 1.3) in the terminal 40 ms.[93] Nondipolar voltage alone explained only 6% of the total QT variance. (The T wave NDPV values were obtained from a program that produced so-called singular value decomposition, also called principal component analysis.)

Among the factors suggesting that the nondipolar components of the T wave may possibly influence QTD measurements was the observation in the above-cited study that the proportion of QTD exceeding 60 ms was significantly higher ($p < 0.001$) among subjects with NDPV exceeding 7 µV in terminal T wave than among those below this threshold, although this was observed only in the CHD-free subgroup with normal terminal T vector direction. The authors concluded that NDPV magnitude in the T wave is sufficient to potentially influence QTD in some conditions but that the association is weak and that in view of the profound methodological problems in QTD measurement, QTD cannot be considered to have a significant role in practical electrocardiography. A study by Malik et al. reached a similar conclusion.[94]

A recent review of the literature concluded that QTD is based on an unsubstantiated hypothesis.[2] An editorial accompanying the review came to the same conclusion.[3] As commented at the beginning of this chapter, the validity of this claimed relationship can be questioned. Concerning T wave nondipolar components, one retrospective study reported it to be the strongest ECG predictor of total mortality.[96] In principle, nondipolar components in the T wave are at present the only available potential measure of localized repolarization disturbances, but it remains doubtful if they are present in quantities large enough to be distinguished from the dominating influence of dipolar T wave components. The review cited above[2] offered several new alternatives to QTD, including $T_{peak}-T_{end}$ interval, T wave nondipolar components and T wave morphology changes (T wave complexity). The $T_{peak}-T_{end}$ interval is proposed as a measure of transmural dispersion of repolarization. Like the measured QTD, these are all manifestations of the changed sequence of repolarization – not necessarily markers of some substrate initiating malignant arrhythmias.

References

1. Lux RL, Fuller MS, MacLeaod RS et al. Noninvasive indices of repolarization and its dispersion. J Electrocardiol 1999;32:153–7.

2. Shah RR. Drug-induced QT dispersion: does it predict the risk of torsade de pointes? J Electrocardiol 2005;38:10–18.

3. Rautaharju PM. A farewell to QT dispersion. Are the alternatives any better? Invited editorial. J Electrocardiol 2005;38:7–9.

4. Lee RJ, Liem LB, Cohen TJ, Franz MR. Relation between repolarization and refractoriness in the human ventricle: cycle length dependence and effect of procainamid. J Am Coll Cardiol 1992;19:614–18.

5. Kuo C-S, Munakata K, Reddy CP, Surawicz B. Characteristics and possible mechanism of ventricular arrhythmia dependent on the dispersion of action potential durations. Circulation 1983;67:1356–67.

6. Vassallo JA, Cassidy DM, Kindwall KA et al. Nonuniform recovery of excitability in the left ventricle. Circulation 1988;78:1365–72.

7. Cranefield PF. Action potentials, afterpotentials, and arrhythmias. Circ Res 1977;41:415–23.

8. Rosen MR, Reder RF. Does triggered activity have a role in the genesis of cardiac arrhythmias? Ann Intern Med 1981;94:794–801.

9. Sicouri S, Fish J, Antzelevitch C. Distribution of M cells in the canine ventricle. J Cardiovasc Electrophysiol 1994;5:824–37.

10. Sicouri S, Antzelevitch C. A subpopulation of cells with unique electrophysiological properties in the deep subendocardium of the canine ventricle. The M cell. Circ Res 1991;68:1729–41.

11. Bazett HC. An analysis of the time-relations of electrocardiograms. Heart 1920;7:353–70.

12. Simonson. E. Differentiation between Normal and Abnormal in Electrocardiography. St. Louis: The CV Mosby Company, 1961, p 158.

13. Rautaharju PM, Warren JW, Calhoun HP. Estimation of QT prolongation: a persistent, avoidable error in computer electrocardiography. J Electrocardiol 1991;23:111–17.

14. Hnatkova K, Malik M. "Optimum" formulae for heart rate correction of the QT interval. Pacing Clin Electrophysiol 1999;22:1683–7.

15. Rautaharju PM, Zhang ZM. Linearly scaled, rate-invariant normal limits for QT interval. Eight decades of incorrect application of power functions. J Cardiovasc Electrophysiol 2002;13:1211–18.

16. Karjalainen J, Viitasalo M, Mänttäri M, Manninen V. Relation between QT intervals and heart rates from 40 to 120 beats/min in rest electrocardiograms of men and a simple method to adjust QT interval values. J Am Coll Cardiol 1994;23:1547–53.

17. Sagie A, Larson MG, Goldberg RJ et al. An improved method for adjusting the QT interval for heart rate

(the Framingham Heart Study). Am J Cardiol 1992; 70:797–801.

18. Vitelli LL, Crow RS, Shahar E et al. Electrocardiographic findings in a healthy biracial population. Am J Cardiol 1998;81:453–9.

19. Rautaharju PM, Prineas R, Kadish A et al. Normal standards for QT and QT subintervals derived from a large ethnically diverse population of women aged 50 to 79 years (the Women's Health Initiative [WHI]). Am J Cardiol 2006;97:730–7.

20. Surawicz B, Parikh SR. Differences between ventricular repolarization in men and women: description, mechanism and implications. Ann Noninvasive Electrocardiol 2003;8:333–40.

21. US Food and Drug Administration/Health Canada. The clinical evaluation of QT/QTc interval prolongation and proarrhythmic potential for non-antiarrhythmic drugs. Preliminary Concept Paper, 15 November 2002.

22. Rautaharju PM, Zhou SH, Wong S. Differences in the evolution of the electrocardiographic QT interval with age. Can J Cardiol 1992;8:690–5.

23. Rautaharju PM, Zhang ZM, Prineas R, Heiss G. Assessment of prolonged QT and JT intervals in ventricular conduction defects. Am J Cardiol 2004; 93:1017–21.

24. Das G. QT interval and repolarization time in patients with intraventricular conduction delay. J Electrocardiol 1990;23:49–52.

25. Crow RS, Hannan PJ. Prognostic significance of corrected QT and corrected JT interval for incident CHD in a general population sample stratified by presence or absence of wide QRS complex: the ARIC Study with 13 years follow-up. Circulation 1993;108:1985–9.

26. Rautaharju PM, Manolio TA, Psaty BM et al. Correlates of QT prolongation in older adults (the Cardiovascular Health Study). Am J Cardiol 1994;73:999–1002.

27. Rautaharju PM, Warren JW, Jain U et al. Cardiac infarction injury score: an electrocardiographic coding scheme for ischemic heart disease. Circulation 1981;64:249–66.

28. Rautaharju PM, Park LP, Gottdiener JS et al. Race- and gender-specific ECG models for ECG-LVM in older populations. Factors influencing overestimation of left ventricular hypertrophy prevalence by ECG criteria in African-Americans. J Electrocardiol 2000;33:205–18.

29. Rautaharju PM, Manolio TA, Siscovick D et al. for the Cardiovascular Health Study Collaborative Research Group. Utility of new electrocardiographic models for left ventricular mass in older adults. Hypertension 1996;28:8–15.

30. El-Gamal A, Callagher D, Nawras A et al. Effects of obesity on QT, RR, and QTc intervals. Am J Cardiol 1995;75:956–9.

31. Frank S, Colliver JA, Frank A. The electrocardiogram in obesity: statistical analysis of 1,029 patients. J Am Coll Cardiol 1986;7:295–9.

32. Peiris AN, Thakur RK, Sothmann MS et al. Relationship of regional fat distribution to electrocardiographic parameters in healthy premenopausal women. Southern Med J 1991;84:961–91.

33. Isner JM, Sours HE, Paris AL et al. Sudden, unexpected death in avid dieters using liquid-protein-modified fast diet. Circulation 1979;60:1401–12.

34. Carella MJ, Mantz SL, Rovner DR et al. Obesity, adiposity, and lengthening of the QT interval: improvement after weight loss. Int J Obes Relat Metab Disord 1996;20:938–42.

35. Werner M, Tolls RE, Hultin JV, Melleker J. Influence of sex and age on the nominal range of eleven serum constituents. Z Klin Chem Klin Biochem 1970;8:105–15.

36. Gray A, Feldman HA, McKinlay JB, Longcope C. Age, disease, and changing sex hormone levels in middle-aged men: results of the Massachusetts Male Aging Study. J Clin Endocrinol Metab 1991; 73:1016–25.

37. Mohamed R, Forcey PR, Davies MK, Neuberger JM. Effect of liver transplantation on QT prolongation and autonomic dysfunction in end-stage liver disease. Hepatology 1996;23:1128–34.

38. Bidoggia H, Maciel JP, Capalozza N et al. Sex differences on the electrocardiographic pattern of cardiac repolarization: possible role of testosterone. Am Heart J 2000;140:678–83.

39. Bidoggia H, Maciel JP, Capalozza N et al. Sex-dependent electrocardiographic pattern of cardiac repolarization. Am Heart J 2000;140:430–6.

40. Drici MD, Burklow TR, Haridasse V et al. Sex hormones prolong the QT interval and downregulate potassium channel expression in the rabbit heart. Circulation 1996;94:1471–4.

41. Hara M, Danilo P Jr, Rosen MR. Effects of gonadal steroids on ventricular repolarization and on the response to E4031. J Pharmacol Exper Therap 1998; 285:1068–72.

42. McGill HC Jr, Anselmo VC, Buchanan JM, Sheridan PJ. The heart is a target organ for androgen. Science 1980;207:775–7.

43. March JD, Lehmann MH, Ritchie RH et al. Androgen receptors mediate hypertrophy in cardiac myocytes. Circulation 1998;98:256–61.

44. Lin AL, Schultz JJ, Brenner RM, Shain SA. Sexual dimorphism characterizes baboon myocardial androgen receptors but not myocardial estrogen

and progesterone receptors. J Steroid Biochem Mol Biol 1990;37:85–95.

45. Carnethon MR, Anthony MS, Cascio WE et al. A prospective evaluation of the risk of QT prolongation with hormone replacement therapy: the Atherosclerosis Risk in Communities Study. Ann Epidemiol 2003;13:530–6.

46. Larsen JA, Tung RH, Sadanandra R et al. Effects of hormone replacement therapy on QT interval. Am J Cardiol 1998;82:993–5.

47. Kadish AH, Greenland P, Limacher MC et al. Estrogen and progestin use and the QT interval in postmenopausal women. Ann Noninvasive Electrocardiol 2004;9:366–74.

48. Vrtovec B, Starc V, Meden-Vrtovec H. Effect of estrogen replacement therapy on ventricular repolarization dynamics in healthy postmenopausal women. J Electrocardiol 2001;34:277–83.

49. Kahn JK, Sisson JC, Vinik AI. QT interval prolongation and sudden death in diabetic neuropathy. J Clin Endocrinol Metab 1987;64:751–4.

50. Bellavere F, Ferri M, Guarini L et al. Prolonged QT period in diabetic autonomic neuropathy: a possible role in sudden cardiac death? Br Heart J 1988;59:379–83.

51. Ewing DJ, Boland O, Neilson JM et al. Autonomic neuropathy, QT interval lengthening, and unexpected deaths in male diabetic patients. Diabetologia 1991;34:182–5.

52. Tentolouris N, Katsilambros N, Papazachos D et al. Corrected QT interval in relation to the severity of diabetic autonomic neuropathy. Eur J Clin Invest 1997;27:1049–54.

53. Katsuoka H, Mimori Y, Kurokawa K et al. QTc interval, and autonomic and somatic nerve function in diabetic neuropathy. Clin Autonomic Res 1998;8:139–43.

54. Sivieri R, Veglio M, Chinaglia A et al. Prevalence of QT prolongation in a type 1 diabetic population and its association with autonomic neuropathy. The Neuropathy Study Group of the Italian Society for the Study of Diabetes. Diabetic Med 1993;10: 920–4.

55. Kirvelä M, Toivonen L, Lindgren L. Cardiac repolarization interval in end-stage diabetic and non-diabetic renal disease. Clin Cardiol 1997;20:791–6.

56. Bravenboer B, Hendriksen PH, Oey LP et al. Is the corrected QT interval a reliable indicator of the severity of diabetic autonomic neuropathy? Diabetes Care 1993;16:1249–53.

57. Marques JL, George E, Peacey SR et al. Altered ventricular repolarization during hypoglycaemia in patients with diabetes. Diabetic Med 1997; 14:648–54.

58. Dekker JM, Feskens EJ, Schouten EG et al. QTc duration is associated with levels of insulin and glucose tolerance. The Zutphen Study. Diabetes 1996;45:376–80.

59. Fauchier L, Maison-Blanche P, Forhan A et al. Association between heart rate-corrected QT interval and coronary risk factors in 2,894 healthy subjects (The DESIR Study). Am J Cardiol 2000;86:557–9.

60. Festa A, D'Agostino R Jr, Rautaharju P et al. Determinants of QT interval duration in non-diabetic and diabetic subjects. Am J Cardiol 2000;86:1117–22.

61. Suzuki R, Tsumura K, Inoue T et al. QT interval prolongation in patients receiving maintenance hemodialysis. Clin Nephrology 1998;49:240–4.

62. Mohamed R, Forsey PR, Davies MK, Neuberger JM. Effect of liver transplantation on QT interval prolongation and autonomic dysfunction in end-stage liver disease. Hepatology 1996;23:1128–34.

63. Rautaharju PM, Ge S, Clark Nelson J et al. Comparison of mortality risk for electrocardiographic abnormalities in men and women with and without coronary heart disease (from the Cardiovascular Health Study). Am J Cardiol 2006;97:309–15.

64. Rautaharju PM, Kooperberg C, Larson JC, LaCroix A. Electrocardiographic abnormalities that predict coronary heart disease events and mortality in postmenopausal women: the Women's Health Initiative. Circulation 2006;113:473–80.

65. Dekker JM, Schouten EG, Klootwijk P et al. Association between QT interval and coronary heart disease in middle-aged and elderly men. The Zutphen Study. Circulation 1994;90:779–85.

66. Schouten EG, Dekker JM, Meppelink P et al. QT-interval prolongation predicts cardiovascular mortality in an apparently healthy population. Circulation 1991;84:1516–23.

67. de Bruyne MC, Hoes AW, Kors JA et al. Prolonged QT interval predicts cardiac and all-cause mortality in the elderly. The Rotterdam Study. Eur Heart J 1999;20:278–84.

68. Karjalainen J, Raunanen A, Ristola P, Viitasalo M. QT interval as a cardiac risk factor in a middle aged population. Heart 1997;77:543–8.

69. Reunanen A, Aromaa A, Pyörälä K et al. The Social Insurance Institution's Coronary Heart Disease Study. Acta Med Scand 1983;673(Suppl): 1–120.

70. Elming H, Holm E, Jun L et al. The prognostic value of the QT interval and QT interval dispersion in all-cause and cardiac mortality and morbidity in a population of Danish citizens. Eur Heart J 1998;19:1391–400.

71. Goldberg RJ, Bengtson J, Chen Z et al. Duration of the QT interval and total and cardiovascular mortality in healthy persons (the Framingham Heart Study Experience). Am J Cardiol 1991;67: 55–8.

72. Robbins J, Clark Nelson J, Rautaharju PM, Gottdiener JS. The association between the length of the QT interval and mortality in the Cardiovascular Health Study. Am J Med 2003;115:689–94.

73. Schwartz PJ, Wolf S. QT interval prolongation as predictor of sudden death in patients with myocardial infarction. Circulation 1978;57:1074–7.

74. Juul-Møller S. Corrected QT-interval during one year follow-up after an acute myocardial infarction. Eur Heart J 1986;7:299–304.

75. Ahnve S, Gilpin E, Madsen EB et al. Prognostic importance of QTc interval at discharge after acute myocardial infarction: a multicenter study of 865 patients. Am Heart J 1984;108:395–400.

76. Fioretti P, Tijssen JG, Azar AJ et al. Prognostic value of predischarge 12 lead electrocardiogram after myocardial infarction compared with other routine clinical variables. Br Heart J 1987;57:306–12.

77. Pohjola-Sintonen S, Siltanen P, Haapakoski J. Usefulness of QTc interval on the discharge electrocardiogram for predicting survival after acute myocardial infarction. Am J Cardiol 1986;57:1066–8.

78. Wheelan K, Mukharji J, Rude RE et al. Sudden death and its relation to QT-interval prolongation after acute myocardial infarction: two-year follow-up. Am J Cardiol 1986;57:745–50.

79. Peters RW, Byington RP, Barker A, Yusuf S. Prognostic value of prolonged ventricular repolarization following myocardial infarction: the BHAT experience. J Clin Epidem 1990;43:167–72.

80. Bednar MM, Harrigan EP, Anziano RJ et al. The QT interval. Prog Cardiovasc Dis 2001;43(Suppl):1–45.

81. Shah RR. The significance of QT interval in drug development. Br J Clin Pharmacol 2002;54:188–202.

82. Drici MD, Knollmann BC, Wang WX, Woosly RL. Cardiac actions of erythromycin: influence of female sex. JAMA 1998;280:1774–6.

83. Nattel S, Singh BN. Evolution, mechanisms, and classification of antiarrhythmic drugs: focus on class III actions. Am J Cardiol 1999;84:11R–19R.

84. Zehender M, Hohnloser S, Just H. QT-interval prolonging drugs: mechanisms and clinical relevance of their arrhythmogenic hazards. Cardiovasc Drugs Ther 1991;5:515–30.

85. Sawicki PT, Dahne R, Bender R, Berger M. Prolonged QT interval as a predictor of mortality in diabetic nephropathy. Diabetologia 1996;39:77–81.

86. Siscovick DS, Raghunathan TE, Rautaharju P et al. Clinically silent electrocardiographic abnormalities and risk of primary cardiac arrest among hypertensive patients. Circulation 1996;94:1329–33.

87. Moss AJ, Zareba W, Benhorin J et al. ECG T-wave patterns in genetically distinct forms of the hereditary long QT syndrome. Circulation 1995;92:2929–34.

88. Lehmann MH, Suzuki F, Fromm BS et al. T wave "humps" as a potential electrocardiographic marker of the long QT syndrome. J Am Coll Cardiol 1994;24: 746–54.

89. Priori SG, Mortara DW, Napolitano C et al. Evaluation of the spatial aspects of T-wave complexity in the long-QT syndrome. Circulation 1997;96:3006–12.

90. Lupoglazoff JM, Denjoy I, Berthet M et al. Notched T waves on Holter recordings enhance detection of patients with LQT2 (HERG) mutations. Circulation 2001;103:1095–101.

91. Yan G-X, Antzelevich C. Cellular basis for the normal T wave and the electrocardiographic manifestations of the long QT syndrome. Circulation 1998;98:1928–36.

92. Swan H, Saarinen K, Kontula K, Toivonen L, Viitasalo M. Evaluation of QT interval duration and dispersion and proposed clinical criteria in diagnosis of long QT syndrome in patients with genetically uniform type of LQT1. J Am Coll Cardiol 1998;32: 486–91.

93. Rautaharju PM. Why did QT dispersion die? Cardiac Electrophys Review 2002;6:295–301.

94. Malik M, Acar B, Yap YG, Gang Y. QT dispersion does not express spatial heterogeneity of ventricular refractoriness in 12 lead ECG. Circulation 1999;100(Suppl):1–245.

95. Zabel M, Malik M, Hnatkova K, Papademetriou V, Pittaras A, Fletcher RD, Franz MR. Analysis of T-wave morphology from the 12-lead electrocardiogram for prediction of long-term prognosis in male US veterans. Circulation 2002;105:1066–70.

Part 2
Normal ECG Standards for Adults by Gender, Age, and Ethnicity

Section A
ECG Intervals: Tables

TABLE A1 Mean values, standard deviations and the lower to upper (" → ") second and fifth percentiles of heart rate, PR, QRS, and unadjusted QT intervals by race, age and gender.

| Ethnic group | White | | | | | | African–American | | | | | |
| Age group | 40–59 years | | 60 years and older | | | | 40–59 years | | 60 years and older | | | |
Gender	Males (N = 1,478)	Females (N = 2,252)	Males (N = 2,337)	Females (N = 3,312)			Males (N = 452)	Females (N = 778)	Males (N = 459)	Females (N = 639)		
Heart rate (cpm)												
Mean; SD	66; 10.4	68; 9.6	65; 11.0	67; 10.4			67; 10.9	68; 10.3	68; 10.6	68; 11.4		
2% → 98%	48 → 91	60 → 90	46 → 92	49 → 92			49 → 93	50 → 92	48 → 95	48 → 94		
5% → 95%	51 → 84	54 → 84	49 → 85	52 → 86			52 → 87	53 → 87	51 → 90	51 → 87		
PR interval (ms)*												
Mean; SD	163; 20.5	155; 21.9	170; 24.6	163; 23.0			167; 24.6	166; 23.9	170; 23.9	168; 21.3		
2% → 98%	126 → 210	124 → 202	128 → 226	120 → 218			124 → 220	124 → 216	126 → 226	122 → 226		
5% → 95%	132 → 198	136 → 192	134 → 216	128 → 206			132 → 210	130 → 206	132 → 216	132 → 213		
QRS interval (ms)												
Mean; SD	96; 8.9	87; 7.8	93; 9.9	86; 8.5			93; 8.9	86; 8.2	92; 9.6	86; 9.1		
2% → 98%	78 → 114	80 → 106	74 → 114	70 → 106			76 → 112	70 → 104	72 → 114	70 → 106		
5% → 95%	82 → 110	76 → 100	78 → 110	74 → 100			80 → 108	74 → 100	76 → 108	72 → 102		
QT interval† (ms)												
Mean; SD	396; 28.8	398; 26.4	408; 33.0	407; 30.3			392; 30.2	398; 29.4	400; 30.7	405; 33.9		
2% → 98%	344 → 462	376 → 456	344 → 482	346 → 472			336 → 456	344 → 461	333 → 474	340 → 474		
5% → 95%	352 → 446	356 → 444	356 → 464	358 → 458			348 → 441	352 → 450	348 → 456	352 → 464		

* Excluding 196 subjects (1.7%) with PR ≥ 240 ms.
† Unadjusted QT.

TABLE A2 QT and JT adjustment functions for white men and women, the R-square values for the corresponding prediction function, and the lower to upper ("→") second and fifth percentile normal limits.

Race/gender group	Adjustment function	R^2	Mean; SD	2% → 98%	5% → 95%
White men	QTrr = QT + 185 * [1 − (60/HR)] + 6	0.78	419; 15.0	393 → 457	398 → 447
White women	QTrr = QT + 182 * [1 − (60/HR)]	0.70	420; 16.1	392 → 459	397 → 450
White men	QTsqr = QT + 360 * [1 − (60/HR)$^{0.5}$] + 6	0.77	420; 15.2	394 → 458	400 → 448
White women	QTsqr = QT + 348* [1 − (60/HR)$^{0.5}$]	0.69	420; 16.1	393 → 460	398 → 450
White men	QT$_{0.42}$ = QT + 426 * [1 − (60/HR)$^{0.42}$] + 6	0.77	420; 15.2	394 → 458	400 → 449
White women	QT$_{0.42}$ = QT + 411 * [1 − (60/HR)$^{0.42}$]	0.69	420; 16.2	393 → 460	398 → 451
White men	JTrr = JT + 176 * [1 − (60/HR)] + 14	0.72	332; 16.9	301 → 372	307 → 362
White women	JTrr = JT + 175 * [1 − (60/HR)]	0.66	333; 16.7	303 → 371	308 → 364
White men[†]	JTrr, qrs = JT + 184 * [1 − (60/HR)] + 0.83 * (94 − QRS) + 14	0.78	333; 21.8	290 → 378	297 → 370
White women[†]	JTrr, qrs = JT + 180 * [1 − (60/HR)]+ 0.66 * (86 − QRS)	0.69	333; 19.2	294 → 375	303 → 367

QTrr QT adjusted for RR, *HR* heart rate. Note that (60/HR) = RR interval (s). Adjusted intervals are in milliseconds (ms).

[†] Adjustment for rate and QRS duration; QRS does not improve QT prediction in normal ventricular conduction and it is included as a covariate with RR for JT adjustment only.

Note that when using JT adjustment functions, it is preferable to include the adjustment for QRS as a covariate. In general, it is better to use the simpler QT adjustment functions.

TABLE A3 QT and JT adjustment functions for African–American men and women, the R-square values for the corresponding prediction function, and the lower to upper ("→") second and fifth percentile normal limits.

Race/gender group	Adjustment function[†]	R^2	Mean; SD	2% → 98%	5% → 95%
Black men	QTrr = QT + 181 * [1 − (60/HR)] + 7	0.72	418; 17.0	389 → 461	395 → 449
Black women	QTrr = QT + 188 * [1 − (60/HR)]	0.72	418; 16.7	391 → 460	395 → 450
Black men	QTsqr = QT + 343 * [1 − (60/HR)$^{0.5}$] + 7	0.71	419; 17.2	389 → 462	396 → 451
Black women	QTsqr = QT + 360 * [1 − (60/HR)$^{0.5}$]	0.72	419; 16.8	392 → 460	396 → 450
Black men	QT$_{0.42}$ = QT + 405 * [1 − (60/HR)$^{0.42}$] + 7	0.71	419; 17.3	389 → 463	396 → 451
Black women	QT$_{0.42}$ = QT + 426 * [1 − (60/HR)$^{0.42}$]	0.72	419; 16.8	461 → 393	396 → 451
Black men	JTrr = JT + 171 * [1 − (60/HR)] + 13	0.66	331; 18.4	298 → 376	305 → 365
Black women	JTrr = JT + 179 * [1 − (60/HR)]	0.68	331; 17.7	300 → 374	306 → 364
Black men[†]	JTrr, qrs = JT + 179 * [1 − (60/HR)] + 0.79 * (92 − QRS) + 13	0.72	332; 22.5	290 → 385	298 → 368
Black women	JTrr, qrs = JT + 186 * [1 − (60/HR)] + 0.76 * (86 − QRS)	0.72	332; 21.1	290 → 378	299 → 367

QTrr QT adjusted for RR, *HR* heart rate. Note that (60/HR) = RR interval(s). Adjusted intervals are in milliseconds (ms).

[†] Adjustment for rate and QRS duration; QRS does not improve QT prediction in normal ventricular conduction and it is included as a covariate with RR for JT adjustment only.

Note that when using JT adjustment functions, it is preferable to include the adjustment for QRS as a covariate. In general, it is better to use the simpler QT adjustment functions.

TABLE A4 Common rate- and gender-adjusted QT and JT adjustment functions for white and African–American men and women.

Adjustment function	R^2	Mean; SD	98%	95%
QTrr = QT + 182 * (1 − 60/HR) for women; add 6 ms in men	0.72	419; 15.9	459	449
JTrr[†] = JT + 171 * (1 − 60/HR) for women; add 13 in men	0.64	332; 17.1	372	363
JTrr,qrs = JT + 181 * (1 − 60/HR − 0.91 * (89 − QRS) for women; add 6 ms in men	0.72	330; 15.8	369	360

TABLE A5 Formulas for QT subinterval adjustment for rate and gender in white and African–American men and women, the R-square value for the corresponding prediction function, and the lower to upper (" → ") second and fifth percentile normal limits.

Race/gender group	Adjustment function	R^2	Mean; SD	2% → 98%	5% → 95%
White men	QTF1rr = QT + 129 * [1 − (60/HR)] + 16	0.51	284; 19.4	245 → 325	263 → 315
White women	QTF1rr = QT + 144 * [1 − (60/HR)]	0.45	283; 21.1	241 → 333	252 → 319
Black men	QTF1rr = QT + 132 * [1 − (60/HR)] + 14	0.42	277; 23.1	233 → 334	243 → 317
Black women	QTF1rr = QT + 138 * (1 − 60/HR)	0.42	277; 25.7	224 → 334	239 → 319
White men	QTprr = QT + 135 * [1 − (60/HR)] + 17	0.77	330; 18.5	295 → 371	301 → 361
White women	QTprr = QT + 148 * [1 − (60/HR)]	0.69	329; 18.7	292 → 369	300 → 359
Black men	QTprr = QT + 136 * [1 − (60/HR)] + 17	0.47	324; 21.7	283 → 373	291 → 362
Black women	QTprr = QT + 146 * [1 − (60/HR)]	0.48	324; 23.3	277 → 368	287 → 359
White men	QTF2rr = QT + 135 * [1 − (60/HR)] + 16	0.69	372; 18.6	338 → 415	345 → 405
White women	QTF2rr = QT + 147 * [1 − (60/HR)]	0.55	373; 18.1	338 → 411	345 → 403
Black men	QTF2rr = QT + 134 * [1 − (60/HR)] + 16	0.72	372; 22.1	332 → 420	339 → 407
Black women	QTF2rr = QT + 150 * [1 − (60/HR)]	0.66	371; 19.9	330 → 414	339 → 403

HR heart rate. Note that (60/HR) = RR interval (s). Adjusted intervals are in milliseconds (ms).

QTF1rr QRS onset to T upstroke inflection point interval adjusted for RR and gender, *QTprr* QRS onset to Tpeak interval adjusted for RR and gender, *QTF2rr* QRS onset to T downstroke interval adjusted for RR and gender.

Note that the R-square values are considerably lower than those for QT adjustment in Tables A3 and A4, and it is preferable in general to use QT adjustment functions as the primary choice.

TABLE A6 QT and JT adjustment functions for use in evaluating prolongation of repolarization in bundle branch blocks.

Adjustment function	R^2	Mean; SD	98%	95%
QTrr,qrs = QT − 155 * (60/HR − 1) − 0.93 * (QRS − 139) + k, k = −22 for men, −34 for women	0.69	420; 20.0	460	450
JTrr[†] = JT − 155 * (60/HR − 1) + k, k = 34 ms for men, 22 ms for women	0.63	333; 19.0	370	350

Modified from data in Rautaharju et al. Am J Cardiol 2004;93:1017–21.

TABLE A7 Statistics for T wave subintervals by ethnicity, age and gender.

Ethnic group	White						African–American					
	40–59 years		60 years and older				40–59 years		60 years and older		
Age group Gender	Males (N = 1,478)	Females (N = 2,252)	Males (N = 2,337)	Females (N = 3,312)			Males (N = 452)	Females (N = 778)	Males (N = 459)	Females (N = 639)
Interval (ms)										
Infl1–Tpeak										
Mean; SD	46; 12.0	46; 12.0	46; 12.2	46; 14.7			44; 11.6	45; 13.5	44; 13.2	47; 18.5
2% → 98%	30 → 74	24 → 74	26 → 74	20 → 80			22 → 76	18 → 74	20 → 80	12 → 104
5% → 95%	32 → 64	28 → 66	30 → 64	26 → 68			26 → 61	26 → 95	26 → 64	22 → 78
Tpeak–Infl2										
Mean; SD	44; 8.5	43; 7.5	45; 9.6	44; 9.6			47; 11.8	46; 12.1	48; 10.0	48; 14.5
2% → 98%	40 → 70	40 → 68	40 → 77	40 → 76			40 → 86	40 → 86	40 → 92	35 → 92
5% → 95%	40 → 60	40 → 56	40 → 62	40 → 61			40 → 74	40 → 72	40 → 74	40 → 82
Infl1–Infl2										
Mean; SD	90; 13.4	89; 14.4	91; 16.0	90; 17.3			91; 16.0	91; 16.8	92; 16.7	95; 23.5
2% → 98%	70 → 126	64 → 124	68 → 136	62 → 136			66 → 134	63 → 134	62 → 154	56 → 163
5% → 95%	74 → 114	70 → 114	72 → 120	68 → 122			70 → 123	70 → 124	68 → 128	66 → 136
Tpeak–Tend										
Mean; SD	97; 15.0	85; 14.1	98; 17.9	89; 17.7			100; 18.1	88; 17.9	99; 18.2	93; 23.1
2% → 98%	70 → 132	60 → 118	66 → 142	60 → 128			70 → 144	58 → 132	60 → 146	46 → 150
5% → 95%	76 → 122	64 → 108	72 → 130	66 → 118			76 → 132	64 → 120	68 → 138	62 → 136

Infl1 inflection point at T wave upstroke, *Tpeak* T wave peak, *Infl2* inflection point at T wave downstroke, *Tend* end of the T wave.
All time points are global, i.e. estimated from the T spatial magnitude function.

Section B
ECG Wave Amplitudes*: Tables

---

* Normal standards for ECG variables commonly used in LVH criteria were listed in Section 7B of Part 1

TABLE B1 P wave amplitudes and durations, and the lower to upper ("→") second and fifth percentile normal limits for variables used in ECG criteria for right and left atrial enlargement.

		White				African–American			
Ethnicity		40–59		60+		40–59		60+	
Age group		Males	Females	Males	Females	Males	Females	Males	Females
Gender		(N = 1,478)	(N = 2,252)	(N = 2,337)	(N = 3,312)	(N = 452)	(N = 778)	(N = 459)	(N = 639)
PII Dur (ms)	% Obs*	99	100	98	99	100	100	98	99
	Mean; SD	109; 11.8	103; 11.8	112; 14.9	107; 14.9	113; 12.6	108; 12.2	113; 14.2	112; 13.4
	2%→98%	86 → 132	80 → 126	73 → 140	66 → 134	90 → 138	86 → 132	86 → 144	85 → 138
	5%→95%	92 → 128	86 → 122	88 → 134	86 → 128	96 → 132	90 → 128	92 → 135	92 → 134
PII Amp >0 (µV)	% Obs	99	100	97	98	100	99	97	98
	Mean; SD	110; 34.4	118; 40.3	102; 39.1	113; 41.7	123; 41.6	122; 41.5	120; 48.2	127; 46.4
	2%→98%	43 → 185	43 → 205	34 → 185	39 → 200	43 → 219	43 → 209	39 → 239	41 → 222
	5%→95%	58 → 168	58 → 185	43 → 166	53 → 180	58 → 195	58 → 190	58 → 200	63 → 200
PV1 Dur (ms)	% Obs	100	99	97	99	99	99	98	99
	Mean; SD	61; 23.9	59; 25.9	56; 21.2	53; 22.9	63; 27.2	59; 26.8	55; 21.9	52; 21.0
	2%→98%	32 → 120	28 → 118	30 → 118	27 → 118	30 → 124	30 → 124	28 → 122	28 → 118
	5%→95%	36 → 114	32 → 110	34 → 110	31 → 110	34 → 120	34 → 114	34 → 112	31 → 106
PV1 Amp >0 (µV)	% Obs	98	95	93	91	98	98	93	95
	Mean; SD	50; 21.1	45; 19.2	45; 22.7	44; 22.3	61; 26.1	51; 20.5	48; 23.2	47; 25.5
	2%→98%	14 → 97	14 → 87	9 → 102	9 → 132	18 → 119	14 → 101	14 → 104	14 → 102
	5%→95%	19 → 83	19 → 78	14 → 87	14 → 87	24 → 102	19 → 92	14 → 92	14 → 92
PPV1 Dur	% Obs	61	55	75	75	59	60	81	81
	Mean; SD	60; 12.2	60; 11.8	65; 12.5	64; 12.7	63; 14.6	63; 12.2	67; 12.6	67; 12.5
	2%→98%	30 → 83	29 → 82	36 → 91	33 → 83	24 → 93	39 → 87	40 → 96	39 → 92
	5%→95%	40 → 79	40 → 78	45 → 85	42 → 83	36 → 84	44 → 82	47 → 88	46 → 87
PPV1 Amp <0 (µV)	% Obs	59	60	80	81	59	60	80	81
	Mean; SD	−38; 15.0	−41; 15.1	−47; 18.9	−47; 19.5	−42; 21.6	−41; 17.3	−52; 21.4	−54; 23.2
	2%→98%	−83 → −24	−83 → −24	−97 → −24	−97 → −24	−110 → −24	−97 → −24	−105 → −24	−117 → −24
	5%→95%	−68 → −24	−68 → −24	−83 → −24	−83 → −24	−73 → −24	−78 → −24	−92 → −24	−92 → −24

* Per cent subjects with corresponding P wave component.

TABLE B2 Limb lead Q wave duration statistics including small Q waves* by ethnicity, gender, and age.

	White				African–American			
Ethnic group	40–59 years		60+ years		40–59 years		60+ years	
Age group Gender	Males (N = 1,478)	Females (N = 2,252)	Males (N = 2,337)	Females (N = 3,312)	Males (N = 452)	Females (N = 778)	Males (N = 459)	Females (N = 639)
aVL								
% Obs†	44	31	48	45	50	46	52	57
Mean; SD	21; 4.1	20; 4.1	21; 4.6	19; 4.5	20; 3.7	19; 3.8	20; 5.0	19; 4.6
2% → 98%	14 → 30	13 → 29	13 → 32	11 → 30	13 → 27	12 → 27	11 → 31	12 → 35
5% → 95%	15 → 28	14 → 27	14 → 28	13 → 27	15 → 26	13 → 26	13 → 29	13 → 28
I								
% Obs	52	44	47	47	46	45	42	47
Mean; SD	20; 3.5	18; 3.3	19; 3.7	18; 3.6	19; 3.2	17; 3.4	18; 3.6	17; 3.5
2% → 98%	13 → 27	12 → 26	13 → 28	12 → 27	13 → 25	11 → 24	12 → 26	11 → 37
5% → 95%	14 → 26	13 → 24	14 → 26	13 → 24	14 → 24	12 → 23	13 → 25	12 → 24
Inverted aVR								
% Obs	39	41	27	27	27	26	21	24
Mean; SD	16; 4.4	15; 4.0	15; 4.3	15; 4.2	15; 4.3	14; 3.8	15; 4.3	15; 4.2
2% → 98%	10 → 25	10 → 23	10 → 24	10 → 24	10 → 24	10 → 23	10 → 24	10 → 27
5% → 95%	10 → 23	11 → 22	10 → 23	10 → 22	10 → 23	10 → 21	11 → 22	10 → 22
II								
% Obs	41	49	30	32	25	26	21	20
Mean; SD	19; 4.0	18; 3.7	20; 4.5	18; 4.2	19; 3.8	17; 3.9	19; 4.5	17; 4.0
2% → 98%	12 → 28	11 → 26	12 → 29	11 → 27	12 → 28	10 → 27	12 → 30	10 → 31
5% → 95%	13 → 26	12 → 24	14 → 28	12 → 25	13 → 24	12 → 25	13 → 27	12 → 23
aVF								
% Obs	37	46	26	28	24	25	18	20
Mean; SD	22; 5.7	20; 4.8	23; 6.9	20; 6.3	21; 5.6	19; 4.9	21; 5.1	20; 5.9
2% → 98%	12 → 34	12 → 31	12 → 41	11 → 38	11 → 32	11 → 30	12 → 31	11 → 37
5% → 95%	13 → 32	13 → 28	14 → 36	12 → 31	13 → 32	11 → 28	13 → 28	12 → 31
III								
% Obs	33	44	25	26	22	27	19	18
Mean; SD	28; 8.9	24; 8.3	31; 10.8	27; 10.3	26; 9.3	26; 8.9	28; 11.4	28; 9.6
2% → 98%	13 → 49	12 → 44	13 → 54	12 → 51	11 → 47	12 → 45	13 → 53	11 → 50
5% → 95%	15 → 44	13 → 40	14 → 50	13 → 46	14 → 43	13 → 43	14 → 48	13 → 43

* Q amplitude ≥25 μV and R amplitude ≥100 μV; R amplitude ≥300 μV for aVL.
† Per cent subjects with small Q waves excluding QS.

TABLE B3 Limb lead Q wave duration statistics for larger Q waves* each by ethnicity, gender, and age.

		White				African–American			
Ethnic group		40–59 years		60+ years		40–59 years		60+ years	
Age group		Males	Females	Males	Females	Males	Females	Males	Females
Lead	Gender	(N = 1,478)	(N = 2,252)	(N = 2,337)	(N = 3,312)	(N = 452)	(N = 778)	(N = 459)	(N = 639)
aVL[††]	% Obs	11	7	11	12	15	14	16	26
	Mean; SD	24; 3.1	23; 3.3	24; 4.0	23; 3.7	22; 3.3	22; 3.4	24; 4.6	23; 4.3
	2% → 98%	19 → 30	16 → 29	17 → 33	17 → 32	17 → 29	15 → 28	16 → 32	16 → 33
	5% → 95%	19 → 29	18 → 29	18 → 32	18 → 30	17 → 28	17 → 27	18 → 31	17 → 31
I	% Obs[†]	8	6	7	8	8	9	6	16
	Mean; SD	23; 2.6	22; 2.7	23; 3.2	22; 2.8	22; 2.4	21; 3.2	22; 2.2	21; 3.3
	2% → 98%	19 → 28	17 → 27	17 → 29	16 → 28	17 → 27	15 → 28	19 → 26	16 → 28
	5% → 95%	19 → 28	18 → 27	18 → 28	17 → 27	19 → 26	16 → 26	20 → 26	17 → 28
Inverted aVR	% Obs	3	4	2	2	2	2	1	1
	Mean; SD	19; 5.7	19; 4.3	16; 5.1	16; 4.6	17; 5.0	18; 5.0	18; 5.2	17; 5.8
	2% → 98%	11 → 29	10 → 25	10 → 24	10 → 24	11 → 24	11 → 23	12 → 22	10 → 27
	5% → 95%	11 → 26	11 → 24	11 → 23	10 → 23	11 → 24	11 → 23	13 → 22	11 → 25
II	% Obs	7	10	4	4	4	4	4	11
	Mean; SD	23; 3.4	21; 2.8	24; 3.7	21; 4.2	22; 3.3	21; 3.8	22; 3.2	22; 2.9
	2% → 98%	16 → 29	18 → 27	18 → 30	15 → 28	18 → 29	16 → 29	18 → 30	16 → 29
	5% → 95%	17 → 28	17 → 26	18 → 29	16 → 27	19 → 28	16 → 27	19 → 29	17 → 25
aVF	% Obs	6	9	5	5	3	5	4	12
	Mean; SD	24; 4.0	23; 3.5	28; 6.1	25; 7.6	24; 4.0	23; 3.8	24; 3.7	27; 5.3
	2% → 98%	17 → 32	17 → 31	19 → 43	16 → 45	19 → 32	16 → 31	19 → 31	18 → 44
	5% → 95%	18 → 31	18 → 30	20 → 38	17 → 42	21 → 32	18 → 30	20 → 30	19 → 36
III	% Obs	16	17	13	15	10	12	8	9
	Mean; SD	36; 8.4	29; 8.0	37; 9.3	34; 5.2	31; 7.7	31; 7.7	36; 11.9	33; 7.7
	2% → 98%	18 → 52	17 → 48	20 → 57	18 → 54	18 → 50	18 → 47	20 → 60	19 → 54
	5% → 95%	20 → 48	19 → 43	22 → 52	10 → 50	19 → 47	20 → 45	21 → 53	21 → 48

* Q amplitude ≥ 100 μV and R amplitude ≥ 100 μV.

† Per cent subjects with Q and R ≥ 100 μV each (Minnesota Code Q wave).

†† Q amplitude ≥ 100 μV and R ≥ 300 μV for aVL.

TABLE B4 Chest lead V4–V6 Q wave duration statistics for smaller and larger Q waves* by ethnicity, gender, and age.

		White					African–American			
Ethnic group		40–59 years		60+ years		40–59 years		60+ years	
Age group		Males	Females	Males	Females	Males	Females	Males	Females
Lead	Gender	(N = 1,478)	(N = 2,252)	(N = 2,337)	(N = 3,312)	(N = 452)	(N = 778)	(N = 459)	(N = 639)
Smaller Q waves									
V4	% Obs†	23	20	21	25	23	16	20	23
	Mean; SD	18; 3.5	17; 3.4	17; 3.8	16; 3.6	17; 3.2	16; 3.5	15; 3.7	15; 3.4
	2% → 98%	11 → 25	11 → 24	10 → 25	10 → 24	10 → 23	10 → 22	9 → 23	10 → 25
	5% → 95%	12 → 24	12 → 23	11 → 24	11 → 22	12 → 22	10 → 22	10 → 22	11 → 22
V5	% Obs	50	41	39	41	43	32	35	34
	Mean; SD	18; 3.7	17; 3.4	17; 3.8	16; 3.6	18; 3.4	16; 3.6	17; 3.4	15; 3.5
	2% → 98%	12 → 27	11 → 25	11 → 26	10 → 25	11 → 25	11 → 24	11 → 24	10 → 36
	5% → 95%	13 → 25	12 → 24	12 → 24	11 → 23	12 → 23	11 → 22	11 → 23	11 → 21
V6	% Obs	59	60	46	51	48	45	37	40
	Mean; SD	20; 3.7	18; 3.4	19; 3.8	17; 3.6	19; 3.5	17; 3.4	18; 3.5	17; 3.5
	2% → 98%	13 → 28	12 → 26	12 → 27	11 → 25	13 → 27	12 → 25	12 → 25	11 → 41
	5% → 95%	14 → 26	13 → 25	13 → 26	12 → 24	14 → 24	13 → 23	13 → 24	12 → 23
Larger Q waves									
V4 Q ≥ 100 µV	% Obs	4	3	5	6	7	3	6	5
	Mean; SD	21; 3.0	21; 2.9	21; 3.4	20; 3.2	19; 2.6	19; 2.6	19; 2.8	19; 3.9
	2% → 98%	15 → 27	16 → 27	14 → 28	14 → 26	16 → 25	15 → 23	15 → 24	13 → 27
	5% → 95%	16 → 26	17 → 25	16 → 26	15 → 25	16 → 24	16 → 22	15 → 23	13 → 25
V5 Q ≥ 100 µV	% Obs	12	8	10	10	13	7	7	7
	Mean; SD	22; 3.0	21; 2.8	21; 3.3	20; 2.9	21; 2.5	20; 2.9	20; 3.0	19; 3.7
	2% → 98%	17 → 28	16 → 28	16 → 28	15 → 26	16 → 25	15 → 25	15 → 25	14 → 28
	5% → 95%	17 → 27	17 → 25	16 → 27	16 → 25	17 → 25	15 → 24	16 → 24	14 → 26
V6 Q ≥ 100 µV	% Obs	12	12	9	11	12	10	7	7
	Mean; SD	23; 3.1	22; 2.7	22; 3.4	21; 3.0	22; 2.7	21; 3.1	21; 2.9	21; 3.7
	2% → 98%	18 → 30	17 → 28	16 → 29	15 → 27	18 → 28	16 → 27	16 → 26	15 → 29
	5% → 95%	19 → 29	18 → 26	17 → 28	16 → 26	18 → 27	17 → 25	17 → 26	16 → 27

* Smaller Q waves: Q amplitude 25–99 µV and R amplitude ≥100 µV; larger Q waves: Q amplitude ≥100 µV and R amplitude ≥100 µV.
† Per cent subjects with a corresponding qualifying Q wave (QS waves excluded).

TABLE B5 Limb lead Q wave amplitude statistics including small Q waves* by ethnicity, gender, and age.

| | | White | | | | | | African–American | | | | | |
| | | 40–59 years | | 60+ years | | 40–59 years | | 60+ years | | | |
Lead	Ethnic group Age group Gender	Males (N = 1,478)	Females (N = 2,252)	Males (N = 2,337)	Females (N = 3,312)	Males (N = 452)	Females (N = 778)	Males (N = 459)	Females (N = 639)
aVL	% Obs[†]	44	31	48	45	50	46	52	57
	Mean; SD	79; 44.6	76; 44.1	78; 46.0	80; 47.9	84; 47.6	86; 50	82; 53.6	92; 59
	2% → 98%	29 → 195	29 → 191	29 → 205	29 → 219	29 → 219	29 → 214	29 → 235	29 → 266
	5% → 95%	29 → 170	29 → 161	29 → 168	29 → 170	29 → 175	34 → 175	29 → 166	30 → 200
I	% Obs	51	43	47	47	46	44	41	47
	Mean; SD	68; 36.7	65; 36	67; 36.8	70; 39.4	69; 37.3	69; 37.4	61; 32.9	72; 43.2
	2% → 98%	29 → 169	29 → 175	29 → 175	29 → 180	29 → 180	29 → 166	29 → 157	29 → 180
	5% → 95%	29 → 141	29 → 136	29 → 141	29 → 146	29 → 154	29 → 131	29 → 122	29 → 161
Inverted aVR	% Obs	53	52	42	44	40	39	34	38
	Mean; SD	55; 24.8	56; 28.6	54; 28.4	55; 27.3	53; 25.8	53; 28.5	49; 19.9	53; 29.1
	2% → 98	27 → 137	27 → 136	27 → 130	27 → 131	27 → 123	27 → 131	27 → 102	27 → 137
	5% → 95%	27 → 109	27 → 113	27 → 107	27 → 110	27 → 99	27 → 107	27 → 83	27 → 113
II	% Obs	41	49	30	32	25	26	21	20
	Mean; SD	69; 43.4	72; 41.3	64; 36	64; 35.1	68; 38.5	66; 40.2	67; 30.1	67; 42.6
	2% → 98%	29 → 209	29 → 195	29 → 161	29 → 161	29 → 187	29 → 185	29 → 126	29 → 199
	5% → 95%	29 → 142	29 → 156	29 → 135	29 → 131	29 → 138	29 → 141	29 → 122	29 → 159
aVF	% Obs	36	46	26	28	24	25	18	20
	Mean; SD	71; 45.3	72; 41.7	70; 44.5	67; 39.7	73; 40.3	68; 39.7	78; 42.8	71; 50.3
	2% → 98%	29 → 215	29 → 185	29 → 199	29 → 173	29 → 184	29 → 170	29 → 180	29 → 207
	5% → 95%	29 → 166	29 → 156	29 → 149	29 → 141	29 → 151	29 → 155	34 → 161	29 → 169
III	% Obs	33	44	25	26	21	27	19	18
	Mean; SD	132; 103.3	105; 77.1	150; 121.1	127; 111.9	128; 92.9	125; 101.0	140; 153.4	149; 122.3
	2% → 98%	29 → 445	29 → 341	29 → 473	29 → 424	34 → 380	29 → 416	29 → 588	31 → 447
	5% → 95%	34 → 361	34 → 263	34 → 397	29 → 346	34 → 313	34 → 345	34 → 435	39 → 367

* Includes Q waves with amplitude ≥25 µV and R amplitude ≥100 µV (R amplitude ≥300 µV for aVL).
[†] Per cent subjects with qualifying Q wave.

TABLE B6 Chest lead V4–V6 Q Wave Amplitude Statistics* by Ethnicity, Gender, and Age.

		White				African–American			
		40–59 years		60+ years		40–59 years		60+ years	
Lead	Ethnic group / Age group / Gender	Males (N = 1,478)	Females (N = 2,252)	Males (N = 2,337)	Females (N = 3,312)	Males (N = 452)	Females (N = 778)	Males (N = 459)	Females (N = 639)
V4 Any Q	% Obs†	23	20	21	25	23	16	20	23
	Mean; SD	70; 41.7	68; 45.9	76; 51.5	78; 58.2	81; 56.2	68; 46.4	80; 50.4	73; 42.5
	2% → 98%	29 → 195	29 → 190	29 → 234	29 → 222	29 → 249	29 → 187	29 → 184	29 → 220
	5% → 95%	29 → 151	29 → 151	29 → 175	29 → 194	29 → 174	29 → 168	29 → 168	34 → 156
V5 Any Q	% Obs	50	41	39	41	43	32	35	34
	Mean; SD	78; 46.3	71; 43.7	80; 55.4	81; 55.2	83; 55.3	72; 47.2	76; 52.1	75; 45.4
	2% → 98%	29 → 200	29 → 182	29 → 233	29 → 234	29 → 220	29 → 180	29 → 260	29 → 235
	5% → 95%	29 → 175	29 → 161	29 → 183	29 → 190	29 → 199	29 → 148	29 → 175	29 → 157
V6 Any Q	% Obs	59	60	46	51	48	45	37	40
	Mean; SD	75; 40.8	72; 40	72; 44.5	75; 46.6	78; 48.6	72; 42.7	70; 44.1	70; 40.6
	2% → 98%	29 → 185	29 → 190	29 → 200	29 → 206	29 → 234	29 → 185	29 → 195	29 → 203
	5% → 95%	29 → 156	29 → 151	29 → 157	29 → 165	33 → 175	29 → 143	29 → 144	29 → 154
V4 ≥ 100 μV Q	% Obs	4	3	5	6	7	3	6	5
	Mean; SD	141; 40.2	152; 54.9	152; 52.0	160; 66.5	151; 57.3	152; 48.3	144; 40.3	141; 40.5
	2% → 98%	102 → 243	102 → 347	102 → 288	102 → 318	102 → 312	104 → 250	107 → 245	102 → 315
	5% → 95%	102 → 209	102 → 248	102 → 269	107 → 271	104 → 270	107 → 208	107 → 193	102 → 217
V5 ≥ 100 μV Q	% Obs	12	8	10	10	13	7	7	7
	Mean; SD	144; 41.7	143; 46.6	151; 60.9	157; 58.8	153; 53.0	141; 47.7	158; 61.1	146; 45.2
	2% → 98%	102 → 243	102 → 265	102 → 333	102 → 307	102 → 330	102 → 277	102 → 314	102 → 313
	5% → 95%	102 → 223	102 → 210	102 → 250	102 → 255	102 → 229	102 → 255	102 → 299	102 → 247
V6 ≥ 100 μV Q	% Obs	12	12	9	11	12	10	7	7
	Mean; SD	138; 38.5	137; 36.7	143; 46.9	144; 47.2	148; 44.4	137; 37.8	141; 48.3	143; 37.3
	2% → 98%	102 → 231	102 → 239	102 → 286	102 → 273	102 → 258	102 → 250	102 → 276	102 → 262
	5% → 95%	102 → 211	102 → 205	102 → 219	102 → 239	102 → 253	102 → 217	102 → 241	103 → 213

* Q amplitude ≥25 μV and R amplitude ≥100 μV.
† Per cent subjects with a Q qualifying Q wave (QS waves excluded).

TABLE B7 Limb lead Q/R amplitude ratio statistics in selected leads including smaller Q waves* by ethnicity, gender, and age.

| | White | | | | | | African–American | | | | | |
| | 40–59 years | | 60+ years | | 40–59 years | | 60+ years | |
Ethnic group Age group Gender	Males (N = 1,478)	Females (N = 2,252)	Males (N = 2,337)	Females (N = 3,312)	Males (N = 452)	Females (N = 778)	Males (N = 459)	Females (N = 639)
Lead								
aVL								
% Obs†	44	31	48	45	50	46	52	57
Mean; SD	12.4; 6.4	13; 7.1	11.4; 6.2	12.1; 6.7	12.1; 6.9	12.5; 7.1	11.1; 6.7	11.3; 7.4
2% → 98%	4 → 29	4 → 31	3 → 28	3 → 31	3 → 29	3 → 32	3 → 30	3 → 41
5% → 95%	5 → 24	4 → 26	4 → 23	4 → 24	4 → 24	4 → 25	4 → 25	3 → 24
I								
% Obs	51	44	47	47	46	44	42	47
Mean; SD	8; 4.1	8.2; 1.4	8.1; 4.4	8.1; 4.3	6.9; 3.9	6.9; 3.9	6.8; 3.7	6.5; 3.2
2% → 98%	2 → 17	3 → 19	3 → 18	2 → 19	2 → 15	2 → 15	2 → 16	2 → 33
5% → 95%	3 → 15	3 → 16	3 → 16	3 → 15	3 → 12	2 → 14	2 → 13	2 → 12
Inverted aVR								
% Obs	53	52	42	44	40	39	34	38
Mean; SD	10.7; 5.5	12.2; 6.2	11.3; 7.5	11.1; 6.1	8.2; 4.2	8.7; 4.5	9.7; 5.4	8.2; 4.7
2% → 98%	4 → 27	4 → 28	4 → 29	4 → 28	3 → 20	3 → 22	3 → 26	3 → 37
5% → 95%	4 → 22	5 → 24	4 → 22	4 → 22	3 → 15	3 → 18	3 → 19	4 → 16
II								
% Obs	41	49	30	32	25	26	21	20
Mean; SD	7; 4.2	7.2; 3.5	9.4; 7.5	8.7; 8.7	5.6; 6.0	5.7; 3.1	7.5; 4.7	7.2; 4.9
2% → 98%	2 → 17	2 → 16	3 → 30	3 → 29	2 → 13	2 → 15	2 → 19	2 → 30
5% → 95%	2 → 14	3 → 14	3 → 23	3 → 19	2 → 11	2 → 11	2 → 14	2 → 17
aVF								
% Obs	36	46	26	28	24	25	18	20
Mean; SD	11; 9.9	11; 12.0	17; 23.0	16; 19.4	10.2; 11.1	9.7; 8.8	15.1; 20.2	15.8; 21
2% → 98%	3 → 39	4 → 39	4 → 77	4 → 71	3 → 45	2 → 31	3 → 90	3 → 69
5% → 95%	4 → 25	4 → 22	5 → 48	5 → 42	3 → 28	3 → 20	3 → 40	3 → 49
III								
% Obs	33	44	25	26	21	27	19	18
Mean; SD	33; 45.7	27; 37.7	52; 66.2	46; 69.2	28.4; 40.8	37.5; 52.9	44.3; 79.5	45.2; 55.0
2% → 98%	4 → 168	4 → 155	5 → 247	5 → 256	3.6 → 154	3 → 228	4 → 366	4 → 248
5% → 95%	5 → 110	5 → 97	6 → 196	6 → 173	5 → 101	5 → 136	4 → 153	5 → 150

* Q amplitude ≥25 μV and R amplitude ≥100 μV.
† Per cent subjects with a Q-R wave combination.

TABLE B8 Q/R Amplitude ratios (%) in chest leads V4–V6 for smaller* and larger[†] wave combinations by ethnicity, gender, and age.

| Ethnic group | White | | | | African–American | | | |
| Age group | 40–59 years | | 60+ years | | 40–59 years | | 60+ years | |
Lead / Gender	Males (N = 1,478)	Females (N = 2,252)	Males (N = 2,337)	Females (N = 3,312)	Males (N = 452)	Females (N = 778)	Males (N = 459)	Females (N = 639)
Smaller Q waves								
V4								
% Obs[††]	23	20	21	25	23	16	20	23
Mean; SD	4; 2.1	5; 2.5	4; 3.3	5; 3.3	3; 2.1	4; 2.6	4; 2.0	4; 2.2
2% → 98%	$1 \rightarrow 10$	$2 \rightarrow 12$	$1 \rightarrow 12$	$2 \rightarrow 13$	$1 \rightarrow 8$	$1 \rightarrow 11$	$1 \rightarrow 9$	$1 \rightarrow 21$
5% → 95%	$2 \rightarrow 8$	$2 \rightarrow 10$	$2 \rightarrow 9$	$2 \rightarrow 11$	$1 \rightarrow 7$	$2 \rightarrow 8$	$1 \rightarrow 7$	$2 \rightarrow 9$
V5								
% Obs	50	41	39	41	43	32	35	34
Mean; SD	5; 2.8	5; 2.8	5; 3.0	6; 3.4	4; 2.7	5; 2.8	4; 2.3	4; 2.5
2% → 98%	$2 \rightarrow 12$	$2 \rightarrow 13$	$2 \rightarrow 14$	$2 \rightarrow 15$	$1 \rightarrow 11$	$1 \rightarrow 12$	$1 \rightarrow 10$	$1 \rightarrow 36$
5% → 95%	$2 \rightarrow 10$	$2 \rightarrow 11$	$2 \rightarrow 11$	$2 \rightarrow 12$	$2 \rightarrow 10$	$2 \rightarrow 9$	$2 \rightarrow 9$	$2 \rightarrow 9$
V6								
% Obs	59	60	46	51	48	45	37	40
Mean; SD	7; 3.4	7; 3.4	7; 3.6	7; 3.8	6; 3.4	6; 3.1	6; 2.9	6; 2.9
2% → 98%	$2 \rightarrow 16$	$2 \rightarrow 16$	$2 \rightarrow 16$	$2 \rightarrow 17$	$2 \rightarrow 16$	$2 \rightarrow 13$	$2 \rightarrow 14$	$2 \rightarrow 41$
5% → 95%	$3 \rightarrow 13$	$3 \rightarrow 14$	$2 \rightarrow 14$	$3 \rightarrow 14$	$2 \rightarrow 12$	$2 \rightarrow 11$	$2 \rightarrow 11$	$2 \rightarrow 11$
Larger Q waves								
V4								
% Obs	4	3	5	6	7	3	6	5
Mean; SD	7; 2.4	9; 2.3	7; 2.7	9; 4.0	6; 2.1	8; 3.4	6; 1.7	7; 2.4
2% → 98%	$4 \rightarrow 14$	$5 \rightarrow 14$	$4 \rightarrow 14$	$4 \rightarrow 16$	$3 \rightarrow 11$	$4 \rightarrow 16$	$3 \rightarrow 10$	$4 \rightarrow 15$
5% → 95%	$4 \rightarrow 11$	$5 \rightarrow 13$	$4 \rightarrow 12$	$4 \rightarrow 14$	$3 \rightarrow 9$	$4 \rightarrow 12$	$4 \rightarrow 8$	$4 \rightarrow 12$
V5								
% Obs	12	8	10	10	13	7	7	7
Mean; SD	8; 2.8	9; 2.7	9; 3.1	10; 3.7	7; 2.8	8; 3.2	7; 2.5	7; 2.8
2% → 98%	$4 \rightarrow 15$	$5 \rightarrow 17$	$4 \rightarrow 17$	$5 \rightarrow 18$	$4 \rightarrow 14$	$4 \rightarrow 15$	$4 \rightarrow 13$	$3 \rightarrow 17$
5% → 95%	$5 \rightarrow 14$	$6 \rightarrow 15$	$5 \rightarrow 15$	$5 \rightarrow 16$	$4 \rightarrow 13$	$4 \rightarrow 12$	$4 \rightarrow 12$	$4 \rightarrow 11$
V6								
% Obs	12	12	9	11	12	10	7	7
Mean; SD	11; 3.5	11; 3.2	11; 3.7	11; 4	10; 3.8	9; 3.4	9; 2.7	9; 3.1
2% → 98%	$6 \rightarrow 20$	$6 \rightarrow 19$	$5 \rightarrow 20$	$5 \rightarrow 21$	$6 \rightarrow 21$	$5 \rightarrow 17$	$5 \rightarrow 16$	$5 \rightarrow 20$
5% → 95%	$6 \rightarrow 17$	$7 \rightarrow 17$	$6 \rightarrow 18$	$6 \rightarrow 19$	$6 \rightarrow 18$	$6 \rightarrow 15$	$6 \rightarrow 14$	$6 \rightarrow 15$

* Q amplitude ≥25 μV, R amplitude ≥100 μV.

[†] Q and R amplitudes ≥100 μV each.

[††] Per cent subjects with qualifying Q/R wave combination.

TABLE B9 Limb lead R wave amplitude statistics for R waves* by ethnicity, gender, and age.

		White				African–American			
	Ethnic group	40–59 years		60+ years		40–59 years		60+ years	
Lead	Age group / Gender	Males (N = 1,478)	Females (N = 2,252)	Males (N = 2,337)	Females (N = 3,312)	Males (N = 452)	Females (N = 778)	Males (N = 459)	Females (N = 639)
aVL	% Obs	89	82	93	93	92	92	93	97
	Mean; SD	517; 288.9	426; 252.3	568; 298.3	561; 301.2	577; 339.8	574; 310.4	642; 336.3	725; 369
	2% → 98%	119 → 1,213	112 → 1,065	126 → 1,259	122 → 1,299	131 → 1,454	123 → 1,313	126 → 1,371	179 → 1,598
	5% → 95%	146 → 1,070	126 → 922	166 → 1,137	156 → 1,125	160 → 1,210	166 → 1,162	167 → 1,230	244 → 1,451
I	% Obs†	100	100	100	100	100	100	100	100
	Mean; SD	784; 297.1	701; 289.3	763; 298.4	835; 302.7	909; 334.3	924; 326.8	875; 343.8	1,010; 360
	2% → 98%	263 → 1,511	219 → 1,411	224 → 1,464	268 → 1,512	361 → 1,655	339 → 1,625	274 → 1,625	425 → 1,821
	5% → 95%	355 → 1,290	288 → 1,220	315 → 1,279	351 → 1,337	429 → 1,466	427 → 1,488	375 → 1,496	507 → 1,684
Inverted aVR	% Obs	100	100	100	100	100	100	100	100
	Mean; SD	501; 169.5	444; 166.9	461; 170.5	431; 170.8	580; 197.6	559; 184.3	523; 197.7	586; 209.2
	2% → 98%	195 → 913	166 → 842	163 → 871	180 → 886	244 → 1,029	225 → 961	184 → 939	262 → 1,087
	5% → 95%	249 → 794	200 → 744	210 → 770	227 → 780	279 → 933	281 → 880	251 → 877	300 → 968
II	% Obs	99	100	97	99	98	99	97	99
	Mean; SD	821; 341.5	881; 305	636; 300.2	707; 300.9	973; 384	973; 349.7	772; 371.1	812; 371
	2% → 98%	239 → 1,629	332 → 1,602	146 → 1,360	193 → 1,435	287 → 1,907	291 → 1,832	178 → 1,667	198 → 1,716
	5% → 95%	327 → 1,445	420 → 1,425	209 → 1,171	261 → 1,250	411 → 1,698	387 → 1,591	220 → 1,419	258 → 1,484
aVF	% Obs	86	94	76	83	87	93	84	85
	Mean; SD	561; 335.4	604; 305.5	422; 263.4	443; 267.1	634; 375.2	597; 322.8	490; 321.8	471; 295.1
	2% → 98%	112 → 1,396	131 → 1,331	107 → 1,134	112 → 1,149	130 → 1,655	126 → 1,431	112 → 1,296	112 → 1,289
	5% → 95%	136 → 1,179	170 → 1,163	117 → 913	122 → 942	155 → 1,379	156 → 1,211	126 → 1,058	122 → 1,025
III	% Obs	66	74	57	58	69	71	63	63
	Mean; SD	445; 323.4	470; 294.6	335; 238.8	337; 246.4	452; 353.1	393; 288.6	361; 285.7	325; 239.1
	2% → 98%	102 → 1,259	107 → 1,186	102 → 976	102 → 1,051	107 → 1,428	102 → 1,156	107 → 1,140	102 → 1,110
	5% → 95%	107 → 1,054	122 → 1,035	107 → 802	112 → 834	112 → 1,219	112 → 1,000	112 → 923	107 → 756

* Includes R waves ≥100 μV.

† Per cent subjects with an R wave.

TABLE B10 Chest lead R wave amplitude statistics for R waves* by ethnicity, gender, and age.

Ethnic group	White				African–American			
Age group	40–59 years		60+ years		40–59 years		60+ years	
Gender	Males (N = 1,478)	Females (N = 2,252)	Males (N = 2,337)	Females (N = 3,312)	Males (N = 452)	Females (N = 778)	Males (N = 459)	Females (N = 639)
V1								
% Obs†	97	96	89	90	94	96	86	87
Mean; SD	224; 140.2	193; 120.2	174; 128.9	172; 128.8	266; 198.9	199; 124.4	194; 172.7	184; 146.5
2% → 98%	43 → 566	39 → 502	34 → 522	34 → 527	34 → 853	34 → 522	34 → 669	34 → 632
5% → 95%	58 → 478	48 → 410	39 → 415	39 → 410	49 → 648	48 → 439	39 → 531	42 → 479
V2								
% Obs	100	100	99	98	100	99	98	98
Mean; SD	638; 350.3	452; 261.9	553; 369.0	510; 344.9	715; 419.9	482; 298.7	631; 446.8	633; 452.8
2% → 98%	107 → 1,497	87 → 1,147	63 → 1,536	63 → 1,425	92 → 1,762	87 → 1,206	58 → 1,718	58 → 1,808
5% → 95%	164 → 1,289	126 → 937	97 → 1,264	97 → 1,191	151 → 1,460	141 → 1,017	97 → 1,460	117 → 1,423
V3								
% Obs	100	99	99	99	100	99	98	99
Mean; SD	1,051; 489.7	792; 403.2	1,020; 542.5	968; 515.5	1,281; 630.9	886; 454.1	1,240; 682.2	1,187; 627.0
2% → 98%	239 → 2,172	175 → 1,743	185 → 2,303	127 → 2,230	288 → 2,928	200 → 1,937	219 → 2,824	219 → 2,597
5% → 95%	341 → 1,915	249 → 1,554	263 → 2,003	249 → 1,835	388 → 2,431	287 → 1,696	317 → 2,468	330 → 2,311
V4								
% Obs	100	100	100	100	100	100	100	100
Mean; SD	1,558; 538.4	1,198; 418.8	1,520; 587.9	1,379; 539.8	1,961; 656.2	1,362; 479.2	1,888; 702.7	1,570; 603.3
2% → 98%	605 → 2,763	415 → 2,172	453 → 2,880	451 → 2,651	748 → 3,393	466 → 2,519	598 → 3,606	544 → 3,078
5% → 95%	776 → 2,510	556 → 1,926	671 → 2,608	610 → 2,346	969 → 3,129	640 → 2,386	859 → 3,175	672 → 2,586
V5								
% Obs	100	100	100	100	100	100	100	100
Mean; SD	1,440; 463.1	1,210; 360.2	1,429; 520.8	1,363; 498.9	1,701; 497.7	1,408; 421.6	1,683; 637.6	1,555; 550.4
2% → 98%	678 → 2,638	532 → 2,041	576 → 2,695	528 → 2,641	771 → 2,846	677 → 2,570	739 → 3,419	660 → 2,829
5% → 95%	775 → 2,270	688 → 1,855	712 → 2,359	673 → 2,250	933 → 2,540	804 → 2,266	854 → 2,860	834 → 2,510
V6								
% Obs	100	100	100	100	100	100	100	100
Mean; SD	1,051; 344.8	1,010; 290.4	1,022; 386.6	1,067; 397.3	1,217; 357.8	1,203; 367.1	1,154; 440.1	1,198; 442.1
2% → 98%	468 → 1,845	498 → 1,704	374 → 1,967	429 → 2,049	537 → 2,001	605 → 2,052	463 → 2,200	510 → 2,309
5% → 95%	545 → 1,660	571 → 1,533	483 → 1,714	522 → 1,777	660 → 1,840	683 → 1,875	556 → 1,966	581 → 1,997

* Includes for V1 and V2 R waves ≥25 V and for V3–V6 R waves ≥100 µV.
† Per cent subjects with an R wave measurement.

TABLE B11 Limb lead S wave amplitude statistics excluding small S waves* by ethnicity, gender, and age.

		White						African–American					
Ethnic group		40–59 years		60+ years				40–59 years		60+ years			
Age group		Males	Females	Males	Females			Males	Females	Males	Females		
Lead	Gender	(N = 1,478)	(N = 2,252)	(N = 2,337)	(N = 3,312)			(N = 452)	(N = 778)	(N = 459)	(N = 639)		
aVL	% Obs	39	28	25	19			34	23	24	18		
	Mean; SD	258; 143.1	242; 130.4	217; 106.8	224; 132.7			261; 150.7	228; 120.6	232; 134.1	228; 126.2		
	2% → 98%	102 → 651	102 → 634	102 → 499	102 → 582			102 → 649	102 → 606	107 → 575	102 → 568		
	5% → 95%	112 → 532	107 → 511	107 → 426	107 → 463			112 → 553	107 → 495	114 → 470	105 → 498		
I	% Obs†	39	23	23	15			28	15	16	11		
	Mean; SD	196; 89.1	177; 71.4	175; 67.4	180; 92.7			207; 89.7	181; 68.5	183; 69.7	193; 88.4		
	2% → 98%	102 → 439	102 → 413	102 → 341	102 → 375			104 → 429	103 → 373	102 → 352	102 → 382		
	5% → 95%	107 → 347	107 → 324	103 → 302	102 → 318			107 → 360	107 → 310	102 → 300	107 → 358		
Inverted aVR	% Obs	42	27	36	28			34	20	37	30		
	Mean; SD	180; 79.6	160; 59.2	182; 72.0	176; 69.7			194; 89.2	167; 64.8	196; 86.5	191; 86.3		
	2% → 98%	100 → 412	100 → 324	102 → 386	100 → 355			102 → 411	100 → 346	103 → 443	100 → 452		
	5% → 95%	105 → 312	102 → 290	105 → 326	103 → 308			106 → 360	103 → 298	107 → 363	106 → 364		
II	% Obs	38	32	40	36			34	25	40	35		
	Mean; SD	231; 123.8	204; 102.4	257; 142.4	246; 135.1			263; 160.1	228; 127.7	303; 167.4	298; 173.1		
	2% → 98%	102 → 566	102 → 516	102 → 670	102 → 620			107 → 678	102 → 573	105 → 711	105 → 771		
	5% → 95%	107 → 482	107 → 395	107 → 527	107 → 517			107 → 622	107 → 454	112 → 616	113 → 619		
aVF	% Obs	29	31	32	35			34	31	41	41		
	Mean; SD	265; 155.6	226; 136.7	338; 219.7	323; 222.6			307; 203.1	296; 195.6	403; 244.7	422; 291.8		
	2% → 98%	105 → 685	102 → 595	102 → 912	102 → 937			107 → 922	102 → 796	107 → 1,018	108 → 1,214		
	5% → 95%	110 → 559	107 → 496	112 → 771	112 → 795			112 → 784	107 → 684	118 → 901	117 → 980		
III	% Obs	27	26	28	30			35	34	50	40		
	Mean; SD	502; 336.6	347; 264.5	609; 384.9	557; 389.3			543; 377.0	514; 373.2	650; 396.0	764; 474.5		
	2% → 98%	107 → 1,314	102 → 1,108	107 → 1,445	107 → 1,496			108 → 1,504	107 → 1,403	105 → 1,509	122 → 2,000		
	5% → 95%	112 → 1,126	107 → 870	122 → 1,287	122 → 1,318			125 → 1,318	117 → 1,245	122 → 1,316	155 → 1,683		

* Includes S waves ≥100 μV when R amplitude ≥100 μV.
† Per cent subjects with an S wave.

TABLE B12 Chest lead S wave amplitude statistics for larger S waves* by ethnicity, gender, and age.

		White				African–American			
Ethnic group		40–59 years		60+ years		40–59 years		60+ years	
Age group Gender		Males (N = 1,478)	Females (N = 2,252)	Males (N = 2,337)	Females (N = 3,312)	Males (N = 452)	Females (N = 778)	Males (N = 459)	Females (N = 639)
Lead									
V1	% Obs[†]	80	75	60	60	76	75	55	59
	Mean; SD	808; 346.2	848; 315.1	812; 364.3	821; 341.4	1,161; 507.1	1,087; 392.2	1,094; 507.6	1,061; 440.2
	2% → 98%	242 → 1,699	292 → 1,616	213 → 1,658	272 → 1,624	317 → 2,384	398 → 2,015	293 → 2,524	361 → 2,028
	5% → 95%	322 → 1,440	375 → 1,401	312 → 1,466	346 → 1,404	450 → 2,080	475 → 1,787	383 → 2,056	416 → 1,760
V2	% Obs	98	96	94	93	96	96	92	94
	Mean; SD	1,204; 476.7	1,025; 411.7	1,096; 471.8	992; 426.4	1,466; 610.9	1,119; 466.1	1,267; 588.1	1,059; 529.3
	2% → 98%	361 → 2,291	317 → 1,990	288 → 2,223	255 → 2,011	348 → 2,707	379 → 2,232	296 → 2,598	253 → 2,373
	5% → 95%	512 → 2,060	456 → 1,801	401 → 1,952	380 → 1,747	530 → 2,552	458 → 1,966	449 → 2,353	346 → 1,937
V3	% Obs	98	97	97	96	94	94	94	93
	Mean; SD	874; 405.6	638; 315.7	913; 429.3	720; 360	980; 484.3	655; 339.4	962; 508.7	710; 405.9
	2% → 98%	200 → 1,847	161 → 1,401	211 → 1,972	161 → 1,584	200 → 2,131	141 → 1,426	200 → 2,307	146 → 1,770
	5% → 95%	297 → 1,601	209 → 1,254	292 → 1,681	209 → 1,362	289 → 1,881	195 → 1,280	320 → 1,964	208 → 1,358
V4	% Obs	91	89	93	87	83	82	87	83
	Mean; SD	529; 291.9	408; 221.5	620; 339.2	477; 265.6	589; 332.2	428; 252.1	625; 377.9	472; 299
	2% → 98%	117 → 1,309	117 → 937	131 → 1,502	117 → 1,135	126 → 1,403	117 → 1,026	141 → 1,791	112 → 1,255
	5% → 95%	161 → 1,059	136 → 830	166 → 1,250	141 → 976	156 → 1,230	131 → 874	170 → 1,337	133 → 977
V5	% Obs	62	65	68	58	55	59	58	57
	Mean; SD	294; 167.9	265; 141.1	341; 199.3	301; 171	305; 190	293; 163.9	342; 196.1	319; 210.1
	2% → 98%	109 → 752	102 → 629	107 → 889	102 → 756	107 → 876	107 → 702	109 → 812	107 → 958
	5% → 95%	117 → 605	112 → 551	122 → 727	112 → 642	117 → 654	112 → 615	117 → 721	113 → 693
V6	% Obs	27	21	29	20	22	20	23	18
	Mean; SD	196; 112.0	182; 86.4	212; 105.9	216; 104.8	199; 105.4	207; 106.6	216; 95.7	234; 142.4
	2% → 98%	107 → 459	102 → 428	102 → 504.4	102 → 512	102 → 513	102 → 510	102 → 443	107 → 682
	5% → 95%	107 → 385	102 → 664	107 → 407.1	107 → 439	112 → 392	122 → 416	102 → 402	112 → 524

* Includes S waves ≥100 μV with R ≥ 100 μV.

† Per cent subjects with an S wave.

TABLE B13 Limb lead R/S ratio statistics for larger R and S wave combinations by ethnicity, gender, and age.

		White				African–American			
		40–59 years		60+ years		40–59 years		60+ years	
Ethnic group Age group		Males	Females	Males	Females	Males	Females	Males	Females
Lead	Gender	(N = 1,478)	(N = 2,252)	(N = 2,337)	(N = 3,312)	(N = 452)	(N = 778)	(N = 459)	(N = 639)
aVL	% Obs	47	40	30	23	40	28	27	19
	Mean; SD	1.9; 1.85	1.3; 1.46	2.1; 1.82	2; 2.03	1.8; 1.62	1.9; 1.79	2.5; 2.10	2.8; 2.25
	2% → 98%	0.1 → 6.8	0.1 → 5.7	0.1 → 7.3	0.1 → 7.3	0.1 → 6.8	0.1 → 6.3	0.1 → 7.3	0.2 → 8.4
	5% → 95%	0.1 → 5.8	0.1 → 4.2	0.2 → 5.6	0.1 → 5.9	0.2 → 5.1	0.1 → 5.2	0.1 → 6.7	0.3 → 7.0
I	% Obs[†]	39	23	22	15	28	15	16	11
	Mean; SD	4.4; 2.46	3.9; 2.08	4.4; 2.24	4.3; 2.38	4.5; 5.57	4.7; 2.20	5.2; 2.68	5.5; 3.05
	2% → 98%	1.0 → 10.6	0.9 → 9.1	1.0 → 9.5	1.1 → 10.7	1.0 → 10.5	1.2 → 9.4	1.4 → 11.8	1.4 → 11.4
	5% → 95%	1.3 → 8.9	1.4 → 7.6	1.4 → 8.6	1.4 → 8.7	1.4 → 9.1	1.7 → 8.8	1.9 → 9.8	1.6 → 10.8
Inverted aVR	% Obs	42	27	36.2	28	34	20	37	30
	Mean; SD	3.0; 1.48	2.8; 1.36	2.7; 1.40	2.9; 1.42	3.2; 1.61	3.5; 1.69	2.9; 1.55	3.4; 1.68
	2% → 98%	0.6 → 6.7	0.8 → 6.0	0.7 → 6.1	0.8 → 6.7	0.8 → 7.0	1.1 → 7.8	0.7 → 6.6	1.0 → 7.4
	5% → 95%	0.9 → 5.6	0.9 → 5.1	0.9 → 5.3	1.1 → 5.6	1.1 → 6.6	1.3 → 6.3	0.9 → 5.9	1.2 → 6.5
II	% Obs	38	32	40	36	34	25	40	35
	Mean; SD	2.2; 2.27	4.5; 2.66	2.6; 2.02	3.1; 2.26	4.0; 2.55	4.3; 2.77	2.7; 2.21	2.8; 2.44
	2% → 98%	0.4 → 10.1	0.7 → 11.0	0.3 → 8.0	0.4 → 9.2	0.5 → 10.6	0.5 → 10.5	0.3 → 8.7	0.4 → 10.5
	5% → 95%	0.8 → 9.0	1.0 → 9.4	0.4 → 6.6	0.5 → 7.4	0.6 → 8.3	0.8 → 9.3	0.4 → 7.4	0.5 → 7.9
aVF	% Obs	29	31	32	35	34	31	41	41
	Mean; SD	1.1; 1.72	2.8; 2.25	1.3; 1.36	1.6 1.64	2.4; 2.48	2.2; 1.93	1.4; 1.62	1.3; 1.35
	2% → 98%	0.2 → 9.1	0.3 → 9.0	0.2 → 5.0	0.2 → 6.2	0.2 → 9.3	0.3 → 7.0	0.2 → 6.2	0.2 → 5.5
	5% → 95%	0.3 → 7.0	0.4 → 7.4	0.2 → 4.1	0.2 → 4.9	0.3 → 7.4	0.3 → 6.0	0.2 → 4.9	0.2 → 4.0
III	% Obs	27	26	28	30	35	34	40	40
	Mean; SD	1.1; 1.72	1.7; 1.87	0.7; 1.10	0.8 1.19	1.2; 2.06	1.0; 1.29	0.8; 1.60	0.5; 0.84
	2% → 98%	0.1 → 6.5	0.1 → 7.3	0.1 → 4.3	0.1 → 4.7	0.1 → 8.3	0.1 → 5.2	0.1 → 4.7	0.1 → 3.3
	5% → 95%	0.1 → 4.9	0.2 → 5.5	0.1 → 2.9	0.1 → 3.1	0.1 → 5.3	0.1 → 3.8	0.1 → 3.8	0.1 → 1.9

* Includes R and S waves ≥100 μV each.
† Per cent subjects with an R and S ≥ 100 μV each.

TABLE B14 Chest lead R/S ratio statistics for larger R and S wave combinations* by ethnicity, gender, and age.

		White				African–American			
	Ethnic group	40–59 years		60+ years		40–59 years		60+ years	
	Age group	Males	Females	Males	Females	Males	Females	Males	Females
Lead	Gender	(N = 1,478)	(N = 2,252)	(N = 2,337)	(N = 3,312)	(N = 452)	(N = 778)	(N = 459)	(N = 639)
V1	% Obs[†]	80	75	60	60	76	75	55	59
	Mean; SD	0.4; 0.30	0.3; 0.28	0.3; 0.26	0.3; 0.25	0.3; 0.31	0.2; 0.16	0.3; 0.31	0.3; 0.17
	2% → 98%	0.1 → 1.3	0.1 → 0.9	0.1 → 1.1	0.1 → 1.0	0.1 → 1.2	0.1 → 0.7	0.1 → 1.2	0.1 → 0.7
	5% → 95%	0.1 → 0.9	0.1 → 0.6	0.1 → 0.8	0.1 → 0.7	0.1 → 0.9	0.1 → 0.5	0.1 → 0.7	0.1 → 0.6
V2	% Obs	98	96	94	93	96	96	92	94
	Mean; SD	0.7; 0.77	0.6; 0.56	0.7; 0.72	0.7; 0.79	0.7; 0.90	0.6; 0.72	0.7; 0.82	0.9; 1.21
	2% → 98%	0.1 → 2.3	0.1 → 1.9	0.1 → 2.9	0.1 → 2.9	0.1 → 3.0	0.1 → 1.9	0.1 → 3.2	0.1 → 4.5
	5% → 95%	0.1 → 1.6	0.1 → 1.4	0.1 → 1.9	0.1 → 1.8	0.1 → 1.7	0.1 → 1.4	0.1 → 2.2	0.1 → 2.7
V3	% Obs	98	97	97	96	94	94	94	93
	Mean; SD	1.7; 1.70	1.7; 1.78	1.6; 1.77	1.9; 1.98	1.9; 2.10	1.9; 2.00	1.9; 1.94	2.4; 2.68
	2% → 98%	0.2 → 6.3	0.2 → 7.8	0.2 → 7.1	0.2 → 7.8	0.2 → 8.0	0.2 → 8.4	0.2 → 8.8	0.2 → 10.1
	5% → 95%	0.3 → 4.7	0.3 → 5.0	0.3 → 4.6	0.3 → 5.7	0.3 → 5.8	0.4 → 6.2	0.3 → 5.7	0.4 → 7.5
V4	% Obs	91	89	93	87	83	82	87	83
	Mean; SD	4.2; 3.50	3.9; 3.00	3.6; 3.44	4.1; 3.50	4.7; 4.20	4.4; 3.48	4.4; 3.91	4.8; 3.93
	2% → 98%	0.7 → 14.8	0.6 → 13.2	0.6 → 15.1	0.6 → 14.8	0.9 → 17.1	0.7 → 15.0	0.7 → 17.1	0.7 → 17.5
	5% → 95%	1.0 → 11.7	0.9 → 10.1	0.8 → 10.5	0.9 → 11.2	1.1 → 11.8	1.0 → 11.9	1.0 → 12.6	1.0 → 13.5
V5	% Obs	62	65	68	58	55	59	58	57
	Mean; SD	6.2; 3.89	5.6; 3.30	5.5; 3.89	5.7; 3.80	7.1; 4.46	6.1; 3.93	6.5; 4.53	6.3; 3.69
	2% → 98%	1.3 → 16.7	1.2 → 14.2	1.1 → 15.7	1.1 → 15.7	1.9 → 15.6	1.6 → 16.6	1.6 → 19.5	1.3 → 13.3
	5% → 95%	1.7 → 14.1	1.6 → 11.8	1.4 → 13.3	1.5 → 13.1	2.3 → 14.0	2.5 → 13.1	0.1 → 2.25	1.7 → 12.0
V6	% Obs	27	21	29	20	22	20	23	18
	Mean; SD	5.8; 3.12	6.0; 2.83	5.2; 3.01	5.5; 3.10	14.1; 13.01	15.1; 12.99	12.7; 11.72	12.8; 12.09
	2% → 98%	1.2 → 14.1	1.6 → 12.3	1.1 → 13.1	1.2 → 14.1	1.9 → 15.6	1.6 → 16.6	1.6 → 19.5	1.3 → 13.3
	5% → 95%	1.7 → 11.1	1.9 → 11.0	1.6 → 11.3	1.6 → 11.0	2.3 → 14.0	2.5 → 13.1	1.8 → 13.8	1.7 → 12.0

* Includes R and S waves ≥100 µV each.
† Per cent subjects with qualifying R and S wave combination.

TABLE B15 Limb lead J-point amplitude statistics by ethnicity, gender, and age.

Lead	Ethnic group	White				African–American			
	Age group	40–59 years		60+ years		40–59 years		60+ years	
	Gender	Males (N = 1,478)	Females (N = 2,252)	Males (N = 2,337)	Females (N = 3,312)	Males (N = 452)	Females (N = 778)	Males (N = 459)	Females (N = 639)
aVL	% Obs*	100	100	100	100	100	100	100	100
	Mean; SD	7; 23.3	5; 20.4	8; 25.2	6; 24.8	20; 27.5	17; 24.4	17; 27.9	17; 28.4
	2% → 98%	−40 → 58	−35 → 48	−40 → 63	−44 → 63	−35 → 78	−30 → 68	−30 → 78	−35 → 83
	5% → 95%	−30 → 48	−25 → 39	−30 → 53	−30 → 48	−20 → 68	−21 → 58	−20 → 68	−25 → 68
I	% Obs	100	100	100	100	100	100	100	100
	Mean; SD	18; 21.9	11; 18.8	14; 23.7	12; 23.3	32; 23.7	27; 22.0	22; 25.8	21; 27.7
	2% → 98%	−25 → 68	−25 → 53	−35 → 68	−40 → 63	−15 → 87	−20 → 78	−25 → 78	−35 → 83
	5% → 95%	−15 → 58	−20 → 43	−25 → 53	−25 → 48	−5 → 70	−10 → 63	−16 → 68	−20 → 68
Inverted aVR	% Obs	85	76	71	73	89	90	75	74
	Mean; SD	24; 21.9	16; 19.0	15; 22.2	15; 21.0	31; 23.5	27; 20.3	18; 24.4	18; 25.1
	2% → 98%	−24 → 69	−24 → 54	−29 → 59	−29 → 59	−14 → 79	−14 → 69	−33 → 68	−35 → 74
	5% → 95%	−9 → 59	−14 → 44	−19 → 54	−19 → 49	−4 → 69	−9 → 60	−24 → 54	−24 → 59
II	% Obs	100	100	100	100	100	100	100	100
	Mean; SD	25; 32.0	15; 28.3	13; 32.1	13; 30.0	26; 36.7	23; 30.1	11; 35.8	10; 34.8
	2% → 98%	−40 → 89	−44 → 73	−59 → 78	−53 → 73	−44 → 107	−40 → 89	−69 → 78	−64 → 79
	5% → 95%	−25 → 78	−30 → 63	−40 → 63	−40 → 63	−30 → 83	−25 → 73	−49 → 68	−49 → 64
aVF	% Obs	100	100	100	100	100	100	100	100
	Mean; SD	16; 30.9	9; 27.4	6; 31.4	7; 29.8	10; 36.7	9; 30.3	0; 35.3	−1; 33.8
	2% → 98%	−49 → 80	−49 → 63	−60 → 68	−59 → 63	−59 → 92	−54 → 73	−69 → 68	−69 → 64
	5% → 95%	−30 → 63	−35 → 53	−44 → 58	−44 → 53	−46 → 68	−41 → 58	−54 → 58	−54 → 48
III	% Obs	100	100	100	100	100	100	100	100
	Mean; SD	6; 33.3	3; 29.6	−1; 34.9	1; 33.7	−6; 40.3	−5; 34.0	−12; 39.2	−12; 38.1
	2% → 98%	−64 → 73	−59 → 63	−74 → 64	−74 → 68	−88 → 78	−79 → 63	−93 → 63	−93 → 58
	5% → 95%	−44 → 63	−46 → 48	−59 → 53	−59 → 53	−74 → 53	−64 → 48	−74 → 48	−75 → 43

* Per cent subjects with amplitude measurement.

TABLE B16 Chest lead J-point amplitude statistics by ethnicity, gender, and age.

| | | White | | | | | | African–American | | | | | |
| | | 40–59 years | | 60+ years | | | 40–59 years | | 60+ years | | |
Lead	Ethnic group Age group Gender	Males (N = 1,478)	Females (N = 2,252)	Males (N = 2,337)	Females (N = 3,312)		Males (N = 452)	Females (N = 778)	Males (N = 459)	Females (N = 639)
V1	% Obs*	100	100	100	100		100	100	100	100
	Mean; SD	11; 30.5	−2; 25.4	8; 32.4	−1; 28.7		22; 42.8	−3; 27.5	18; 37.7	−1; 31.2
	2% → 98%	−44 → 83	−44 → 53	−50 → 83	−59 → 68		−49 → 131	−54 → 63	−49 → 102	−64 → 63
	5% → 95%	−35 → 64	−40 → 39	−40 → 63	−44 → 48		−35 → 94	−49 → 48	−36 → 78	−49 → 53
V2	% Obs	100	100	100	100		100	100	100	100
	Mean; SD	45; 47.0	11; 37.1	32; 49.6	10; 42.6		79; 59.1	25; 41.8	59; 58.3	25; 45.7
	2% → 98%	−35 → 151	−54 → 102	−59 → 146	−69 → 112		−30 → 205	−49 → 131	−40 → 199	−59 → 146
	5% → 95%	−25 → 126	−44 → 78	−40 → 117	−54 → 83		−10 → 177	−35 → 107	−20 → 157	−44 → 107
V3	% Obs	100	100	100	100		100	100	100	100
	Mean; SD	40; 43.8	7; 32.1	21; 47.3	2; 38.8		77; 56.8	29; 36.1	48; 52.5	18; 43.4
	2% → 98%	−35 → 138	−54 → 83	−69 → 126	−78 → 87		−25 → 214	−37 → 122	−48 → 169	−74 → 124
	5% → 95%	−25 → 117	−44 → 63	−49 → 102	−54 → 68		−5 → 180	−25 → 97	−25 → 137	−49 → 88
V4	% Obs	100	100	100	100		100	100	100	100
	Mean; SD	28; 38.8	6; 29.7	6; 42.8	−3; 35.9		57; 50.8	29; 33.3	30; 47.4	13; 41.2
	2% → 98%	−42 → 117	−49 → 73	−79 → 97	−79 → 73		−30 → 175	−40 → 99	−64 → 140	−74 → 102
	5% → 95%	−30 → 97	−40 → 55	−64 → 78	−59 → 53		−15 → 146	−25 → 87	−35 → 113	−49 → 78
V5	% Obs	100	100	100	100		100	100	100	100
	Mean; SD	22; 31.3	7; 25.8	5; 36.3	2; 31.6		38; 35.6	27; 28.7	18; 38.6	13; 37.0
	2% → 98%	−40 → 92	−40 → 68	−69 → 83	−64 → 68		−20 → 122	−27 → 87	−58 → 97	−59 → 92
	5% → 95%	−25 → 78	−30 → 48	−54 → 68	−46 → 53		−10 → 97	−15 → 78	−40 → 83	−44 → 74
V6	% Obs	100	100	100	100		100	100	100	100
	Mean; SD	21; 25.1	11; 20.5	11; 28.6	12; 26.1		28; 26.5	25; 23.1	17; 30.3	16; 29.7
	2% → 98%	−25 → 73	−30 → 53	−49 → 73	−44 → 63		−20 → 87	−20 → 80	−53 → 78	−44 → 74
	5% → 95%	−15 → 63	−20 → 43	−35 → 58	−30 → 53		−10 → 75	−10 → 63	−35 → 68	−35 → 63

* Per cent subjects with amplitude measurement.

TABLE B17 Limb lead ST 60 ms amplitude statistics by ethnicity, gender, and age.

		White					African–American			
		40–59 years		60+ years			40–59 years		60+ years	
Lead	Ethnic group Age group Gender	Males (N = 1,478)	Females (N = 2,252)	Males (N = 2,337)	Females (N = 3,312)		Males (N = 452)	Females (N = 778)	Males (N = 459)	Females (N = 639)
aVL	% Obs*	100	100	100	100		100	100	100	100
	Mean; SD	15; 18.6	5; 13.9	7; 18.8	0; 17.2		28; 21.0	16; 16.9	14; 20.3	8; 20.9
	2% → 98%	−22 → 57	−21 → 36	−30 → 48	−39 → 35		−13 → 73	−20 → 53	−29 → 57	−35 → 58
	5% → 95%	−13 → 47	−15 → 29	−21 → 38	−28 → 27		−5 → 66	−10 → 44	−15 → 49	−23 → 42
I	% Obs	100	100	100	100		100	100	100	100
	Mean; SD	33; 22.9	16; 17.5	16; 23.0	7; 20.9		47; 24.2	29; 19.4	24; 24.6	14; 24.7
	2% → 98%	−9 → 83	−20 → 54	−34 → 63	−43 → 48		2 → 102	−12 → 68	−28 → 76	−41 → 63
	5% → 95%	0 → 72	−11 → 44	−22 → 53	−28 → 38		10 → 91	0 → 61	−16 → 66	−28 → 52
Inverted aVR	% Obs	95	85	77	71		96	93	81	78
	Mean; SD	35; 22.3	18; 18.3	16; 22.4	10; 20.3		43; 25.1	28; 18.9	21; 25.6	14; 23.2
	2% → 98%	−8 → 84	−20 → 58	−32 → 62	−36 → 50		−3 → 96	−12 → 66	−34 → 76	−40 → 71
	5% → 95%	2 → 71	−11 → 48	−21 → 52	−23 → 42		7 → 84	−4 → 57	−20 → 62	−27 → 49
II	% Obs	100	100	100	100		100	100	100	100
	Mean; SD	37; 27.4	21; 23.4	17; 27.5	14; 25.1		39; 33.4	26; 24.3	19; 33.1	13; 28.4
	2% → 98%	−17 → 95	−28 → 70	−43 → 74	−44 → 65		−24 → 114	−21 → 77	−48 → 92	−45 → 72
	5% → 95%	−4 → 83	−18 → 58	−26 → 60	−25 → 55		−8 → 92	−10 → 68	−33 → 70	−35 → 60
aVF	% Obs	100	100	100	100		100	100	100	100
	Mean; SD	20; 22.8	13; 19.4	9; 22.9	11; 21		15; 28.9	12; 21.1	7; 27.9	6; 24.1
	2% → 98%	−25 → 71	−27 → 54	−39 → 57	−34 → 54		−40 → 81	−32 → 57	−51 → 64	−48 → 64
	5% → 95%	−14 → 59	−19 → 44	−28 → 46	−22 → 45		−27 → 63	−21 → 49	−37 → 53	−35 → 46
III	% Obs	100	100	100	100		100	100	100	100
	Mean; SD	3; 23.4	5; 18.9	1; 23.7	7; 21.8		−8; 29.3	−3; 22.2	−5; 27.7	−125.9
	2% → 98%	−45 → 55	−36 → 43	−48 → 49	−37 → 53		−65 → 51	−52 → 45	−60 → 52	−55 → 54
	5% → 95%	−35 → 43	−26 → 35	−37 → 38	−26 → 43		−51 → 43	−39 → 32	−48 → 42	−45 → 41

* Percent subjects with amplitude measurement.

TABLE B18 Chest lead ST 60 ms amplitude statistics by ethnicity, gender, and age.

Lead	Ethnic group	White				African–American			
	Age group	40–59 years		60+ years		40–59 years		60+ years	
	Gender	Males (N = 1,478)	Females (N = 2,252)	Males (N = 2,337)	Females (N = 3,312)	Males (N = 452)	Females (N = 778)	Males (N = 459)	Females (N = 639)
V1	% Obs*	100	100	100	100	100	100	100	100
	Mean; SD	53; 37.2	32; 24.1	44; 37.3	33; 30.2	79; 51.2	40; 29.2	63; 42.2	41; 35.5
	2% → 98%	$-9 \to 145$	$-10 \to 92$	$-15 \to 136$	$-18 \to 109$	$-4 \to 200$	$-9 \to 126$	$0 \to 182$	$-14 \to 126$
	5% → 95%	$0 \to 120$	$-4 \to 74$	$-4 \to 111$	$-8 \to 85$	$10 \to 178$	$0 \to 91$	$9 \to 146$	$-4 \to 107$
V2	% Obs	100	100	100	100	100	100	100	100
	Mean; SD	147; 71.5	71; 42.1	108; 63.8	67; 49.4	201; 81.9	95; 47.8	146; 71.3	89; 54.6
	2% → 98%	$27 \to 316$	$-1 \to 176$	$0 \to 266$	$-18 \to 187$	$40 \to 360$	$16 \to 238$	$32 \to 324$	$-4 \to 247$
	5% → 95%	$45 \to 272$	$11 \to 146$	$16 \to 223$	$0 \to 155$	$67 \to 338$	$29 \to 191$	$45 \to 266$	$16 \to 191$
V3	% Obs	100	100	100	100	100	100	100	100
	Mean; SD	126; 64.8	53; 38.0	90; 59.4	48; 45.0	171; 73.5	77; 42.4	122; 65.7	64; 49.8
	2% → 98%	$15 \to 286$	$-14 \to 141$	$-19 \to 227$	$-35 \to 155$	$38 \to 339$	$4 \to 198$	$8 \to 276$	$-29 \to 215$
	5% → 95%	$34 \to 245$	$-2 \to 120$	$3 \to 194$	$-14 \to 127$	$66 \to 298$	$19 \to 172$	$24 \to 246$	$-9 \to 146$
V4	% Obs	100	100	100	100	100	100	100	100
	Mean; SD	82; 49.4	33; 31.2	50; 49.0	24; 37.4	114; 59.1	56; 35.8	74; 54.9	40; 44.0
	2% → 98%	$-3 \to 204$	$-25 \to 104$	$-47 \to 156$	$-53 \to 105$	$15 \to 249$	$-10 \to 144$	$-22 \to 207$	$-51 \to 150$
	5% → 95%	$9 \to 171$	$-14 \to 86$	$-25 \to 135$	$-33 \to 84$	$31 \to 218$	$0 \to 122$	$-8 \to 163$	$-27 \to 107$
V5	% Obs	100	100	100	100	100	100	100	100
	Mean; SD	48; 35.1	21; 26.3	23; 38.0	11; 31.7	64; 40.5	41; 29.5	34; 41.3	23; 37.5
	2% → 98%	$-15 \to 129$	$-29 \to 78$	$-58 \to 101$	$-63 \to 74$	$-6 \to 157$	$-16 \to 105$	$-39 \to 121$	$-55 \to 106$
	5% → 95%	$-2 \to 107$	$-18 \to 66$	$-39 \to 85$	$-37 \to 58$	$7 \to 135$	$-6 \to 90$	$-26 \to 106$	$-30 \to 80$
V6	% Obs	100	100	100	100	100	100	100	100
	Mean; SD	30; 25.3	12; 19.0	13; 28.6	5; 24.9	36; 28.2	25; 22.4	17; 30.9	10; 27.7
	2% → 98%	$-16 \to 85$	$-26 \to 54$	$-49 \to 68$	$-55 \to 53$	$-15 \to 97$	$-24 \to 74$	$-52 \to 83$	$-54 \to 73$
	5% → 95%	$-6 \to 72$	$-19 \to 44$	$-34 \to 57$	$-34 \to 42$	$-4 \to 84$	$-11 \to 63$	$-34 \to 63$	$-33 \to 51$

* Per cent subjects with amplitude measurement.

TABLE B19 Limb lead T wave amplitude statistics by ethnicity, gender, and age.

		White				African–American			
		40–59 years		60+ years		40–59 years		60+ years	
Lead	Ethnic group / Age group / Gender	Males (N = 1,478)	Females (N = 2,252)	Males (N = 2,337)	Females (N = 3,312)	Males (N = 452)	Females (N = 778)	Males (N = 459)	Females (N = 639)
aVL	% Obs	100	100	100	100	100	100	100	100
	Mean; SD	101; 88.2	82; 74.3	65; 93.5	62; 89.1	110; 91.5	101; 79.2	57; 92.2	61; 97.3
	2% → 98%	−78 → 302	−63 → 249	−123 → 263	−107 → 252	−87 → 297	−68 → 278	−136 → 249	−152 → 274
	5% → 95%	−43 → 249	−39 → 209	−83 → 219	−73 → 209	−39 → 268	−39 → 229	−93 → 210	−93 → 215
I	% Obs*	100	100	100	100	100	100	100	100
	Mean; SD	218; 99.7	195; 84.9	168; 103	173; 101.6	213; 105.2	197; 95.6	138; 109	140; 116.5
	2% → 98%	0 → 439	0 → 395	−49 → 380	−57 → 385	29 → 444	−6 → 405	−97 → 393	−127 → 395
	5% → 95%	78 → 390	73 → 346	0 → 337	−14 → 338	73 → 392	68 → 351	−29 → 313	−44 → 322
Inverted aVR	% Obs	98	99	96	96	97	97	90	90
	Mean; SD	233; 89.5	218; 76.6	191; 89.5	200; 89.2	217; 103.2	202; 86.0	155; 105.5	152; 100.7
	2% → 98%	63 → 419	73 → 380	−29 → 371	−24 → 380	0 → 434	0 → 380	−76 → 379	−89 → 374
	5% → 95%	102 → 380	102 → 343	48 → 336	63 → 341	66 → 382	78 → 336	−15 → 327	−30 → 302
II	% Obs	100	100	100	100	100	100	100	100
	Mean; SD	247; 106	238; 95.7	212; 106	224; 105.3	220; 133.2	205; 99.5	174; 128.5	164; 110.6
	2% → 98%	68 → 488	0 → 454	−20 → 445	−29 → 449	−29 → 517	0 → 424	−99 → 449	−87 → 426
	5% → 95%	102 → 435	97 → 395	43 → 390	53 → 395	0 → 434	38 → 375	−35 → 391	−30 → 346
aVF	% Obs	100	100	100	100	100	100	100	100
	Mean; SD	143; 94.8	142; 88	132; 94.9	139; 92	116; 118	108; 87.8	106; 112.1	96; 93.4
	2% → 98%	−39 → 358	−39 → 332	−54 → 346	−48 → 336	−92 → 405	−58 → 309	−111 → 340	−97 → 317
	5% → 95%	−9 → 302	−19 → 288	−25 → 292	−24 → 292	−65 → 314	−34 → 253	−78 → 292	−63 → 249
III	% Obs	100	100	100	100	100	100	100	100
	Mean; SD	27; 114.2	38; 100.1	46; 113.6	52; 104.2	1; 126.8	1; 98.4	33; 120.5	20; 109.4
	2% → 98%	−195 → 265	−156 → 244	−170 → 279	−156 → 263	−224 → 292	−175 → 226	−185 → 273	−206 → 269
	5% → 95%	−146 → 209	−109 → 205	−131 → 224	−112 → 219	−185 → 207	−142 → 180	−151 → 234	−142 → 200

* Per cent subjects with a T wave amplitude measurement.

TABLE B20 Chest lead T wave amplitude statistics by ethnicity, gender, and age.

| | | White | | | | | | African–American | | | |
| | | 40–59 years | | 60+ years | | 40–59 years | | 60+ years | |
Lead	Ethnic group Age group Gender	Males (N = 1,478)	Females (N = 2,252)	Males (N = 2,337)	Females (N = 3,312)	Males (N = 452)	Females (N = 778)	Males (N = 459)	Females (N = 639)
V1	% Obs*	100	100	100	100	100	100	100	100
	Mean; SD	117; 139.9	−6; 105.9	118; 141	23; 125	145; 167	−12; 117	134; 147.1	27; 129.1
	2% → 98%	−131 → 421	−190 → 214	−131 → 463	−205 → 297	−166 → 517	−207 → 312	−130 → 477	−185 → 341
	5% → 95%	−97 → 356	−166 → 170	−97 → 361	−166 → 229	−117 → 424	−176 → 234	−97 → 367	−146 → 240
V2	% Obs	100	100	100	100	100	100	100	100
	Mean; SD	539; 232	287; 168.4	492; 237.3	330; 207.1	565; 251.8	260; 178	479; 222.3	296; 194.8
	2% → 98%	124 → 1,054	−58 → 683	92 → 1,040	−67 → 805	136 → 1,151	−107 → 771	93 → 960	−78 → 856
	5% → 95%	200 → 948	53 → 585	156 → 914	34 → 703	185 → 961	−53 → 630	151 → 855	19 → 649
V3	% Obs	100	100	100	100	100	100	100	100
	Mean; SD	539; 235.1	346; 175.2	512; 245.2	378; 218.5	523; 247.3	302; 179.1	456; 238.1	301; 216.9
	2% → 98%	141 → 1,071	0 → 751	107 → 1,059	−38 → 869	107 → 1,054	−50 → 810	0 → 980	−133 → 836
	5% → 95%	199 → 966	92 → 654	175 → 938	78 → 742	154 → 961	63 → 689	131 → 864	0 → 650
V4	% Obs	100	100	100	100	100	100	100	100
	Mean; SD	446; 220.5	334; 164.6	413; 233.8	339; 207.1	418; 250	296; 174.3	344; 252.4	251; 213.6
	2% → 98%	87 → 971	0 → 708	0 → 942	−53 → 809	−28 → 999	−43 → 729	−204 → 901	−210 → 744
	5% → 95%	141 → 839	97 → 610	97 → 801	29 → 683	97 → 844	72 → 625	0 → 776	−87 → 576
V5	% Obs	100	100	100	100	100	100	100	100
	Mean; SD	331; 172.6	292; 138.5	292; 185.8	280; 173.6	297; 198	265; 152.6	219; 216.2	199; 186
	2% → 98%	2 → 719	0 → 610	−98 → 683	−63 → 673	−111 → 712	−60 → 607	−248 → 688	−212 → 624
	5% → 95%	97 → 629	87 → 522	0 → 595	0 → 576	56 → 644	57 → 541	−114 → 571	−113 → 473
V6	% Obs	100	100	100	100	100	100	100	100
	Mean; SD	235; 122.2	224; 102.1	203; 131.5	214; 129.6	206; 142.7	205; 118.9	149; 149.4	140; 133.2
	2% → 98%	0 → 507	0 → 458	−74 → 474	−58 → 507	−91 → 512	−48 → 458	−181 → 482	−170 → 449
	5% → 95%	68 → 439	83 → 400	0 → 424	0 → 424	−2 → 444	0 → 396	−102 → 396	−103 → 361

* Per cent subjects with a T wave measurement.

Section C
ECG Vector Components and Spatial Magnitudes at Normalized Time Scale: Tables

TABLE C1 P wave X, Y and Z amplitudes at ten equally spaced time points in white men and women.

		X		Y		Z	
		Men	Women	Men	Women	Men	Women
Ponset	Mean; SD	18; 10.3	18; 10.5	25; 17.2	27; 17.1	0; 10.3	0; 9.9
	2% → 98%	−1 → 41	−1 → 42	−10 → 63	−8 → 65	−20 → 24	−20 → 21
1/10	Mean; SD	25; 11.7	24; 11.9	45; 23.0	47; 22.9	9; 12.2	8; 11.9
	2% → 98%	3 → 51	2 → 52	−4 → 94	−1 → 95	−16 → 35	−17 → 33
2/10	Mean; SD	32; 13.9	31; 14.0	63; 28	65; 27.7	18; 15.9	17; 15.5
	2% → 98%	6 → 63	5 → 63	1 → 121	4 → 122	−14 → 52	−16 → 50
3/10	Mean; SD	40; 16.4	39; 16.7	73; 33.4	75; 33.2	22; 19.8	20; 19.4
	2% → 98%	10 → 77	8 → 77	3 → 144	6 → 147	−21 → 63	−23 → 60
4/10	Mean; SD	53; 19.8	53; 19.9	82; 41.4	86; 42.0	11; 25.0	9; 24.4
	2% → 98%	18 → 99	16 → 99	−1 → 170	1 → 177	−46 → 61	−45 → 57
5/10	Mean; SD	62; 21.0	61; 21.3	84; 46	88; 45.7	−4; 23.6	15; 23.2
	2% → 98%	22 → 107	20 → 109	−7 → 179	−3 → 186	−57 → 43	−12 → 39
6/10	Mean; SD	61; 20.5	61; 21.3	73; 47.7	76; 48.1	−18; 22.2	22; 21.9
	2% → 98%	22 → 106	20 → 109	−17 → 175	−13 → 181	−67 → 25	22 → 22
7/10	Mean; SD	55; 18.2	55; 18.5	54; 41.3	56; 41.1	−19; 19.1	−19; 18.5
	2% → 98%	20 → 95	19 → 96	−21 → 147	−19 → 151	−61 → 16	−58 → 17
8/10	Mean; SD	40; 15.6	38; 15.3	36; 29.3	37; 28.2	−14; 15.7	−13; 15.0
	2% → 98%	10 → 74	10 → 72	−20 → 103	−16 → 102	−47 → 14	−45 → 14
9/10	Mean; SD	19; 10.9	18; 10.2	17; 18.4	18; 17.5	−11; 12.1	−10; 11.3
	2% → 98%	0 → 74	−1 → 41	−20 → 58	−17 → 59	−35 → 9	−33 → 8
10/10	Mean; SD	7; 8.8	7; 8.1	4; 13.8	5; 13.2	−11; 10.6	−11; 9.7
	2% → 98%	−9 → 24	−10 → 25	−28 → 33	−23 → 34	−31 → 4	−30 → 3

TABLE C2 QRS X, Y and Z components and vector magnitude at ten equally spaced time points in white men and women.

		X		Y		Z		Vector magnitude	
		Men	Women	Men	Women	Men	Women	Men	Women
1/10	Mean; SD	$-17; 49.0$	$-18; 46.4$	$-2; 45.4$	$-5; 44.9$	$72; 49.0$	$70; 44.7$	$112; 54.7$	$99; 46.5$
	2% → 98%	$-115 \to 93$	$-111 \to 88$	$-91 \to 103$	$-95 \to 100$	$-16 \to 194$	$-9 \to 178$	$36 \to 253$	$32 \to 226$
2/10	Mean; SD	$114; 153.5$	$105; 146.8$	$23; 76.4$	$26; 75.5$	$189; 129.3$	$179; 120.0$	$335; 173.8$	$281; 135.2$
	2% → 98%	$-155 \to 508$	$-156 \to 460$	$-124 \to 203$	$-122 \to 211$	$-56 \to 486$	$-39 \to 460$	$99 \to 752$	$83 \to 658$
3/10	Mean; SD	$577; 277.1$	$545; 270.4$	$140; 151.1$	$152; 148.1$	$184; 279.2$	$160; 264.8$	$358; 336.9$	$714; 268$
	2% → 98%	$105 \to 1,266$	$86 \to 1,204$	$-119 \to 522$	$-110 \to 511$	$-468 \to 735$	$-467 \to 677$	$312 \to 1,738$	$251 \to 1,371$
4/10	Mean; SD	$1,035; 369.3$	$1,001; 359.1$	$350; 285.7$	$368; 269.1$	$-129; 450.9$	$-149; 413.8$	$1,475; 464.5$	$1,206; 386$
	2% → 98%	$312 \to 1,865$	$363 \to 1,883$	$-196 \to 990$	$-165 \to 969$	$-1,189 \to 724$	$-1,069 \to 651$	$689 \to 2,617$	$496 \to 2,164$
5/10	Mean; SD	$813; 564.8$	$833; 529.0$	$346; 366.7$	$381; 357.7$	$-505; 458.1$	$-505; 429.6$	$1,474; 539.7$	$1,180; 468.9$
	2% → 98%	$-287 \to 1,974$	$-222 \to 1,931$	$-394 \to 1,154$	$-362 \to 1,159$	$-1,465 \to 477$	$-1,391 \to 377$	$479 \to 2,745$	$381 \to 2,353$
6/10	Mean; SD	$223; 439$	$266; 434$	$167; 298$	$185; 297$	$-626; 313$	$-606; 304$	$994; 365$	$867; 313.5$
	2% → 98%	$-452 \to 1,299$	$-415 \to 1,290$	$-434 \to 818$	$-428 \to 828$	$-1,311 \to 35$	$-1,239 \to 58$	$413 \to 1,917$	$343 \to 1,683$
7/10	Mean; SD	$-32; 190.4$	$-12; 189.7$	$45; 186.5$	$48; 184.4$	$-434; 177.7$	$-421; 169.8$	$565; 230.4$	$530; 177.3$
	2% → 98%	$-375 \to 430$	$-353 \to 464$	$-360 \to 432$	$-349 \to 431$	$-849 \to -72$	$-800 \to -75$	$208 \to 1,154$	$228 \to 967$
8/10	Mean; SD	$-27; 87.7$	$-24; 83.8$	$12; 102.8$	$10; 101.7$	$-186; 98.5$	$-184; 94.0$	$243; 121.2$	$243; 94.9$
	2% → 98%	$-211 \to 154$	$-204 \to 146$	$-214 \to 215$	$-215 \to 203$	$-406 \to 13$	$-388 \to 16$	$63 \to 566$	$81 \to 475$
9/10	Mean; SD	$3; 43.3$	$2; 41.0$	$11; 50.4$	$10; 50.8$	$-41; 46.2$	$-44; 44.9$	$89; 44.4$	$84; 38.7$
	2% → 98%	$-82 \to 99$	$-84 \to 87$	$-105 \to 109$	$-106 \to 105$	$-132 \to 65$	$-130 \to 61$	$20 \to 202$	$21 \to 176$
10/10	Mean; SD	$11; 27.2$	$8; 25.7$	$10; 27.3$	$9; 26.7$	$13; 30.9$	$7; 29.2$	$65; 34.8$	$49; 25.9$
	2% → 98%	$-43 \to 73$	$-44 \to 63$	$-48 \to 63$	$-49 \to 62$	$-41 \to 88$	$-44 \to 76$	$14 \to 154$	$11 \to 120$
Rmax	Mean; SD	$1,315; 582.9$	$1,070; 485.7$	$491; 456.3$	$429; 389$	$-465; 588.3$	$-359; 504$	$1,662; 491.5$	$1,350; 411.4$
	2% → 98%	$-293 \to 2,424$	$-237 \to 2,075$	$-338 \to 1,608$	$-282 \to 1,324$	$-1,579 \to 777$	$-1,303 \to 672$	$781 \to 2,800$	$670 \to 2,415$

Rmax time point of maximum QRS vector magnitude.

TABLE C3 ST X, Y and Z amplitudes at ten equally spaced time points in white men and women.

		X		Y		Z	
		Men	Women	Men	Women	Men	Women
1/10	Mean; SD	9; 23.6	6; 22.0	7; 20.8	7; 19.8	32; 29.6	26; 27.0
	2% → 98%	−41 → 60	−42 → 52	−38 → 48	−37 → 46	−17 → 108	−19 → 94
2/10	Mean; SD	10; 24.4	6; 22.6	6; 19.9	6; 18.8	42; 31.6	35; 28.5
	2% → 98%	−42 → 62	−41 → 54	−39 → 45	−35 → 44	−9 → 122	−11 → 109
3/10	Mean; SD	13; 26.1	8; 23.9	6; 20.0	6; 19.2	49; 33.9	41; 30.5
	2% → 98%	−42 → 69	−42 → 59	−38 → 46	−37 → 44	−5 → 137	−9 → 120
4/10	Mean; SD	16; 28.2	11; 25.6	6; 20.7	6; 19.9	55; 36.4	46; 32.6
	2% → 98%	−42 → 77	−43 → 66	−39 → 48	−37 → 47	−4 → 148	−8 → 129
5/10	Mean; SD	20; 30.4	14; 27.6	7; 21.6	7; 20.8	61; 39.2	51; 35.0
	2% → 98%	−43 → 86	−44 → 74	−42 → 50	38 → 50	−3 → 163	−6 → 141
6/10	Mean; SD	24; 33.1	18; 29.8	8; 22.7	8; 21.9	67; 42.3	56; 37.7
	2% → 98%	−43 → 97	−45 → 83	−42 → 54	−39 → 53	−2 → 176	−5 → 153
7/10	Mean; SD	29; 36.1	23; 32.3	10; 24.2	10; 23.3	74; 45.9	62; 40.9
	2% → 98%	−42 → 110	−43 → 94	−42 → 60	−40 → 57	−2 → 190	−5 → 166
8/10	Mean; SD	36; 39.5	29; 35.3	12; 25.7	12; 25.1	83; 50.0	69; 44.9
	2% → 98%	−40 → 126	−42 → 108	−43 → 67	−40 → 63	−1 → 208	−5 → 183
9/10	Mean; SD	45; 43.8	38; 39.1	15; 28.2	16; 27.5	93; 55.0	78; 49.7
	2% → 98%	−40 → 145	−41 → 126	−46 → 74	−41 → 73	−2 → 234	−7 → 205
10/10	Mean; SD	58; 49.5	51; 44.4	20; 31.4	22; 30.8	106; 61.4	90; 56.0
	2% → 98%	−43 → 165	−39 → 149	−47 → 88	−42 → 88	−2 → 258	−11 → 227

TABLE C4 T wave X, Y and Z amplitudes at ten equally spaced time points and T vector spatial magnitude in white men and women.

		X		Y		Z		Vector magnitude	
		Men	Women	Men	Women	Men	Women	Men	Women
1/10	Mean; SD	83; 61.7	76; 56.2	31; 38.1	33; 37.5	132; 77.4	111; 70.9	222; 84.8	196; 75.8
	2% → 98%	−43 → 217	−39 → 197	−47 → 114	−43 → 111	−10 → 322	−20 → 285	80 → 424	73 → 379
2/10	Mean; SD	119; 81.4	113; 75.3	47; 48.4	51; 47.6	166; 100.6	138; 92.6	275; 107	258; 98.3
	2% → 98%	−46 → 297	−34 → 276	−51 → 153	−45 → 153	−18 → 410	−33 → 363	92 → 530	98 → 493
3/10	Mean; SD	166; 107.8	159; 100.8	70; 61.2	76; 60.7	198; 126.2	163; 116.9	335; 134	329; 125.8
	2% → 98%	−50 → 408	−37 → 380	−52 → 205	−43 → 209	−30 → 499	−48 → 436	106 → 660	120 → 620
4/10	Mean; SD	208; 132.6	202; 124.1	93; 72.8	100; 71.9	216; 145.0	175; 135.1	379; 157.2	385; 149.5
	2% → 98%	−54 → 503	−32 → 473	−50 → 256	−40 → 259	−42 → 559	−66 → 491	117 → 732	136 → 734
5/10	Mean; SD	232; 145.6	226; 136.5	111; 79.6	118; 78.5	208; 146.3	169; 137.5	387; 165.5	402; 156.1
	2% → 98%	−61 → 553	−35 → 524	−46 → 286	−39 → 291	−55 → 549	−76 → 499	109 → 766	139 → 757
6/10	Mean; SD	222; 133.1	217; 125.0	115; 74.8	121; 73.9	167; 120.8	137; 114.6	341; 145.9	356; 134.1
	2% → 98%	−50 → 506	−36 → 477	−36 → 279	−30 → 285	−55 → 443	−69 → 405	95 → 661	123 → 665
7/10	Mean; SD	168; 93.2	165; 88.1	97; 57.0	101; 56.5	108; 78.7	91; 74.5	342; 100.1	253; 90.2
	2% → 98%	−35 → 364	−19 → 341	−21 → 279	−14 → 225	−42 → 282	−49 → 259	71 → 470	90 → 462
8/10	Mean; SD	103; 52.6	101; 50.1	67; 38.0	70; 38.0	59; 44.3	50; 41.2	145; 56.3	151; 51.3
	2% → 98%	−10 → 208	−1 → 202	−9 → 148	−5 → 152	−28 → 156	−31 → 142	51 → 282	58 → 270
9/10	Mean; SD	60; 27.7	58; 26.8	44; 26.8	46; 26.9	31; 26.3	27; 24.0	84; 32.2	90; 29.5
	2% → 98%	3 → 117	7 → 113	−10 → 101	−7 → 104	−21 → 90	−20 → 79	28 → 158	36 → 156
Tend	Mean; SD	40; 18.9	38; 18.7	31; 23.1	33; 23.4	20; 20.5	16; 18.8	59; 25	63; 22.4
	2% → 98%	2 → 80	2 → 79	−15 → 80	−13 → 83	−20 → 67	−21 → 58	17 → 113	22 → 115
TSM	Mean; SD	202; 168.9	241; 148.2	83; 99.5	105; 81.5	273; 150.4	267; 143.7	395; 164.5	407; 155.9
	2% → 98%	−138 → 566	−44 → 563	−100 → 306	−47 → 293	−9 → 626	8 → 587	126 → 768	145 → 765

TSM T vector spatial magnitude at time point of maximum. Amplitudes are in μV.

TABLE C5 P wave X, Y and Z amplitudes at ten equally spaced time points in African–American men and women.

		X		Y		Z	
		Men	Women	Men	Women	Men	Women
Ponset	Mean; SD	18; 10.1	17; 10.2	25; 17.7	24; 17.2	1; 10.5	1; 10.0
	2% → 98%	$-1 \to 41$	$-1 \to 41$	$-10 \to 67$	$-9 \to 63$	$-20 \to 24$	$-18 \to 26$
1/10	Mean; SD	24; 11.5	24; 11.6	45; 23.7	44; 23.0	10; 12.0	11; 11.7
	2% → 98%	$2 \to 51$	$2 \to 49$	$-4 \to 98$	$-3 \to 94$	$-16 \to 35$	$-13 \to 35$
2/10	Mean; SD	31; 13.9	30; 14.2	63; 28.9	61; 27.6	19; 15.7	20; 15.3
	2% → 98%	$5 \to 62$	$5 \to 61$	$-3 \to 125$	$0 \to 115$	$-15 \to 49$	$-10 \to 53$
3/10	Mean; SD	39; 16.4	38; 17.3	73; 34.0	71; 32.9	23; 19.7	24; 19.4
	2% → 98%	$8 \to 74$	$8 \to 78$	$0 \to 146$	$3 \to 140$	$-21 \to 61$	$-15 \to 65$
4/10	Mean; SD	53; 20.2	53; 20.5	85; 42.5	84; 41.3	11; 25.6	12; 24.1
	2% → 98%	$15 \to 94$	$16 \to 98$	$-1 \to 181$	$0 \to 169$	$-52 \to 60$	$-40 \to 61$
5/10	Mean; SD	62; 21.8	62; 21.9	88; 46.5	87; 44.8	-3; 24.5	-1; 23.2
	2% → 98%	$20 \to 105$	$24 \to 107$	$-3 \to 192$	$-6 \to 180$	$-62 \to 43$	$-49 \to 43$
6/10	Mean; SD	63; 21.1	62; 21.9	78; 49.0	78; 47.4	-17; 23.5	-15; 22.4
	2% → 98%	$18 \to 105$	$25 \to 107$	$-9 \to 188$	$-10 \to 181$	$-72 \to 27$	$-59 \to 26$
7/10	Mean; SD	56; 18.5	56; 19.7	58; 42.0	57; 41.0	-19; 19.2	-17; 19.5
	2% → 98%	$14 \to 93$	$22 \to 96$	$-15 \to 155$	$-17 \to 151$	$-60 \to 17$	$-59 \to 17$
8/10	Mean; SD	40; 15.4	39; 17.3	38; 28.6	38; 28.8	-14; 15.3	-13; 16.2
	2% → 98%	$9 \to 74$	$9 \to 71$	$-12 \to 101$	$-18 \to 103$	$-49 \to 15$	$-44 \to 13$
9/10	Mean; SD	19; 9.9	19; 13.4	18; 17.9	18; 17.9	-11; 10.7	-10; 13.0
	2% → 98%	$0 \to 41$	$0 \to 43$	$-15 \to 56$	$-16 \to 56$	$-35 \to 8$	$-34 \to 9$
10/10	Mean; SD	7; 7.5	7; 11.9	5; 13.8	4; 13.6	-13; 8.7	-11; 11.6
	2% → 98%	$-8 \to 24$	$-9 \to 24$	$-26 \to 33$	$-24 \to 33$	$-32 \to 3$	$-31 \to 3$

TABLE C6 QRS X, Y and Z components and vector magnitude at ten equally spaced time points in African–American men and women.

		X		Y		Z		Vector magnitude	
		Men	Women	Men	Women	Men	Women	Men	Women
1/10	Mean; SD	−16; 49	−15; 48	1; 47	3; 44	74; 52	71; 45	102; 45.7	96; 43
	2% → 98%	−108 → 102	−111 → 100	−95 → 93	−83 → 105	−18 → 202	−13 → 183	36 → 223	31 → 205
2/10	Mean; SD	124; 158	116; 148	31; 85	33; 76	199; 142	184; 118	282; 133.3	249; 121
	2% → 98%	−165 → 529	−142 → 495	−129 → 242	−107 → 210	−86 → 527	−30 → 451	84 → 637	74 → 556
3/10	Mean; SD	606; 293	563; 264	154; 166	154; 152	200; 302	164; 274	713; 285.7	618; 259
	2% → 98%	74 → 1,328	136 → 1,236	−109 → 571	−114 → 517	−539 → 743	−523 → 653	268 → 1,415	213 → 1,273
4/10	Mean; SD	1,103; 389	1,046; 336	382; 293	376; 280	−140; 468	−161; 439	1,313; 399.7	1,131; 347.1
	2% → 98%	449 → 1,996	439 → 1,851	−131 → 1,061	−154 → 988	−1,175 → 678	−1,129 → 648	633 → 2,257	530 → 1,979
5/10	Mean; SD	905; 579	897; 548	383; 381	386; 365	−535; 496	−523; 451	1,383; 475.7	1,191; 422.5
	2% → 98%	−312 → 2,072	−242 → 2,001	−301 → 1,262	−323 → 1,199	−1,562 → 445	−1,413 → 441	521 → 2,471	427 → 2,155
6/10	Mean; SD	270; 438	306; 450	178; 301	178; 291	−657; 641	−624; 313	917; 328.2	841; 301.5
	2% → 98%	−391 → 1,370	−439 → 1,363	−388 → 865	−418 → 836	−1,314 → 148	−1,290 → 70	391 → 1,721	322 → 1,592
7/10	Mean; SD	−13; 193	2; 184	48; 184	55; 178	−456; 193	−437; 175	500; 171.4	485; 157
	2% → 98%	−335 → 389	−340 → 426	−337 → 451	−335 → 446	−886 → −51	−823 → −103	228 → 925	214 → 860
8/10	Mean; SD	−15; 87	−10; 82	11; 103	17; 96	−191; 110	−185; 97	220; 89.1	226; 77.7
	2% → 98%	−199 → 161	−188 → 145	−216 → 217	−192 → 213	−440 → 22	−410 → 0	83 → 454	92 → 413
9/10	Mean; SD	9; 45	11; 41	9; 52	12; 48	−38; 50	−42; 43	83; 34.3	84; 32.5
	2% → 98%	−77 → 105	−72 → 94	−106 → 103	−96 → 105	−140 → 73	−128 → 53	23 → 165	26 → 161
Rend	Mean; SD	14; 30	14; 26	8; 28	10; 26	18; 34	10; 29	47; 23.1	39; 19.8
	2% → 98%	−41 → 83	−39 → 65	−53 → 62	−45 → 63	−40 → 98	−38 → 81	12 → 101	9 → 88
Rmax	Mean; SD	1,229; 437	1,050; 405.8	494; 380.3	488; 350	−430; 449	−391; 403.8	1,512; 424.8	1,310; 373.7
	2% → 98%	274 → 2,181	7 → 1,924	−286 → 1,388	−142 → 1,319	−1,221 → 562	−1,128 → 514	788 → 2,505	−681 → 2,230

Rmax amplitudes at time point of maximum QRS vector magnitude. Amplitudes are in µV.

TABLE C7 ST X, Y and Z amplitudes at ten equally spaced time points in African–American men and women.

		X		Y		Z	
		Men	Women	Men	Women	Men	Women
1/10	Mean; SD	9; 23.6	6; 22.0	7; 20.8	7; 19.8	32; 29.6	26; 27.0
	2% → 98%	$-41 \to 60$	$-42 \to 52$	$-38 \to 48$	$-37 \to 46$	$-7 \to 108$	$-19 \to 94$
2/10	Mean; SD	10; 24.4	6; 22.6	6; 19.9	6; 18.8	42; 31.6	35; 28.5
	2% → 98%	$-42 \to 62$	$-41 \to 54$	$-39 \to 45$	$-35 \to 44$	$-9 \to 122$	$-11 \to 109$
3/10	Mean; SD	13; 26.1	8; 23.9	6; 20.0	6; 19.2	49; 33.9	41; 30.5
	2% → 98%	$-42 \to 69$	$-42 \to 59$	$-38 \to 46$	$-37 \to 44$	$-5 \to 137$	$9 \to 120$
4/10	Mean; SD	16; 28.2	111; 25.6	6; 20.7	6; 19.9	55; 36.4	46; 32.6
	2% → 98%	$-42 \to 77$	$-43 \to 66$	$-39 \to 48$	$-37 \to 47$	$-4 \to 148$	$-8 \to 129$
5/10	Mean; SD	20; 30.4	14; 27.6	7; 21.6	7; 20.8	61; 39.2	51; 35.0
	2% → 98%	$-43 \to 86$	$-44 \to 74$	$-42 \to 50$	$-38 \to 50$	$-3 \to 163$	$-6 \to 141$
6/10	Mean; SD	24; 33.1	18; 29.8	8; 22.7	8; 22.7	67; 42.3	56; 37.7
	2% → 98%	$-43 \to 97$	$-45 \to 83$	$-42 \to 54$	$-39 \to 53$	$-2 \to 176$	$-5 \to 153$
7/10	Mean; SD	29; 36.1	23; 32.3	10; 24.2	10; 23.3	74; 45.9	62; 40.9
	2% → 98%	$-42 \to 110$	$-43 \to 94$	$-42 \to 60$	$-40 \to 57$	$-2 \to 190$	$-5 \to 166$
8/10	Mean; SD	36; 39.5	29; 35.3	12; 25.7	12; 25.1	83; 50.0	69; 44.9
	2% → 98%	$-40 \to 126$	$-42 \to 108$	$-43 \to 67$	$-40 \to 63$	$-1 \to 208$	$-5 \to 183$
9/10	Mean; SD	45; 43.8	38; 39.1	15; 28.2	16; 27.5	93; 55.0	78; 49.7
	2% → 98%	$-40 \to 145$	$-41 \to 126$	$-46 \to 74$	$-41 \to 73$	$-2 \to 234$	$-7 \to 205$
10/10	Mean; SD	58; 49.5	51; 44.4	20; 31.4	22; 30.8	106; 61.4	90; 56.0
	2% → 98%	$-43 \to 165$	$-39 \to 149$	$-47 \to 83$	$-42 \to 88$	$-2 \to 258$	$-11 \to 227$

TABLE C8 T wave X, Y and Z amplitudes at ten equally spaced time points in African–American men and women.

		X		Y		Z		Vector magnitude	
		Men	Women	Men	Women	Men	Women	Men	Women
1/10	Mean; SD	11; 26.2	10; 22.0	6; 21.4	7; 19.8	38; 33.4	29; 27.1	143; 55.4	141; 53.1
	2% → 98%	−37 → 68	−38 → 54	−38 → 49	−34 → 50	−17 → 119	−16 → 96	57 → 284	57 → 272
2/10	Mean; SD	12; 26.8	10; 22.3	5; 20.4	6; 18.5	49; 36.1	40; 29.0	183; 71.8	191; 71.4
	2% → 98%	−39 → 73	−35 → 54	−38 → 46	−32 → 45	−8 → 135	−6 → 111	72 → 365	75 → 365
3/10	Mean; SD	15; 28.5	13; 23.9	5; 20.5	7; 19.0	57; 39.0	46; 31.1	229; 94.2	250; 96.3
	2% → 98%	−39 → 82	−36 → 61	−38 → 44	−33 → 47	−6 → 151	−4 → 123	83 → 465	91 → 486
4/10	Mean; SD	18; 30.5	16; 25.5	5; 21.2	7; 19.8	63; 41.9	51; 33.5	267; 114.4	300; 118.9
	2% → 98%	−40 → 89	−38 → 67	−39 → 44	−35 → 47	−5 → 166	−2 → 137	91 → 553	101 → 591
5/10	Mean; SD	22; 32.9	19; 27.5	5; 21.8	8; 20.7	70; 44.9	56; 36.0	282; 125.4	325; 130.5
	2% → 98%	−40 → 100	−37 → 74	−39 → 48	−36 → 52	−3 → 178	0 → 149	87 → 586	106 → 637
6/10	Mean; SD	27; 35.5	23; 29.7	6; 22.8	10; 21.8	76; 48.1	62; 38.7	266; 118.9	305; 119.1
	2% → 98%	−36 → 112	−39 → 83	−40 → 50	−35 → 58	−3 → 190	1 → 162	77 → 537	100 → 574
7/10	Mean; SD	32; 38.5	29; 32.4	9; 24.3	12; 23.0	83; 51.4	68; 41.9	206; 87.8	231; 84.8
	2% → 98%	−39 → 123	−39 → 96	−41 → 57	−34 → 63	0 → 205	2 → 173	61 → 408	79 → 415
8/10	Mean; SD	39; 41.8	35; 35.5	12; 26.1	14; 24.9	92; 56.1	75; 45.1	132; 52.2	145; 49.6
	2% → 98%	−37 → 139	−38 → 108	−41 → 58	−35 → 68	3 → 222	2 → 193	44 → 249	55 → 252
9/10	Mean; SD	48; 45.8	44; 39.3	15; 28.2	18; 26.9	102; 61.1	83; 50.6	79; 30.4	87; 28.6
	2% → 98%	−33 → 153	−39 → 126	−40 → 66	−33 → 77	2 → 244	−1 → 211	30 → 152	36 → 150
Tend	Mean; SD	60; 51.1	56; 44.5	20; 31.3	24; 30.0	114; 67.4	94; 57.9	54; 23.6	60; 21.7
	2% → 98%	−32 → 178	−36 → 151	−42 → 73	−34 → 86	1 → 272	−5 → 236	17 → 109	21; 111
TSM	Mean; SD	191; 141.4	234; 128.3	99; 74.9	130; 73.5	113; 116	134; 117.1	288; 124.5	329; 129.4
	2% → 98%	−127 → 477	−20 → 527	−45 → 260	−16 → 298	−98 → 385	−86 → 400	100 → 590	112 → 637

TSM T vector spatial magnitude at time point of maximum. Amplitudes are in μV.

Section D
ECG Amplitudes at 10 ms Intervals: Tables

TABLE D1 QRS amplitudes in X, Y and Z leads in white men and women at 10-ms increments from the onset and backwards from the offset of QRS.

ms	Statistics	X		Y		Z	
		Men	Women	Men	Women	Men	Women
10*	Mean; SD	−14; 59.9	−14; 59.2	−1; 49.5	−2; 50.9	83; 52.3	85; 53.2
	2% → 98%	−126 → 132	−124 → 128	−98 → 113	−102 → 116	−12 → 209	−14 → 212
20	Mean; SD	191; 194.0	198; 191.2	39; 90.6	51; 92.0	202; 146.2	204; 153.2
	2% → 98%	−144 → 691	−123 → 690	−122 → 266	−114 → 282	−126 → 532	−114 → 538
30	Mean; SD	765; 319.0	768; 310.8	210; 197.5	247; 200.7	112; 339.4	92; 338.4
	2% → 98%	−187 → 1,497	224 → 1,533	−124 → 693	−110 → 725	−693 → 719	−661 → 737
40	Mean; SD	1,042; 442.7	1,015; 432.9	376; 330	411; 326.6	−279; 450.2	−319; 435.9
	2% → 98%	139 → 1,988	91 → 1,970	−265 → 1,125	−253 → 1,097	−1,232 → 654	−1,211 → 596
Roff	Mean; SD	11; 28.0	9; 25.8	9; 27.4	9; 26.7	12; 30.8	9; 30
	2% → 98%	−44 → 73	−44 → 63	−49 → 63	−49 → 62	−41 → 86	−43 → 81
−10	Mean; SD	1; 47.6	1; 45	10; 56.1	10; 56.3	−54; 54.8	−57; 54.1
	2% → 98%	−96 → 103	−91 → 95	−119 → 119	−118 → 119	−165 → 65	−169 → 61
−20	Mean; SD	−28; 108.6	−22; 109.6	16; 122.8	19; 123.2	−239; 130.7	−244; 132.8
	2% → 98%	−253 → 187	−241 → 221	−254 → 261	−250 → 277	−536 → 13	−549 → 61
−30	Mean; SD	62; 312.4	110; 330.1	84; 229.2	104; 239.6	−488; 231.7	−495; 232.3
	2% → 98%	−253 → 187	−365 → 1,003	−369 → 588	−389 → 654	−981 → 21	−998 → −17
−40	Mean; SD	498; 588.3	583; 571.3	244; 334.3	292; 340.3	−532; 397.5	−541; 396.6
	2% → 98%	−417 → 1,706	−388 → 1,719	−433 → 991	−396 → 1,018	−1,309 → 357	−1,325 → 347

* Ronset amplitudes are set to 0 at 0 ms (baseline); *Roff* Roffset (J point). The amplitudes are in μV.

TABLE D2 ST and T amplitudes in X, Y and Z leads in white men and women. ST amplitudes are at 20-ms increments from the J point (QRSoffset) and T amplitudes backwards from Tend.

ms	Statistics	X		Y		Z	
		Men	Women	Men	Women	Men	Women
Jp*	Mean; SD	11; 28.0	9; 25.8	9; 27.4	9; 26.7	12; 30.8	9; 30
	2% → 98%	−44 → 73	−44 → 63	−49 → 63	−49 → 62	−41 → 86	−43 → 81
10	Mean; SD	9; 24.6	7; 22.3	7; 21.5	7; 20.6	28; 30.1	26; 29.2
	2% → 98%	−41 → 62	−42 → 53	−38 → 50	−38 → 48	−20 → 101	−22 → 100
20	Mean; SD	10; 24.9	7; 22.3	5; 20.2	6; 19.2	38; 31.8	35; 30.7
	2% → 98%	−42 → 63	−41 → 53	−38 → 46	−36 → 44	−12 → 116	−14 → 113
30	Mean; SD	12; 26.1	8; 23.1	5; 20.0	6; 19.1	44; 33.7	41; 32.7
	2% → 98%	−42 → 68	−41 → 57	−38 → 45	−37 → 44	−9 → 130	−10 → 122
40	Mean; SD	15; 27.7	10; 24.3	5; 20.3	6; 19.5	49; 35.9	46; 34.7
	2% → 98%	−43 → 74	−42 → 62	−39 → 47	−37 → 45	−6 → 142	−8 → 134
Tend	Mean; SD	40; 19.2	37; 18.8	31; 23.3	33; 23.6	19; 20.1	17; 19.7
	2% → 98%	2 → 81	1 → 79	−15 → 81	−13 → 84	−20 → 64	−22 → 60
−10	Mean; SD	49; 22.6	47; 22	37; 24.8	39; 240.9	24; 22.2	22; 21.8
	2% → 98%	4 → 96	4 → 93	−13 → 90	−9 → 94	−20 → 74	−23 → 70
−20	Mean; SD	63; 30.5	62; 29.4	46; 28.3	48; 28.7	32; 27.1	30; 26.6
	2% → 98%	2 → 123	7 → 120	−11 → 107	−7 → 113	−20 → 94	−26 → 87
−30	Mean; SD	85; 44.2	85; 42.4	57; 34.6	61; 35	45; 36.1	43; 35.7
	2% → 98%	−5 → 170	2 → 168	−11 → 133	−6 → 139	−25 → 126	−31 → 119
−40	Mean; SD	115; 63.5	116; 61	72; 43.2	78; 44.1	64; 50.2	60; 49.7
	2% → 98%	−20 → 238	−8 → 234	−10 → 166	−7 → 177	−32 → 176	−42 → 167

Jp = J Point; same as Roff in Table D1. The amplitudes are in µV.

TABLE D3 QRS amplitudes in X, Y and Z leads in African–American men and women at 10-ms increments from the onset and backwards from the offset of QRS.

ms	Statistics	X		Y		Z	
		Men	Women	Men	Women	Men	Women
10*	Mean; SD	−17; 58.2	−15; 60.4	0; 52.7	−2; 49.8	89; 53.5	86; 53.8
	2% → 98%	−127 → 117	−133 → 134	−100 → 109	−105 → 104	−5 → 218	−10 → 226
20	Mean; SD	187; 186.3	189; 191.9	46; 94.9	42; 89.7	207; 149.8	195; 157.9
	2% → 98%	−129 → 656	−138 → 684	−122 → 284	−112 → 260	−99 → 519	−127 → 535
30	Mean; SD	775; 312.9	758; 296.3	233; 209.5	226; 192.6	63; 319.8	51; 343.5
	2% → 98%	231 → 1,510	204 → 1,432	−123 → 741	−104 → 683	−641 → 675	−741 → 683
40	Mean; SD	1,080; 435.0	1,018; 414.7	400; 339	386; 324.9	−360; 429.5	−370; 425.1
	2% → 98%	160 → 1,988	112 → 1,872	−208 → 1,095	−270 → 1,090	−1,196 → 573	−1,268 → 501
Roff	Mean; SD	12; 26.4	11; 25.7	10; 27.6	9; 26.6	11; 30.2	8; 29.5
	2% → 98%	−39 → 73	−44 → 63	−49 → 61	−46 → 62	−40 → 83	−42 → 79
−10	Mean; SD	5; 45.6	3; 44.9	12; 57.1	11; 55.9	−54; 54.3	−59; 53.8
	2% → 98%	−84 → 100	−98 → 94	−113 → 117	−113 → 115	−168 → 58	−174 → 51
−20	Mean; SD	−22; 111	−20; 107.1	20; 122.4	21; 117	−241; 133.5	−249; 134.7
	2% → 98%	−242 → 179	−244 → 193	−234 → 289	−225 → 259	−545 → 11	−555 → −4
−30	Mean; SD	87; 309.8	117; 334.3	98; 235.8	104; 227.7	−494; 229.6	−502; 245.7
	2% → 98%	−345 → 929	−360 → 969	−370 → 577	−360 → 606	−981 → −34	−1,017 → 11
−40	Mean; SD	586; 584.6	594; 571.6	280; 344.1	282; 333.2	−553; 389.5	−557; 395.4
	2% → 98%	−344 → 1,779	−390 → 1,674	−108 → 1,027	−358 → 1,056	−1,331 → 325	−1,313 → 344

* Ronset amplitudes are set to 0 at 0 ms (baseline); *Roff* Roffset (J point). The amplitudes are in µV.

TABLE D4 ST and T amplitudes in X, Y and Z leads in African–American men and women. ST amplitudes are at 20-ms increments from the J point (QRSoffset) and T amplitudes backwards from Tend.

ms	Statistics	X		Y		Z	
		Men	Women	Men	Women	Men	Women
Jp*	Mean; SD	12; 26.4	11; 25.7	10; 27.6	9; 26.6	11; 30.2	8; 29.5
	2% → 98%	−39 → 73	−44 → 63	−49 → 61	−46 → 62	−40 → 83	−42 → 79
10	Mean; SD	10; 23.3	8; 22.5	8; 21.8	7; 20.3	28; 29.1	25; 28.8
	2% → 98%	−37 → 61	−40 → 54	−43 → 49	−34 → 50	−21 → 100	−22 → 99
20	Mean; SD	10; 23.6	7; 22.6	6; 20.1	6; 18.6	37; 30.7	35; 30.6
	2% → 98%	−38 → 60	−38 → 53	−39 → 45	−31 → 45	−12 → 112	−13 → 113
30	Mean; SD	12; 24.8	9; 23.5	6; 19.9	6; 18.4	43; 32.4	41; 32.4
	2% → 98%	−38 → 65	−38 → 56	−38 → 44	−32 → 45	−9 → 124	−8 → 123
40	Mean; SD	14; 26.5	11; 24.9	6; 20.3	6; 18.8	48; 34.3	46; 34.4
	2% → 98%	−37 → 73	−40 → 61	−38 → 46	−34 → 45	−6 → 135	−5 → 134
Tend	Mean; SD	38; 19.9	38; 18.5	33; 22.9	32; 21.9	17; 19.6	16; 18.3
	2% → 98%	−3 → 81	2 → 80	−14 → 81	−13 → 83	−19 → 63	−18 → 57
−10	Mean; SD	47; 23.2	47; 22.2	39; 24.4	39; 23.5	22; 21.5	21; 20.6
	2% → 98%	3 → 97	3 → 95	−9 → 90	−10 → 92	−17 → 71	−18 → 68
−20	Mean; SD	63; 30.7	62; 30	48; 28.4	48; 26.9	30; 26.1	28; 25.4
	2% → 98%	6 → 124	3 → 122	−5 → 110	−6 → 109	−18 → 86	−22 → 82
−30	Mean; SD	86; 43.8	85; 43	61; 34.6	60; 33.4	42; 35.1	40; 34.5
	2% → 98%	6 → 174	−11 → 168	−2 → 138	−4 → 135	−24 → 119	−30 → 114
−40	Mean; SD	118; 62.7	116; 61.2	77; 44.4	77; 42.4	59; 49.4	57; 48.8
	2% → 98%	−9 → 250	−21 → 232	−1 → 176	−4 → 168	−34 → 170	−50 → 161

Jp J Point; same as Roff in Table D1. The amplitudes are in μV.

TABLE D5 Limb lead QRS amplitudes* at 10-ms intervals in white men and women.

Lead		From QRS onset				From end of QRS backwards			
		+10 ms	+20 ms	+30 ms	+40 ms	−10 ms	−20 ms	−30 ms	−40 ms
aVL	M	−23; 50.5	55; 108.5	297; 213.7	416; 342.0	15; 51.3	30; 123.5	108; 261.9	278; 370.9
		−133 → 78	−141 → 314	−86 → 782	−274 → 1,161	−79 → 136	−185 → 346	−319 → 794	−356 → 1,149
	F	−18; 49.1	47; 101.1	257; 211.7	348; 348.3	9; 48.9	15; 116.5	68; 241.6	208; 362.4
		−126 → 81	−146 → 296	−109 → 773	−307 → 1,132	−82 → 124	−192 → 307	−329 → 712	−409 → 1,084
I	M	−18; 45.3	119; 130.5	525; 231.8	735; 329.6	20; 42.9	30; 106.8	152; 260	468; 403.6
		−112 → 82	−97 → 439	126 → 1,063	92 → 1,482	−63 → 117	−165 → 311	−224 → 834	−219 → 1,371
	F	−20; 43	102; 122	479; 224.8	678; 318	14; 41.4	13; 101.1	113; 240.2	404; 385.9
		−112 → 73	−112 → 409	117 → 1,043	92 → 1,400	−68 → 107	−165 → 262	−244 → 771	−229 → 1,293
−aVR	M	−5; 38.3	123; 112.5	490; 197.4	687; 274	16; 40.3	15; 90.9	119; 214.3	425; 348.4
		−78 → 82	−65 → 411	134 → 953	126 → 1,288	−74 → 95	−170 → 204	−218 → 660	−199 → 1,140
	F	−11; 36.1	106; 106.1	461; 187.5	669; 252.8	12; 39.8	4; 88.9	102; 206.4	399; 334.9
		−80 → 73	−80 → 366	125 → 892	142 → 1,207	−73 → 90	−170 → 197	−225 → 652	−204 → 1,085
II	M	9; 56.9	127; 124.1	455; 239.3	639; 372.7	16; 31.7	11; 64.6	−1; 140.1	87; 280.8
		−102 → 136	−82 → 443	39 → 1,015	−86 → 1,459	−53 → 82	−136 → 131	−302 → 283	−443 → 746
	F	−2; 54.9	110; 117.8	443; 229	660; 360.6	17; 31.2	9; 63.3	−5; 137	90; 275.7
		−107 → 122	−102 → 405	39 → 984	−78 → 1,415	−48 → 78	−131 → 131	−297 → 273	−414 → 766
aVF	M	18; 57.4	67; 102.7	193; 219.7	271; 373.6	1; 66.2	−16; 146.4	11; 277.6	147; 389
		−99 → 151	−123 → 329	−209 → 699	−466 → 1,073	−153 → 121	−351 → 265	−616 → 597	−668 → 985
	F	7; 57.4	59; 97.3	203; 215	321; 378.1	2; 64.1	−12; 141.4	33; 268.5	191; 389.9
		−107 → 139	−121 → 292	−201 → 705	−451 → 1,107	−143 → 128	−331 → 270	−524 → 622	−600; 1,021
III	M	24; 65.7	6; 115	−65; 250.1	−76; 447.6	−6; 72.7	−22; 166.6	−43; 312.3	−59; 448.1
		−112 → 175	−239 → 258	−595 → 477	−1,005 → 873	−180 → 126	−434 → 287	−784 → 541	−1,062 → 848
	F	21; 68.2	9; 113.9	−44; 258.6	−38; 449.9	−7; 72.6	−25; 166.8	−41; 325.8	−38; 452.6
		−117 → 175	−234 → 258	−585 → 507	−984 → 882	−175 → 131	−424 → 287	−853 → 585	−1,106 → 849

* Mean values (μV), standard deviation and the range from the lower to the upper second percentile. *M* men, *F* women.

TABLE D6 Limb lead ST-T amplitudes* at 10-ms intervals in white men and women.

		From J point forwards					From end of T backwards			
		J point	J + 10	J + 20	J + 30	J + 40	Toff − 10	Toff − 20	Toff − 30	Toff − 40
aVL	M	9; 25.3	5; 19.3	5; 18.1	5; 17.9	6; 18.4	11; 22.3	15; 25.8	21; 32.3	30; 41.9
		$-39 \to 69$	$-34 \to 48$	$-31 \to 46$	$-31 \to 45$	$-31 \to 46$	$-34 \to 58$	$-36 \to 70$	$-43 \to 92$	$-52 \to 124$
	F	7; 23.6	4; 17.9	4; 16.6	4; 16.6	5; 17	10; 21.8	14; 25.1	20; 31.2	29; 40.4
		$-39 \to 61$	$-31 \to 43$	$-29 \to 39$	$-30 \to 41$	$-29 \to 43$	$-34 \to 58$	$-36 \to 69$	$-41 \to 87$	$-48 \to 119$
I	M	17; 24.1	12; 20.7	11; 20.7	12; 21.4	13; 22.4	40; 21.4	51; 26.1	67; 34.9	90; 47.7
		$-33 \to 68$	$-29 \to 58$	$-34 \to 58$	$-34 \to 58$	$-34 \to 63$	$-3 \to 87$	$0 \to 112$	$0 \to 146$	$-4 \to 200$
	F	15; 22.4	12; 19.2	11; 19.1	12; 19.8	14; 20.7	40; 21	51; 25.4	69; 33.8	92; 46
		$-29 \to 68$	$-29 \to 53$	$-29 \to 53$	$-29 \to 53$	$-29 \to 58$	$0 \to 87$	$4 \to 107$	$9 \to 146$	$14 \to 195$
−aVR	M	16; 22.1	13; 19.6	12; 19.6	13; 20.4	14; 21.3	49; 20.4	61; 25	80; 33.2	105; 45.1
		$-29 \to 61$	$-29 \to 53$	$-30 \to 51$	$-29 \to 56$	$-31 \to 58$	$7 \to 92$	$12 \to 114$	$14 \to 151$	$17 \to 200$
	F	16; 21.4	14; 18.7	13; 18.8	14; 19.4	14; 20.7	50; 19.9	63; 24.3	83; 32.5	109; 43.9
		$-29 \to 61$	$-26 \to 53$	$-29 \to 51$	$-29 \to 56$	$-29 \to 58$	$12 \to 95$	$17 \to 114$	$21 \to 151$	$24 \to 200$
II	M	16; 31.7	14; 25.9	13; 24.9	14; 25.1	15; 25.9	58; 29.6	72; 34.7	93; 43.8	30; 41.9
		$-53 \to 82$	$-39 \to 68$	$-39 \to 63$	$-39 \to 67$	$-39 \to 68$	$0 \to 122$	$4 \to 151$	$9 \to 190$	$-52 \to 124$
	F	17; 31.2	16; 25.1	15; 24.1	16; 24.4	18; 25.9	60; 28.7	75; 33.9	97; 43.1	29; 40.4
		$-48 \to 78$	$-39 \to 68$	$-38 \to 63$	$-39 \to 68$	$-39 \to 68$	$4 \to 122$	$9 \to 146$	$14 \to 190$	$-48 \to 119$
aVF	M	7; 30.9	8; 23.5	7; 21.7	8; 21.3	9; 21.6	38; 28.6	46; 32.6	59; 37.7	90; 47.7
		$-61 \to 68$	$-43 \to 56$	$-39 \to 53$	$-39 \to 51$	$-387 \to 53$	$-19 \to 100$	$-17 \to 119$	$-17 \to 151$	$-4 \to 200$
	F	9; 30.2	9; 22.8	9; 20.9	10; 20.6	10; 20.9	40; 27.7	49; 31.9	63; 39	92; 46
		$-56 \to 70$	$-39 \to 56$	$-36 \to 53$	$-36 \to 53$	$-36 \to 53$	$-17 \to 100$	$-9 \to 119$	$-12 \to 148$	$14 \to 195$
III	M	−1; 34.8	1; 25.5	2; 23.2	2; 22.5	2; 22.8	17; 31.3	21; 35.5	25; 42.9	105; 45.1
		$-82 \to 68$	$-58 \to 53$	$-48 \to 48$	$-48 \to 48$	$-47 \to 48$	$-48 \to 82$	$-48 \to 97$	$-63 \to 121$	$17 \to 200$
	F	1; 33.3	3; 24.4	4; 21.9	4; 21.4	3; 21.6	20; 30.5	24; 34.6	29; 41.8	109; 43.9
		$-73 \to 68$	$-48 \to 53$	$-43 \to 48$	$-43 \to 48$	$-43 \to 48$	$-43 \to 82$	$-43 \to 97$	$-53 \to 122$	$24 \to 200$

* Mean values (µV), standard deviation and the range from the lower to the upper second percentile. *M* men, *F* women.

TABLE D7 Chest lead QRS amplitudes* in white men and women at 10-ms intervals from QRS onset and from end of QRS backwards.

		From QRS onset				From end of QRS backwards			
		+10 ms	+20 ms	+30 ms	+40 ms	−10 ms	−20 ms	−30 ms	−40 ms
V1	M	85; 62.5	104; 173.5	−205; 336.6	−661; 414.7	−59; 61.2	−231; 156.5	−497; 278.7	−696; 384.2
		$-34 \to 229$	$-292 \to 468$	$-987 \to 429$	$-1,634 \to 112$	$-195 \to 63$	$-614 \to 48$	$-1,150 \to 19$	$-1,581 \to 9$
	F	87; 59.5	104; 166.3	−212; 314.5	−644; 371.8	−63; 61.7	−231; 150.5	−486; 263.9	−670; 352.4
		$-24 \to 229$	$-283 \to 439$	$-921 \to 356$	$-1,468 \to 73$	$-195 \to 77$	$-570 \to 68$	$-1,077 \to 43$	$-1,463 \to 4$
V2	M	124; 88.5	342; 258.2	260; 569.6	−332; 745.8	−72; 85.9	−357; 208.6	−719; 372.8	−735; 669.0
		$-29 \to 341$	$-195 \to 921$	$-1,053 \to 1,322$	$-1,839 \to 1,220$	$-253 \to 112$	$-839 \to 24$	$-1,503 \to 107$	$-1,952 \to 873$
	F	126; 83.0	308; 240.7	151; 524.7	−435; 662.8	−78; 83.0	−354; 191.5	−706; 337.4	−746; 592.6
		$-24 \to 326$	$-209 \to 844$	$-1,034 \to 1,156$	$-1,771 \to 1,034$	$-252 \to 107$	$-780 \to 19$	$-1,409 \to 41$	$-1,843 \to 667$
V3	M	83; 82.5	411; 248.3	813; 486.3	590; 757.4	−59; 78.7	−289; 187.8	−469; 451.0	−110; 877.7
		$-68 \to 287$	$-4 \to 1,033$	$-185 \to 1,893$	$-976 \to 2,136$	$-21.9 \to 117$	$-717 \to 82$	$-1,244 \to 741$	$-1,550 \to 1,770$
	F	80; 75.2	374; 229.4	715; 452.4	484; 688.2	−64; 75.9	−289; 172.5	−453; 425.8	−99; 801.8
		$-63 \to 263$	$-9 \to 941$	$-189 \to 1,731$	$-916 \to 1,921$	$-219 \to 102$	$-687 \to 58$	$-1,189 \to 702$	$-1,449 \to 1,609$
V4	M	35; 82.6	383; 269.9	1,074; 452.9	1,165; 712.4	−40; 71.3	−188; 166.2	−204; 464.2	360; 908.6
		$-117 \to 244$	$-53 \to 1,101$	$297 \to 2,191$	$-306 \to 2,693$	$-180 \to 122$	$-546 \to 151$	$-926 \to 1,068$	$-1,083 \to 2,277$
	F	30; 75.7	344; 249.0	983; 423.3	1,065; 652.3	−41; 68.9	−185; 155.7	−182; 453.8	384; 841.5
		$-107 \to 214$	$-63 \to 980$	$239 \to 2,024$	$-278 \to 2,479$	$-180 \to 107$	$-531 \to 146$	$-873 \to 1,070$	$-1,018 \to 2,069$
V5	M	0; 72.7	275; 242.0	952; 407.7	1,187; 575.5	−13; 58.0	−77; 134.8	19; 390.9	563; 725.5
		$-131 \to 180$	$-107 \to 912$	$287 \to 1,981$	$20 \to 2,469$	$-131 \to 112$	$-366 \to 195$	$-566 \to 1,082$	$-610 \to 2,073$
	F	−6; 66.9	251; 226.2	905; 377.0	1,136; 539.9	−13; 56.4	−77; 132.1	33; 388.7	587; 682.6
		$-131 \to 161$	$-122 \to 838$	$234 \to 1,843$	$34 \to 2,361$	$-131 \to 112$	$-345 \to 208$	$-527; 1,092$	$-580 \to 1,952$
V6	M	−18; 54.4	157; 175.1	667; 310.5	937; 403.0	13; 45.7	16; 112.4	164; 296.1	571; 497.1
		$-122 \to 112$	$-117 \to 629$	$170 \to 1,429$	$181 \to 1,849$	$-78 \to 107$	$-209 \to 268$	$-287 \to 926$	$-268 \to 1,663$
	F	−24; 51.5	146; 170.7	660; 298.0	928 → 387.9	14; 44.7	17; 110.7	174; 296.8	595; 476.3
		$-122 \to 101$	$-131 \to 600$	$141 \to 1,375$	$200 \to 1,834$	$-73 \to 107$	$-190 \to 273$	$-278 \to 931$	$-267 \to 1,571$

* Mean values (µV), standard deviation and the lower and upper second percentiles. *M* males, *F* females.

TABLE D8 Chest lead ST-T amplitudes* at 10-ms intervals in white men and women.

		From J point forwards					From end of T backwards			
		J point	J + 10	J + 20	J + 30	J + 40	Toff − 10	Toff − 20	Toff − 30	Toff − 40
V1	M	6; 31.4	22; 29.3	30; 30.5	35; 32.0	38; 33.3	3; 26.8	4; 31.8	5; 40.6	7; 54.0
		$-53 \to 78$	$-29 \to 97$	$-19 \to 107$	$-14 \to 117$	$-14 \to 126$	$-48 \to 63$	$-58 \to 73$	$-73 \to 97$	$-97 \to 130$
	F	2; 29.7	18; 26.2	26; 26.7	30; 28.1	34; 29.1	3; 24.9	2; 29.3	2; 37.0	1; 49.0
		$-53 \to 73$	$-29 \to 82$	$-19 \to 92$	$-19 \to 102$	$-14 \to 107$	$-48 \to 53$	$-58 \to 63$	$-73 \to 82$	$-97 \to 111$
V2	M	28; 50.1	52; 49.6	67; 52.9	77; 56.5	85; 60.2	55; 36.0	73; 44.2	101; 59.8	141; 84.0
		$-58 \to 146$	$-29 \to 175$	$-19 \to 200$	$-14 \to 219$	$-9 \to 239$	$-14 \to 136$	$-14 \to 170$	$-14 \to 234$	$-19 \to 330$
	F	22; 45.6	45; 43.7	58; 46.1	67; 48.8	75; 52.0	48; 31.7	65; 40.3	91; 55.9	129; 79.6
		$-58 \to 131$	$-29 \to 151$	$-19 \to 175$	$-14 \to 190$	$-9 \to 204$	$-14 \to 122$	$-14 \to 156$	$-14 \to 214$	$-19 \to 307$
V3	M	20; 46.6	37; 45.4	48; 48.3	57; 51.3	64; 54.7	69; 37.1	91; 46.6	125; 64.6	172; 91.6
		$-63 \to 131$	$-43 \to 151$	$-34 \to 165$	$-29 \to 185$	$-29 \to 203$	$-4 \to 151$	$0 \to 190$	$0 \to 258$	$-4 \to 365$
	F	17; 43.4	34; 42.2	44; 44.5	52; 47.0	58; 49.9	66; 34.0	89; 43.8	124; 61.7	174; 88.6
		$-63 \to 117$	$-43 \to 136$	$-34 \to 156$	$-29 \to 170$	$-24 \to 185$	$4 \to 141$	$9 \to 185$	$9 \to 253$	$14 \to 365$
V4	M	11; 41.2	18; 37.4	24; 38.4	30; 40.5	36; 43.0	67; 35.3	88; 46.2	120; 65.3	163; 93.0
		$-68 \to 107$	$-53 \to 102$	$-48 \to 112$	$-48 \to 122$	$-43 \to 131$	$-4 \to 141$	$-8 \to 180$	$-14 \to 244$	$-34 \to 346$
	F	10; 39.4	17; 35.9	23; 36.5	28; 38.2	33; 40.6	65; 32.4	88; 43.1	123; 61.8	171; 88.7
		$-73 \to 102$	$-53 \to 102$	$-48 \to 112$	$-47 \to 122$	$-43 \to 131$	$4 \to 136$	$9 \to 175$	$5 \to 248$	$4 \to 346$
V5	M	10; 33.8	10; 29.8	12; 29.8	14; 31.0	18; 32.8	57; 29.5	75; 39.3	101; 56.0	136; 79.6
		$-58 \to 82$	$-53 \to 73$	$-53 \to 73$	$-53 \to 78$	$-48 \to 87$	$0 \to 117$	$-4 \to 151$	$-19 \to 209$	$-39 \to 287$
	F	11; 32.8	11; 28.8	13; 28.7	15; 29.8	18; 31.4	57; 27.2	77; 36.6	106; 52.7	147; 75.4
		$-58 \to 82$	$-53 \to 73$	$-52 \to 73$	$-48 \to 78$	$-48 \to 82$	$4 \to 117$	$9 \to 151$	$9 \to 209$	$0 \to 297$
V6	M	14; 26.3	10; 22.9	8; 22.6	8; 23.2	9; 24.3	46; 22.8	59; 29.6	79; 41.5	105; 58.4
		$-39 \to 68$	$-39 \to 53$	$-43 \to 53$	$-43 \to 53$	$-43 \to 58$	$0 \to 97$	$0 \to 122$	$-4 \to 165$	$-14 \to 224$
	F	16; 25.8	12; 22.1	10; 21.9	10; 22.4	11; 23.4	47; 21.6	62; 28.3	84; 40.1	115; 56.6
		$-39 \to 73$	$-39 \to 58$	$-39 \to 53$	$-39 \to 53$	$-42 \to 58$	$4 \to 92$	$9 \to 122$	$9 \to 165$	$9 \to 234$

* Mean values (μV), standard deviation and the range from the lower to the upper second percentile. *M* men, *F* women.

TABLE D.9 Limb lead QRS amplitudes* at 10-ms intervals in African–American men and women.

		From QRS onset				From end of QRS backwards			
Lead		+10 ms	+20 ms	+30 ms	+40 ms	−10 ms	−20 ms	−30 ms	−40 ms
aVL	M	−24; 48.3	53; 109.2	298; 219.7	431; 350.5	15; 49.6	25; 115.4	106; 261.6	283; 390.1
		$-128 \to 70$	$-169 \to 328$	$-70 \to 826$	$-220 \to 1,156$	$-84 \to 129$	$-172 \to 321$	$-318 \to 787$	$-388 \to 1,185$
	F	−21; 47.6	45; 97.4	265; 202	373; 333.9	11; 50.7	23; 118.7	86; 241.7	235; 356.9
		$-133 \to 70$	$-142 \to 297$	$-95 \to 723$	$-293 \to 1,074$	$-82 \to 139$	$-186 \to 342$	$-327 \to 682$	$-381 \to 1,044$
I	M	−20; 44.5	112; 130.6	521; 240.4	759; 341.6	20; 42.1	26; 103.5	155; 266	485; 428.7
		$-111 \to 77$	$-112 \to 442$	$113 \to 1,086$	$136 \to 1,464$	$-63 \to 111$	$-179 \to 252$	$-239 \to 848$	$-229 \to 1,433$
	F	−21; 40.6	96; 112.9	469; 214.6	678; 303.9	16; 40.6	21; 99.7	128; 242.3	410; 349.1
		$-112 \to 63$	$-110 \to 380$	$107 \to 977$	$107 \to 1,369$	$-58 \to 112$	$-146 \to 271$	$-219 \to 739$	$-219 \to 1,257$
−aVR	M	−6; 38.8	115; 112.2	484; 202.6	708; 287.4	16; 40.5	14; 91.7	127; 218	444; 364.8
		$-78 \to 78$	$-65 \to 405$	$134 \to 944$	$132 \to 1,316$	$-70 \to 92$	$-169 \to 189$	$-211 \to 677$	$-197 \to 1,215$
	F	−10; 34.3	98; 95.9	348; 178.9	645; 245.9	12; 37.9	8; 85.9	105; 208.3	381; 329.7
		$-82 \to 65$	$-73 \to 323$	$102 \to 870$	$157 \to 1,171$	$-72 \to 84$	$-163 \to 191$	$-212 \to 649$	$-180 \to 1,066$
II	M	9; 56.9	127; 124.1	455; 239.3	639; 372.7	11; 64.6	−1; 140.1	87; 280.3	381; 425.8
		$-102 \to 136$	$-82 \to 443$	$39 \to 1,015$	$-86 \to 1,459$	$-136 \to 131$	$-302 \to 283$	$-443 \to 746$	$-421 \to 1,307$
	F	−2; 54.9	110; 117.8	443; 229	660; 360.6	9; 63.3	−5; 137	90; 275.7	393; 420.1
		$-107 \to 122$	$-102 \to 405$	$39 \to 984$	$-78 \to 1,415$	$-131 \to 131$	$-297 \to 273$	$-414 \to 766$	$-418 \to 1,278$
aVF	M	18; 56.8	61; 103.4	186; 220.4	277; 385.1	1; 65.1	−11; 139.3	21; 270.4	162; 396.4
		$-92 \to 139$	$-116 \to 300$	$-208 \to 712$	$-477 \to 1,085$	$-153 \to 119$	$-326 \to 280$	$-564 \to 568$	$-661 \to 1,067$
	F	11; 56.3	53; 93.3	173; 204.9	272; 369	1; 65.7	−14; 143.6	19; 267.7	146; 385.9
		$-101 \to 135$	$-117 \to 278$	$-198 \to 634$	$-449 \to 1,063$	$-155 \to 123$	$-389 \to 274$	$-548 \to 599$	$-628 \to 1,042$
III	M	29; 65.4	5; 120.5	−74; 260.3	−103; 452	−9; 72.4	−24; 159.3	−56; 323.5	−81; 464.6
		$-97 \to 164$	$-244 \to 261$	$-644 \to 485$	$-997 \to 833$	$-188 \to 125$	$-423 \to 283$	$-789 \to 527$	$-1,156 \to 868$
	F	21; 65.7	5; 109.9	−61; 243.5	−68; 439.6	−7; 74.1	−25; 166.1	−45; 310.5	−59; 444.2
		$-107 \to 173$	$-234 \to 248$	$-561 \to 461$	$-933 \to 856$	$-190 \to 131$	$-470 \to 287$	$-748 \to 569$	$-1,025 \to 861$

* Mean values (μV), standard deviation and the range from the lower to the upper second percentile. *M* men, *F* women.

TABLE D.10 Limb lead ST-T amplitudes* at 10-ms intervals in African–American men and women.

		From J point forwards					From end of T backwards			
		J point	J+10	J+20	J+30	J+40	Toff−10	Toff−20	Toff−30	Toff−40
aVL	M	10; 25.2	6; 19.1	6; 17.4	6; 17.4	7; l7.8	12; 21.8	16; 25	22; 31.7	31; 41.4
		$-39 \rightarrow 67$	$-34 \rightarrow 48$	$-31 \rightarrow 43$	$-31 \rightarrow 43$	$-29 \rightarrow 48$	$-36 \rightarrow 53$	$-41 \rightarrow 68$	$-48 \rightarrow 87$	$-58 \rightarrow 114$
	F	7; 23.8	5; l7.8	4; 16.7	4; 16.6	4; 17.3	10; 20.8	14; 24.4	19; 29.8	27; 38.4
		$-39 \rightarrow 63$	$-31 \rightarrow 43$	$-31 \rightarrow 41$	$-31 \rightarrow 39$	$-31 \rightarrow 43$	$-31 \rightarrow 57$	$-34 \rightarrow 68$	$-41 \rightarrow 85$	$-51 \rightarrow 113$
I	M	18; 24.1	13; 21	12; 20	14; 20.6	15; 21.7	43; 21.3	54; 25.9	70; 35.2	93; 48.1
		$-29 \rightarrow 73$	$-34 \rightarrow 58$	$-29 \rightarrow 53$	$-29 \rightarrow 53$	$-33 \rightarrow 63$	$0 \rightarrow 87$	$4 \rightarrow 112$	$0 \rightarrow 150$	$-3 \rightarrow 190$
	F	15; 22.3	11; 19.3	10; 19.4	10; 20.1	22; 21.1	40; 20.2	50; 25	66; 32.7	88; 44.4
		$-34 \rightarrow 63$	$-29 \rightarrow 53$	$-34 \rightarrow 48$	$-34 \rightarrow 53$	$-34 \rightarrow 58$	$0 \rightarrow 87$	$4 \rightarrow 107$	$9 \rightarrow 141$	$9 \rightarrow 193$
−aVR	M	17; 21.5	14; 19.5	13; 18.9	14; 19.5	16; 20.6	52; 20.4	65; 24.9	84; 33.5	108; 45.5
		$-29 \rightarrow 65$	$-31 \rightarrow 56$	$-28 \rightarrow 53$	$-29 \rightarrow 56$	$-33 \rightarrow 60$	$12 \rightarrow 92$	$17 \rightarrow 112$	$17 \rightarrow 153$	$17 \rightarrow 200$
	F	15; 21.1	12; 18.9	11; 18.8	11; 19.4	13; 20.4	49; 19.2	61; 24	80; 32.1	105; 43.7
		$-30 \rightarrow 57$	$-26 \rightarrow 53$	$-30 \rightarrow 48$	$-29 \rightarrow 53$	$-31 \rightarrow 56$	$12 \rightarrow 90$	$19 \rightarrow 112$	$19 \rightarrow 148$	$22 \rightarrow 196$
II	M	16; 30.6	14; 25.2	14; 23.8	15; 24.1	16; 25.1	62; 29.2	76; 34.2	97; 43.3	123; 56.7
		$-53 \rightarrow 78$	$-39 \rightarrow 68$	$-39 \rightarrow 63$	$-34 \rightarrow 68$	$-38 \rightarrow 73$	$4 \rightarrow 130$	$9 \rightarrow 151$	$14 \rightarrow 190$	$15 \rightarrow 244$
	F	15; 30.9	13; 25.2	12; 23.9	13; 24.1	14; 24.9	59; 27.5	73; 33.2	94; 42.6	122; 56
		$-48 \rightarrow 78$	$-39 \rightarrow 63$	$-37 \rightarrow 63$	$-34 \rightarrow 63$	$-39 \rightarrow 68$	$4 \rightarrow 117$	$9 \rightarrow 146$	$14 \rightarrow 183$	$21 \rightarrow 239$
aVF	M	8; 30.1	8; 22.7	8; 20.7	8; 20.5	9; 21	40; 28	49; 31.7	61; 38.7	77; 49
		$-56 \rightarrow 65$	$-39 \rightarrow 56$	$-38 \rightarrow 50$	$-34 \rightarrow 51$	$-36 \rightarrow 53$	$-14 \rightarrow 108$	$-11 \rightarrow 126$	$-9 \rightarrow 153$	$-14 \rightarrow 187$
	F	−7; 30.1	7; 22.7	7; 20.6	8; 20.3	8; 20.7	39; 26.5	48; 31	61; 38.2	78; 48.6
		$-56 \rightarrow 68$	$-39 \rightarrow 53$	$-34 \rightarrow 51$	$-31 \rightarrow 51$	$-34 \rightarrow 51$	$-14 \rightarrow 92$	$-12 \rightarrow 114$	$-11 \rightarrow 146$	$-9 \rightarrow 187$
III	M	−1; 34.2	1; 24.8	1; 22.1	1; 21.7	1; 22.1	19; 30.5	22; 34.2	26; 41.6	30; 52.2
		$-73 \rightarrow 68$	$-53 \rightarrow 53$	$-48 \rightarrow 43$	$-43 \rightarrow 43$	$-48 \rightarrow 47$	$-39 \rightarrow 96$	$-43 \rightarrow 107$	$-53 \rightarrow 126$	$-73 \rightarrow 151$
	F	0; 33.5	2; 24.2	3; 21.7	3; 21.1	3; 21.6	19; 29.1	23; 33.5	28; 40.4	34; 20.6
		$-73 \rightarrow 68$	$-53 \rightarrow 48$	$-43 \rightarrow 48$	$-39 \rightarrow 46$	$-43 \rightarrow 48$	$-43 \rightarrow 78$	$-48 \rightarrow 92$	$-53 \rightarrow 112$	$-68 \rightarrow 144$

* Mean values (µV), standard deviation and the range from the lower to the upper second percentile. *M* men, *F* women.

TABLE D.11 Chest lead QRS amplitudes* in African–American men and women at 10-ms intervals from QRS onset and from the end of QRS backwards.

		From QRS onset				From end of QRS backwards			
		+10 ms	+20 ms	+30 ms	+40 ms	−10 ms	−20 ms	−30 ms	−40 ms
V1	M	87; 60.8	110; 161.3	−200; 323.7	−678; 391.3	−59; 61.3	−227; 161.9	−505; 289.4	−715; 372.5
		$-24 \rightarrow 224$	$-238 \rightarrow 453$	$-354 \rightarrow 382$	$-1{,}542 \rightarrow 68$	$-189 \rightarrow 68$	$-575 \rightarrow 62$	$-1{,}130 \rightarrow 4$	$-1{,}504 \rightarrow -4$
	F	82; 63.9	94; 175.8	−239; 350.0	−698; 430.4	−58; 62.2	−230; 164.6	−497; 286.9	−714; 393.4
		$-42 \rightarrow 229$	$-312 \rightarrow 483$	$-1{,}078 \rightarrow 388$	$-1{,}756 \rightarrow 117$	$-204 \rightarrow 63$	$-647 \rightarrow 51$	$-1{,}151 \rightarrow -6$	$-1{,}687 \rightarrow 7$
V2	M	129; 89.9	328; 254.8	197; 581.5	−436; 730.6	−73; 89.1	−355; 218.7	−757; 370.1	−833; 609.7
		$-19 \rightarrow 359$	$-201 \rightarrow 904$	$-1{,}250 \rightarrow 1{,}291$	$-1{,}874 \rightarrow 1{,}082$	$-244 \rightarrow 125$	$-829 \rightarrow 57$	$-1{,}526 \rightarrow -40$	$-2{,}085 \rightarrow 565$
	F	125; 95.0	337; 274.1	217; 598.4	−383; 758.0	−68; 89.3	−352; 222.2	−708; 375.8	−742; 684.4
		$-37 \rightarrow 363$	$-231 \rightarrow 956$	$-1{,}138 \rightarrow 1{,}324$	$-1{,}927 \rightarrow 1{,}205$	$-263 \rightarrow 125$	$-886 \rightarrow 58$	$-1{,}503 \rightarrow 139$	$-1{,}988 \rightarrow 896$
V3	M	89; 73.1	379; 221.9	682; 481.2	416; 710.0	−70; 78.1	−300; 185.2	−523; 407.0	−255; 755.6
		$-47 \rightarrow 282$	$34 \rightarrow 897$	$-416 \rightarrow 1{,}752$	$-1{,}084 \rightarrow 1{,}853$	$-229 \rightarrow 107$	$-711 \rightarrow 78$	$-1{,}316 \rightarrow 434$	$-1{,}564 \rightarrow 1{,}351$
	F	84; 90.3	425; 273.2	831; 503.3	603; 765.4	−56; 81.8	−298; 197.9	−451; 448.1	−83; 879.4
		$-73 \rightarrow 333$	$-17 \rightarrow 1{,}083$	$-256 \rightarrow 1{,}984$	$-780 \rightarrow 2{,}147$	$-234 \rightarrow 117$	$-720 \rightarrow 105$	$-1{,}218 \rightarrow 802$	$-1{,}512 \rightarrow 1{,}823$
V4	M	42; 73.4	361; 225.3	959; 429.9	1,018; 676.3	−47; 70.5	−198; 164.8	−252; 423.0	246; 824.8
		$-96 \rightarrow 218$	$-29 \rightarrow 910$	$266 \rightarrow 1{,}974$	$-438 \rightarrow 2{,}489$	$-195 \rightarrow 122$	$-570 \rightarrow 145$	$-1{,}003 \rightarrow 860$	$-1{,}052 \rightarrow 1{,}945$
	F	38; 87.6	403; 293.9	1,111; 481.2	1,196; 716.1	−36; 74.7	−181; 169.8	−182; 456.6	404; 903.6
		$-117 \rightarrow 256$	$-48 \rightarrow 1{,}195$	$292 \rightarrow 2{,}308$	$-296 \rightarrow 2{,}652$	$-190 \rightarrow 125$	$-546 \rightarrow 156$	$-863 \rightarrow 1{,}050$	$-1{,}066 \rightarrow 2{,}267$
V5	M	5; 65.4	262; 200.3	872; 362.5	1,093; 544.0	−20; 57.6	−89; 137.6	−23; 362.8	475; 682.7
		$-117 \rightarrow 164$	$-91 \rightarrow 767$	$293 \rightarrow 1{,}724$	$-27 \rightarrow 2{,}346$	$-126 \rightarrow 117$	$-375 \rightarrow 188$	$-575 \rightarrow 904$	$-618 \rightarrow 1{,}818$
	F	2; 75.0	291; 253.4	985; 432.2	1,217; 603.8	−10; 61.2	−71; 136.9	36; 392.4	595; 738.1
		$-131 \rightarrow 195$	$-97 \rightarrow 958$	$289 \rightarrow 2{,}028$	$-17 \rightarrow 2{,}544$	$-131 \rightarrow 117$	$-373 \rightarrow 195$	$-551 \rightarrow 1{,}037$	$-615 \rightarrow 2{,}093$
V6	M	−14; 52.9	155; 150.6	638; 280.4	909; 398.3	6; 45.9	1; 116.0	128; 285.8	520; 492.0
		$-112 \rightarrow 106$	$-102 \rightarrow 512$	$172 \rightarrow 1{,}320$	$136 \rightarrow 1{,}780$	$-82 \rightarrow 102$	$-218 \rightarrow 222$	$-316 \rightarrow 866$	$-300 \rightarrow 1{,}550$
	F	−17; 54.0	161; 173.0	675; 309.4	943; 414.4	16; 47.5	26; 114.6	180; 294.4	584; 491.1
		$-122 \rightarrow 115$	$-122 \rightarrow 603$	$173 \rightarrow 1{,}430$	$143 \rightarrow 1{,}828$	$-78 \rightarrow 110$	$-200 \rightarrow 297$	$-286 \rightarrow 935$	$-251 \rightarrow 1{,}613$

* Mean values (µV), standard deviation and the lower and upper second percentiles. *M* males, *F* females.

TABLE D.12 Chest lead ST-T amplitudes* at 10-ms intervals in African–American men and women.

		From J point forwards					From end of T backwards			
		J point	J +10	J +20	J +30	J +40	Toff −10	Toff −20	Toff −30	Toff −40
V1	M	4; 30.3	20; 28.4	28; 29.4	33; 30.6	36; 32.0	0; 25.8	0; 31.0	0; 40.1	1; 53.3
		−48 → 68	−28 → 87	−19 → 97	−14 → 107	−14 → 112	−53 → 58	−58 → 73	−77 → 97	−96 → 129
	F	6; 31.9	23; 29.2	31; 30.1	36; 31.2	39; 32.6	2; 28.1	3; 33.7	3; 42.7	5; 55.9
		−48 → 78	−24 → 95	−14 → 110	−14 → 117	−14 → 122	−53 → 63	−63 → 73	−78 → 92	−97 → 126
V2	M	23; 49.5	47; 50.2	62; 54.7	72; 58.8	80; 62.9	46; 36.7	62; 45.4	87; 60.9	122; 84.2
		−58 → 146	−29 → 179	−19 → 203	−9 → 224	−4 → 252	−29 → 125	−29 → 161	−24 → 224	−29 → 312
	F	31; 51.2	55; 48.9	69; 51.7	79; 54.7	87; 57.8	52; 36.0	70; 45.1	97; 61.0	136; 85.6
		−53 → 151	−24 → 175	−14 → 200	−9 → 217	−4 → 232	−14 → 131	−14 → 170	−14 → 229	−19 → 329
V3	M	10; 44.1	28; 44.5	40; 48.2	49; 51.5	56; 55.3	64; 35.3	83; 44.8	112; 63.0	150; 90.1
		−68 → 125	−47 → 151	−39 → 169	−34 → 185	−34 → 209	−4 → 146	−4 → 175	−13 → 239	−19 → 336
	F	23; 46.1	39; 44.5	50; 47.2	59; 50.1	66; 53.4	65; 39.2	87; 50.2	120; 69.6	166; 97.7
		−63 → 131	−39 → 146	−29 → 165	−24 → 188	−24 → 203	−14 → 151	−19 → 185	−29 → 253	−51 → 364
V4	M	5; 40.4	14; 38.3	20; 39.8	26; 42.0	32; 44.5	65; 34.3	85; 44.5	114; 63.1	150; 90.8
		−68 → 102	−58 → 112	−48 → 117	−48 → 131	−43 → 150	0 → 141	−3 → 180	−9 → 239	−29 → 346
	F	13; 41.3	20; 37.3	26; 38.0	32; 40.0	37; 42.3	63; 37.7	83; 50.1	113; 71.2	155; 101.1
		−63 → 110	−48 → 105	−43 → 112	−42 → 122	−39 → 131	−14 → 141	−22 → 175	−51 → 234	−84 → 336
V5	M	5; 34.0	7; 31.2	9; 32.5	12; 34.4	16; 36.3	58; 29.1	74; 37.1	99; 52.9	130; 75.5
		−58 → 86	−52 → 78	−53 → 73	−52 → 82	−48 → 87	−3 → 125	−3 → 156	−13 → 208	−39 → 287
	F	11; 35.0	11; 30.5	13; 30.1	15; 31.3	18; 32.7	54; 32.9	70; 44.1	95; 62.8	128; 88.6
		−58 → 82	−53 → 73	−51 → 73	−53 → 81	−48 → 87	−22 → 117	−43 → 146	−70 → 204	−100 → 287
V6	M	10; 26.6	7; 23.4	6; 23.7	7; 24.7	8; 25.9	49; 25.1	61; 30.7	80; 41.8	105; 58.1
		−43 → 68	−43 → 53	−42 → 53	−43 → 58	−43 → 62	−3 → 107	1 → 126	−9 → 165	−19 → 229
	F	15; 26.7	10; 23.1	8; 22.8	8; 23.4	9; 24.3	43; 24.0	55; 31.3	73; 44.4	97; 62.5
		−39 → 68	−43 → 53	−43 → 51	−43 → 53	−43 → 53	−9 → 92	−14 → 117	−32 → 161	−53 → 214

* Mean values (μV), standard deviation and the range from the lower to the upper second percentile. *M* men, *F* women.

Section E
Repolarization Waveform Vectors: Tables

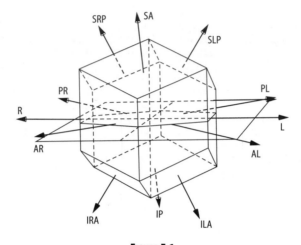

FIGURE E.1

TABLE E.1 Angular directions and unit vectors of the 12 reference directions used to indicate directional distributions of waveform vectors.

| Order | Acronym | Angular directions | | Unit vector components | | |
		Azimuth*	Elevation†	x	y	z
1	L	0	0	1	0	0
2	ILA	30	45	0.497	0.819	0.287
3	AL	60	0	0.5	0	0.866
4	SA	90	135	0	−0.819	0.574
5	AR	120	0	−0.5	0	0.866
6	IRA	150	55	−0.497	0.819	0.287
7	R	180	0	−1	0	0
8	SRP	−30	135	0.497	−0.819	−2.287
9	PR	−120	0	−0.5	0	−0.866
10	IP	−90	45	0	0.819	−0.574
11	PL	−60	0	0.5	0	−0.866
12	SLR	−150	135	−0.497	−0.819	−0.287

* Azimuth: $0° =$ left, $90° =$ anterior, $−90° =$ posterior, and $\pm 180° =$ right.

† Elevation: $0° =$ down, $90° =$ horizontal, and $180° =$ up.

272

TABLE E.2 Mean T waveform vector's spatial magnitude, orientation angles, projections on aVF, V1 and V5 leads, and the spatial angle between QRS and T mean vectors, with lower to upper fifth and second percentile ranges by ethnicity, age, and gender.

Waveform vector	Ethnic group Age group Gender	White				African–American			
		40–59 years		60+ years		40–59 years		60+ years	
		Males	Females	Males	Females	Males	Females	Males	Females
Spatial magnitude (μV)	Mean; SD	196; 64.8	151; 50.4	181; 66.1	151; 56.7	188; 62.5	154; 57.6	170; 64.0	135; 56.2
	5% → 95%	98 → 308	74 → 238	85 → 296	68 → 251	89 → 297	70 → 248	77 → 275	60 → 235
	2% → 98%	80 → 340	61 → 267	67 → 331	56 → 281	73 → 323	57 → 274	58 → 307	47 → 270
Frontal plane angle (°)	Mean; SD	25; 21.1	32; 17.7	22; 34.6	30; 29.6	22; 31.9	31; 25.7	16; 48.8	25; 48.8
	5% → 95%	3 → 51	11 → 56	−16 → 63	3 → 65	−11 → 56	5 → 61	−87 → 71	−35 → 91
	2% → 98%	−8 → 61	2 → 65	−71 → 92	−20 → 94	−38 → 66	−9 → 84	−145 → 116	−151 → 139
Azimuth (°)	Mean; SD	49; 17.8	32; 22.4	51; 24.3	36; 30.6	49; 22.6	36; 26.9	56; 27.7	40; 41.9
	5% → 95%	21 → 75	3 → 63	19 → 86	−9 → 77	19 → 79	−5 → 73	22 → 99	−13 → 100
	2% → 98%	11 → 83	−23 → 73	7 → 101	−30 → 96	7 → 96	−27 → 90	3 → 114	−72 → 125
Elevation (°)	Mean; SD	76; 22.2	65; 17.9	83; 33.7	69; 24.7	84; 33.4	70; 26.3	93; 43.0	79; 37.6
	5% → 95%	55 → 89	44 → 83	52 → 176	44 → 88	57 → 176	44 → 87	49 → 178	39 → 176
	2% → 98%	49 → 177	36 → 88	46 → 178	36 → 174	48 → 179	36 → 173	41 → 179	27 → 178
Projection on aVF (μV)	Mean; SD	42; 34.4	55; 32.5	33; 38.6	48; 35.2	34; 37.3	49; 35.5	27; 42.4	34; 37.7
	5% → 95%	−7 → 103	5 → 110	−26 → 99	−7 → 107	−27 → 99	−5 → 109	−39 → 102	−24 → 98
	2% → 98%	−22 → 118	−9 → 127	−42 → 120	−25 → 125	−41 → 116	−20 → 126	−55 → 121	−42 → 113
Projection on V1 (μV)	Mean; SD	81; 55.3	21; 43.6	80; 61.5	31; 51.5	78; 57.2	31; 52.5	84; 61.8	36; 55.7
	5% → 95%	−6 → 172	−51 → 91	−12 → 187	−52 → 117	−10 → 177	−51 → 110	−2 → 188	−45 → 125
	2% → 98%	−32 → 209	−67 → 113	−31 → 218	−73 → 148	−36 → 207	−71 → 140	−34 → 231	−72 → 166
Projection on V5 (μV)	Mean; SD	164; 69.8	151; 58.8	141; 75.5	141; 69.5	153; 71.8	144; 69.9	119; 84.4	109; 76.8
	5% → 95%	63 → 283	62 → 249	27 → 263	38 → 256	41 → 275	45 → 255	−6 → 260	−10 → 227
	2% → 98%	42 → 317	41 → 274	−8 → 300	−1 → 286	2 → 307	15 → 285	−50 → 295	−71 → 260
QRS/T angle* (°)	Mean; SD	72; 26.8	59; 25.0	79; 30.7	63; 28.8	76; 28.2	63; 27.7	79; 33.1	66; 31.5
	5% → 95%	31 → 119	20 → 101	31 → 132	22 → 115	31 → 123	21 → 112	26 → 140	22 → 123
	2% → 98%	22 → 132	14 → 116	23 → 149	15 → 135	24 → 140	15 → 130	19 → 151	15 → 148

* Spatial angle between the mean QRS and T vectors.

TABLE E.3 T wave convexity vector's spatial magnitude, orientation angles, projections on aVF, V1 and V5 leads, with lower to upper fifth and second percentile ranges by ethnicity, age, and gender.

Waveform vector	Ethnic group Age group Gender	White				African–American			
		40–59 years		60+ years		40–59 years		60+ years	
		Males	Females	Males	Females	Males	Females	Males	Females
Spatial magnitude (μV)	Mean; SD	77; 29.5	60; 23.5	74; 30.0	61; 26.3	77; 29.2	63; 27.1	69; 32.7	52; 27.9
	5% $\to$ 95%	34 $\to$ 130	26 $\to$ 101	30 $\to$ 126	22 $\to$ 108	34 $\to$ 130	23 $\to$ 107	25 $\to$ 123	18 $\to$ 100
	2% $\to$ 98%	28 $\to$ 147	18 $\to$ 113	23 $\to$ 143	16 $\to$ 124	27 $\to$ 145	16 $\to$ 122	19 $\to$ 139	12 $\to$ 117
Frontal plane angle (°)	Mean; SD	22; 25.5	27; 20.9	20; 39.6	27; 33.3	18; 35.4	27; 28.2	11; 59.5	21; 56.5
	5% $\to$ 95%	$-3 \to 49$	$4 \to 51$	$-26 \to 67$	$0 \to 65$	$-15 \to 53$	$1 \to 59$	$-135 \to 90$	$-121 \to 113$
	2% $\to$ 98%	$-24 \to 68$	$-5 \to 67$	$-132 \to 106$	$-48 \to 110$	$-108 \to 67$	$-27 \to 97$	$-157 \to 145$	$-165 \to 155$
Azimuth (°)	Mean; SD	46; 22.4	23; 27.1	49; 28.9	28; 36.0	47; 23.3	28; 32.2	57; 35.8	34; 50.8
	5% $\to$ 95%	$14 \to 80$	$-20 \to 61$	$13 \to 90$	$-26 \to 78$	$11 \to 84$	$-23 \to 74$	$11 \to 108$	$-35 \to 106$
	2% $\to$ 98%	$0 \to 89$	$-42 \to 76$	$-3 \to 108$	$-69 \to 101$	$1 \to 97$	$-53 \to 95$	$-8 \to 139$	$-137 \to 148$
Elevation (°)	Mean; SD	80; 27.4	69; 22.5	85; 34.3	72; 26.3	82; 31.9	70; 24.6	97; 44.1	82; 38.2
	5% $\to$ 95%	$55 \to 173$	$46 \to 87$	$52 \to 176$	$45 \to 152$	$53 \to 176$	$46 \to 89$	$53 \to 177$	$40 \to 175$
	2% $\to$ 98%	$49 \to 178$	$40 \to 174$	$46 \to 178$	$35 \to 176$	$43 \to 179$	$37 \to 175$	$44 \to 179$	$32 \to 178$
Projection on aVF (μV)	Mean; SD	14; 14.5	18; 13.4	12; 15.2	17; 13.9	13; 15.0	18; 13.9	8; 17.9	1; 14.9
	5% $\to$ 95%	$-7 \to 39$	$-2 \to 41$	$-12 \to 36$	$-4 \to 40$	$-8 \to 38$	$-4 \to 41$	$-18 \to 38$	$-10 \to 35$
	2% $\to$ 98%	$-11 \to 47$	$-7 \to 48$	$-18 \to 45$	$-9 \to 47$	$-13 \to 51$	$-9 \to 48$	$-29 \to 47$	$-18 \to 41$
Projection on V1 (μV)	Mean; SD	28; 25.0	1; 19.6	30; 28	6; 23.1	28; 25.0	6; 24.0	34; 31.1	12; 26.1
	5% $\to$ 95%	$-11 \to 70$	$-30 \to 33$	$-11 \to 79$	$-29 \to 47$	$-12 \to 70$	$-29 \to 42$	$-9 \to 84$	$-23 \to 56$
	2% $\to$ 98%	$-20 \to 84$	$-38 \to 42$	$-19 \to 94$	$-37 \to 61$	$-17 \to 86$	$-37 \to 55$	$-20 \to 110$	$-31 \to 75$
Projection on V5 (μV)	Mean; SD	65; 32.7	61; 28.0	57; 35.4	57; 32.4	64; 33.2	60; 32.6	43; 44.0	39; 37.6
	5% $\to$ 95%	$17 \to 122$	$17 \to 106$	$6 \to 116$	$7 \to 113$	$13 \to 1,213$	$10 \to 110$	$-12 \to 107$	$-18 \to 94$
	2% $\to$ 98%	$5 \to 138$	$7 \to 120$	$-13 \to 134$	$-7 \to 129$	$0 \to 134$	$-2 \to 127$	$-44 \to 127$	$-40 \to 109$

Index